GERONTOLOGY AND COMMUNICATION DISORDERS

Edited by
Linda Jacobs-Condit, M.S.
Project Director
Gerontological Training in
Speech-Language Pathology and Audiology

January 1985

American Speech-Language-Hearing Association
10801 Rockville Pike
Rockville, Maryland 20852

General Information

The original publication of the enclosed materials was distributed at the "Gerontological and Communication Disorders" Conference held on October 9-10, 1984, at the ASHA National Office in Rockville, Maryland. Because the demand for attendance was greater than we could accommodate, the manual is being reprinted for broader dissemination of knowledge.

Contained herein is information regarding the inter-relationship between the physical, psychological, and social aspects of aging as they interact with and impact upon communication. The Gerontology and Communication Disorders manual is ultimately designed to effect improved intervention with the elderly within the context of the communication restrictions imposed by the aging process.

The development of this manual was supported in part by grant award number 90-AT-0095 from the Administration on Aging, Office of Human Development Services, Department of Health and Human services, Washington, D.C. 20201. Grantees undertaking projects under government sponsorship are encouraged to express freely their findings and conclusions. Points of view or opinions expressed do not, therefore, necessarily represent official Administration on Aging policy.

Linda Jacobs-Condit, M.S.
Project Director
Gerontological Training in
Speech-Language Pathology
and Audiology

Gerontology and Communication Disorders is published by the American Speech-Language-Hearing Association.

Copies are available upon written requests to:

American Speech-Language-Hearing Association
Publication Sales Office
10801 Rockville Pike
Rockville, Maryland 20852
(301) 897-5700

Table of Contents

Contributors

Jon K. Ashby, Ph.D., Director, Communication Disorders Program, Abilene Christian University, Abilene, Texas.

Terry W. Baggs, M.S., Doctoral Student in Speech-Language Pathology, Memphis Speech & Hearing Center, Memphis State University, Memphis, Tennessee.

Patrice Cruise, M.S., R.N., Assistant Professor of Community Health Nursing, Andrews University, Berrien Springs, Michigan.

Jess Dancer, Ph.D., Associate Professor, Department of Communicative Disorders, University of Arkansas at Little Rock, University of Arkansas for Medical Sciences, Little Rock, Arkansas.

G. Albyn Davis, Ph.D., Associate Professor, Department of Communication Disorders, University of Massachusetts, Amherst, Massachusetts.

Richard M. Flower, Ph.D., Director, Audiology and Speech Clinic, University of California Medical Center, San Francisco, California.

Thomas Hickey, D.P.H., Professor & Director, Health Gerontology Program, School of Public Health; Research Scientist, Institute of Gerontology, University of Michigan, Ann Arbor, Michigan.

Linda Jacobs-Condit, M.S., Project Director, Gerontological Training in Speech-Language Pathology & Audiology, American Speech-Language-Hearing Association, Rockville, Maryland.

Rosemary Lubinski, Ed.D., Associate Professor, Department of Communicative Disorders & Sciences, State University of New York at Buffalo, Amherst, New York.

Mary Louise Ortenzo, M.S., Adjunct Faculty, School of Education & Human Development, George Washington University, Washington, DC.

Alina C. Otal, Project Manager, Gerontological Training in Speech-Language Pathology & Audiology, American Speech-Language-Hearing Association, Rockville, Maryland.

Herbert J. Oyer, Ph.D., Professor & Director, Speech & Hearing Science Section, Department of Communication, Ohio State University, Columbus, Ohio.

Barbara B. Shadden, Ph.D., Associate Professor, Program in Speech Pathology & Audiology, University of Arkansas, Fayetteville, Arkansas.

Lennie-Marie P. Tolliver, Ph.D., Commissioner on Aging, Administration on Aging, Office of Human Development Services, Department of Health & Human Services, Washington, DC.

Barbara E. Weinstein, Ph.D. Assistant Professor of Audiology, Department of Speech Pathology & Audiology, Teachers College, Columbia University, New York, New York.

Preface

Benjamin Franklin said "Wish not so much to live long as to live well."
We are living far longer than Franklin would have imagined, but we still face
the challenge of learning how to live well. One challenge that increasingly
faces the elderly is that of overcoming barriers to communication such as,
hearing loss, illness, and/or environmental factors that may impact upon daily
living. From the normal hearing loss that may accompany the aging process, to
the devastating effects of stroke or dementia, the loss of communication is an
increasing and unfortunate fact of life among our older citizens. We are only
beginning to realize the magnitude of the challenge.

The individual's capacity to communicate is a vital factor in being able
to maintain his or her own quality of life. Daniel Webster once wrote, "If all
my possessions were taken from me with one exception, I would choose to keep
the power of communication, for by it I would soon regain all the rest."

A principal objective of the Administration on Aging is to support
activities which enhance the well-being of older persons. Effective
communication between older persons and the professionals who serve them is
one such activity. Clinical practitioners, administrators, and others will
find within the contents of this text knowledge and insight which will help
them to better understand and to communicate with and serve older clients.
The Administration on Aging is pleased to have supported the development of
this text.

Lennie-Marie P. Tolliver, Ph.D.
U.S. Commissioner on Aging
Department of Health & Human Services
Washington, DC 20201

Foreword

Communication is highly important to self and social adjustment not only in the early and formative years but also through the adult years and on into old age. As time passes many older persons may experience a decline in the support systems provided them by spouses, relatives, and close friends. This is of itself traumatic, as loneliness then besets them, and their existence, once vibrant and bright, may well become flat and lusterless. When this situation is exacerbated by hearing loss, neurological disorders that fractionate language and speech, or other physical or psychosocial problems affecting the older persons' ability to interact successfully with those about them or even passively with the messages of the mass media, an erosion in self-worth occurs which over a period of time, has a dehumanizing effect.

Given this knowledge it behooves speech-language pathologists and audiologists to see clearly their responsibilities for ameliorating the effects of those factors that deteriorate the quality of life for the elderly. The importance of this is further emphasized by the demographics available to us which shows the daily net increase in persons age 65 years and older in the United States to be approximately 1,500 people. In 1900 only about 4% of the population was age 65 years or above, whereas today this figure has risen to approximately 11.5%. Projections are for a steady increment, with the elderly cohort increasing more rapidly than any other cohort of society. With the figures clearly before us, the quality of life in later years becomes an increasing concern.

Although comprehensive education and training programs in speech-language pathology and audiology in the United States have taken into account the older individual, children and younger adults have received the greatest attention by professionals in communicative disorders. Only recently has the magnitude of the problem of providing informed care to those elderly with communicative disorders been realized. With this realization has come a great challenge to do one of two things: (a) incorporate relevant materials on communicative disorders of the aging into education and training programs for students; and (b) increase awareness of administrators and others who provide service within the aging network of the need for and benefits to be derived from the systematic delivery of services by speech-language pathologists and audiologists.

In order that the most informed service be provided the elderly with communicative disorders, those responsible for policy development and implementation must understand the value of care given by speech-language pathologists and audiologists. Services must be delivered by those who not only have knowledge of those disorders, but also have a thorough understanding of the normal aging processes. This is as important as the rendering of service to children against a backdrop of theory and principles of child development. With an understanding of the normal aging processes it soon becomes quite evident that contrary to popular myth, the old are not "all alike." They are in fact, considered to be the most heterogeneous cohort of the population making it imperative to exercise caution in attempting to define aging. The most simplistic and perhaps least accurate or descriptive definition is the chronological one, for people do not age at the same rate. Another common definition is the cultural one in which aging is viewed within the boundaries of specific cultural groups and is related to life expectancy, positions and roles of elders, and cultural traditions within the group. However, the most realistic definition of aging is the functional one wherein the extent to which one is considered old is based upon that which the individual is capable of doing. Thus, an individual age 70 years might in fact be considered substantially younger than one age 60 years because the 70-year-old can walk or run more easily, has more stamina, takes less time off from work, etc., than the 60-year-old.

It is highly gratifying to witness the coalescence of talents and energies by those knowledgeable about the effects of communication disorders as well as of the potentials and problems of aging, making this gerontological training manual in speech-language pathology and audiology possible. This manual, coupled with the extant literature and the increasing number of findings from research in both the areas of gerontology and communicative disorders, should serve as splendid resources from which to draw in order to develop highly knowledgeable clinicians to provide service to the elderly.

To consider in depth the role of older persons in our society, the myths that surround them, the normal aging processes, the importance of communication, the effects of the various disorders of communication that occur more frequently as persons grow older, management approaches, and service delivery models is no small task. All of these considerations have been dealt with most skillfully and with great insight within this manual. It should serve professionals in communicative disorders well as they plan for and work with the elderly. It stands as a tribute to all who have contributed to its substance: American Speech-Language-Hearing Association, Peggy S. Williams, Ph.D., Charles C. Diggs, Ph.D., the Administration on Aging and grant staff, James P. Gelatt, Ph.D., Project Administrator, Linda Jacobs-Condit, M.S., Project Director, and Alina C. Otal, Project Manager.

Herbert J. Oyer, Ph.D.
Professor and Director
Speech and Hearing Science Section
Department of Communication
Ohio State University
Columbus, OH 43221

Acknowledgments

I would like to acknowledge those individuals who have contributed to the conceptualization, development, refinement, and successful implementation of the grant project, "Gerontological Training in Speech-Language Pathology and Audiology." This manual, Gerontology and Communication Disorders, is one aspect of that project.

Peggy S. Williams, Ph.D. and Charles C. Diggs, Ph.D., authors of the original grant proposal, provided guidance, knowledge, and encouragement throughout the project's duration. Other ASHA staff members who provided particular knowledge and support for the grant project include Frederick T. Spahr, Ph.D., Kathleen M. Griffin, Ph.D., and James B. Lingwall, Ph.D. I wish to particularly acknowledge James P. Gelatt, Ph.D. who offered constant guidance and encouragement in his role as Project Administrator. Also, Alina C. Otal gave her support to the project in her role as Project Manager. Finally, Sharyn Schlesinger and Cathy Skinner are acknowledged for their diligent efforts in editing and typing the manuscript, respectively.

Special thanks go to those individuals who served as members of the Advisory Group and provided their invaluable assistance and guidance: Martha Johns, Arthur D. Kay, M.D., Joyce Leanse, M.P.H., Terri Lynch, David M. Resnick, Ph.D., Patricia Riley, and Carol N. Wilder, Ph.D. These individuals assisted with the refinement of the curriculum outline, recommended authors for the manual, and critically reviewed the drafts of the chapters.

Those individuals who contributed material to the manual deserve recognition, since the success of this project would not have been possible without their commitment and involvement: Jon K. Ashby, Ph.D., Terry W. Baggs, M.S., Patrice Cruise, M.S., Jess Dancer, Ph.D., G. Albyn Davis, Ph.D., Richard M. Flower, Ph.D., Thomas Hickey, D.P.H., James F. Maurer, Ph.D., Mary Louise Ortenzo, M.S., Herbert J. Oyer, Ph.D., Elizabeth Robertson-Tchabo, Ph.D., Barbara B. Shadden, Ph.D., and Barbara B. Weinstein, Ph.D.

Great appreciation is also extended to Rosemary B. Lubinski, Ph.D., Barbara B. Shadden, Ph.D., and Barbara C. Sonies, Ph.D. who served as external readers of the manual and provided additional guidance to its development. Also acknowledged is the support of Lennie-Marie P. Tolliver, Ph.D., Commissioner on Aging, and Carolyn Dingeldein, Project Officer, both of the Administration on Aging.

Each of these individuals, as well as the many colleagues and friends too numerous to mention, deserves my thanks.

This manual was developed as part of a grant project conducted by the American Speech-Language-Hearing Association (ASHA) and funded partly by the U.S. Department of Health and Human Services, Administration on Aging (Grant #90-AT-0095). These contents do not necessarily represent the policies of that agency or of the Association. Rather, the information presented here reflects the philosophy and practice of the contributing authors and is intended to provide resource material to the profession.

Linda Jacobs-Condit, M.S.
Project Director
Gerontological Training in
Speech-Language Pathology & Audiology

Introduction

James F. Maurer

Portland State University, Oregon

There is nothing to prepare you for the experience of growing old. Living is a process, an irreversible progression toward old age and eventual death. You see men of eighty still vital and straight as oaks; you see men of fifty reduced to gray shadows in the human landscape. The cellular clock differs for each one of us, and is profoundly affected by our own life experiences, our heredity, and perhaps most important, by the concepts of aging encountered in society and in oneself. (Curtin, 1972, p. 68)

Myths About Aging

The aging in our society are the biologically elite, presenting special problems as well as special strengths that younger persons do not manifest (Jernigan, 1979). Nonetheless, older persons have been portrayed as the antithesis of good health, youthful vigor, and enduring happiness. One need only browse through the formidable collection of gerontology and geriatric literature to conclude that the "problems" of aging dominate the growing spectrum of topics, ranging from economic woes to physical disabilities.

Younger adults particularly perceive the elderly less positively than themselves or even middle-aged individuals, stereotyping them as physically weaker, less able to create changes in society, less knowledgeable, and even less intelligent (Cameron, 1970a, 1970b, 1973). Many older persons view their peers with a negative valence as well. Although the majority of persons over 60 identify with their age cohort, old age identification is less likely among those elderly persons who are unencumbered by handicaps, poverty, dependency, and other problems (Miller, Gurin, & Gurin, 1980). Undoubtedly, the image of aging in society is profoundly affected by the idealization of youth that is perpetuated daily in American living rooms by a body-beautiful oriented media.

Older persons represent a growing enigma to health disciplines, not only because of the magnitude of problems that beset them over other age groups, but because they are increasing in numbers and longevity. Moreover, the difficulties they present to clinicians can no longer be stereotyped and closeted under the dubious heading of chronological age. Their long history of benign neglect is rapidly drawing to a close, and whether due to their accelerating population, their increasing public and political advocacy, or their growing manifest of scientific benefactors, older persons are becoming "au courant." Increasing interest in their communication problems in recent years is no exception.

One of the most positive changes in scientific attitudes concerns the knowledge that the elderly can learn. Their capability for achieving new knowledge has been underestimated for centuries. Perpetuated by public sentiment "You can't teach an old dog new tricks" and lack of opportunity for continuing education, the myth that older persons are uneducable is being destroyed by a virtual influx of senior citizens who are proving the new axiom that learning can continue throughout the lifespan of the healthy aging person.

The elderhostel idea, which began in 1975 by an offering of summer courses to the elderly at a New England university, is now growing rapidly at institutions across the United States. Such lifelong learning programs revitalize the self-concept of older persons, which is an area of concern among gerontologists, who attribute the loss of self-concept among the aging to the transition from independent to dependent living, loss of self-esteem, and other factors (Schuetz, 1980; Wolfe, 1983). Aging individuals are demonstrating that they can compete with youthful peers in acquiring new knowledge, particularly when they can control the pace of the learning task. Demo (1980) has observed that the more education the older person is exposed to, albeit at a slower pace, the more resources he or she can harness to cope with family problems, adjustment to change, and worthy use of leisure time (Demo, 1980).

Another myth of aging has been that the aging are intellectually inferior to other age groups. Early psychometric measures tended to demonstrate an age-related decline in intellectual functions, largely because intelligence scores were based on instruments and normative data developed for the young (Botwinick, 1977; Demming & Pressey, 1957; Schaie, 1978). These authors have

10

pointed out that aging persons have not been recognized as a psychometric entity unto themselves.

Unquestionably, there is need for more comprehensive research on intellectual functioning among older people (Price, Fein, & Feinberg, 1980). As the authors indicate/suggest, pathological levels of performance may not have the same implications for central nervous system functioning among the aging as they do in younger people. The relevance of intellectual changes during the later years of life is open to question. For example, normal-aging individuals generally show declines in both speed of response and certain areas of perceptual integration; however, these performance differences may not make a difference in the daily living performances of the older person (Botwinick, 1977). Given ample rehearsal time, older persons have been shown to demonstrate adequate short-term memory, even equalling the abilities of much younger persons (Adamowicz, 1976). As Butler repeatedly indicates in his classic book Why Survive? Being Old in America (1975) most older people are not senile, forgetful, and confused, and the relative few who generally suffer from very real physical or mental illnesses.

Incidence, Prevalence, and Growth of the Elderly Population

One in nine Americans (11.3%) is 65 years and older, a fact that is commonly attributed to the baby boom prior to World War I and an increase in average life expectancy from 47 years in 1900 to over 73 years today (Harris, 1978; Soldo, 1980; Wetrogan, 1983). This population is projected to increase 8% by 1990 and another 9% by the year 2000 (Wetrogan, 1983). As indicated in Table 1, which expresses the differential growth of age groups within the older population, senior adults 75 years and older constitute the fastest growing segment in our society.

The geriatric boom of the 1980s can be demonstrated by increased caseloads of aging individuals with communication disabilities. A sharper focus on the importance of communication skills among older persons will serve to illustrate the need for involvement among audiologists and speech-language pathologists.

Table 1. Percent distribution of population 65 years and over, by age: 1950-2020.

Age	1950	1970	1976	1980	2000	2020
65-69	40.7	35.0	36.1	34.9	28.9	35.4
70-74	27.8	27.2	25.8	27.3	25.9	26.9
75-79	17.4	19.2	17.7	17.3	20.1	16.8
80-84	9.3	11.5	11.9	11.3	13.3	10.2
85 and over	4.8	7.1	8.6	9.2	11.8	10.6

Note. From "America's elderly in the 1980s" by B. J. Soldo, 1980/November, Population Bulletin, 35(4), p. 11.

Importance of Communication to Aging Persons

Perhaps no behavior is more essential to life satisfaction and self-esteem during the later years of life than the act of communicating with others. The sharing of life experiences, the release from stress afforded by social interaction, the need for social contact to control the environment, keep current on events of the world, and test and cope with the realities of change, all underscore the importance of maintaining communication during the later years of life.

> Our culture has chosen to ignore many of the normal communication
> needs of our older citizens. It may very well be that older
> people in our culture are communication starved. Many experience
> a state of communication deprivation that could be affecting
> other aspects of their lives, including such social psychological
> phenomena as life satisfaction, self esteem, or even the will to
> live. (Carmichael, 1982, p. 155)

One of the major reasons that older persons fail to communicate is depression. Complex interactions between failing body systems, decreasing self-image, diminishing self-worth, attrition of social contacts in the form of relatives and friends, and an increasing feeling of helplessness and dependency all contribute toward a high incidence of depression (Epstein, 1976).

In a more positive vein, the frequency of contact with close friends and relatives appears to be significantly related to life satisfaction among the aging (Spakes, 1979). Moreover, individuals receiving support from social networks are better able to cope with life stresses and disabilities that could lead to depression (Kemp & Vash, 1971; Schulz & Decker, 1983). Thus, studies which have demonstrated relationships between loss of social contact and increasing mental health problems (Hirsch, 1981; McKinlay, 1981) and higher mortality rate among the aging (Berkman & Syme, 1979) underscore the need for maintaining communication skills.

> Members of the older person's social network must possess the ability, knowledge and motivation to provide continuing emotional support. While motivation springs form societal expectations, e.g. children are <u>supposed</u> to care for their frail, elderly parents, etc., ability and knowledge are acquired through social communication. Support is particularly needed when life course events occur, e.g. a stroke or laryngectomy, which are unexpected. Such events are inherently more stressful, both for the aging persons and for the social network, both because there is lack of time to prepare for them and because appropriate abilities and knowledge are lacking, even if motivation is evident. What is needed is greater emphasis by communication disorders specialists on educating and sensitizing the social network to the disorder. (Rau, 1984)

One can only speculate on the effect of a communication disability during the aging years on the handicapped person's social network. As indicated by Schulz and Decker (1983), older individuals who lack mobility because of spinal cord injuries demonstrate much smaller networks than healthy, nondisabled persons of similar age. The reduction in social network likely also applies to stroke victims (Schulz & Rau, 1984). Research is needed in this area, because the loss of a portion of the support system could have a significant influence both on intervention for a communicative disorder and on the rate of physical and mental decline.

Incidence and Prevalence of Communication Disorders

Estimated percentages of speech and hearing impairments for 1982, based on 1977 prevalence rates provided by the National Center for Health Statistics and reported by Fein (1983a), are reproduced in Table 2. Fein noted that the designation "speech" impairments likely included language deficits as well. These data suggest that aging, handicapped persons are not proportionately represented in the caseloads of communication disorders specialists, at least when compared with services for children. The percentages also indicate that the majority of older persons (80%) do not have speech or language impairments, although only 57% of the over 65 group do not have hearing impairments.

Table 2. U. S. population, impaired populations, and clinical caseloads by age.

		Type of population			
		Impaired		Caseloads	
Age	U.S.	Speech	Hearing	Speech-Language Pathologists	Audiologists
0-5	9%	9%	1%	19%	23%
8-12	10%	19%	2%	46%	17%
13-21	15%	14%	4%	15%	11%
22-64	54%	38%	49%	10%	25%
65-	12%	20%	43%	10%	24%
All Ages	100%	100%	100%	100%	100%

Note. From "Population data from the U.S. Census Bureau" by D. J. Fein, 1983/March, Asha, 25, p. 47.
Sources: U.S. population data are 1982 U.S. Census Bureau estimates (U.S. Bureau of Census, 1982). Figures for impairments are 1982 estimates based on 1977 prevalence rates (NCHS, 1981), adjusted to include the long-term care institutionalized population. Caseload data are unpublished data from the 1982 ASHA Self-Study Project survey of clinical practitioners.

Table 3 expresses the rate and number of speech (and language) impairments in the 1977 survey (Fein, 1983b). It is important to note that these data do not include institutionalized persons, among whom an increased prevalence of handicaps exists. Nonetheless, the rate per 100 persons of impairments is second only in magnitude to that of children in the 5-14 year category. Surveys of institutionalized, nursing home residents have indicated that from 60% (Mueller & Peters, 1981) to 92.5% (Chafee, 1967) have communication disabilities that would require speech and hearing services. One of the greatest challenges facing the profession is providing services to institutionalized elderly persons.

Table 3. Number and rate per 100 persons of speech impairments* by age: 1977 U.S. civilian, noninstitutionalized population.

Age	Number	Rate Per 100 Persons
Under 5	140,018	.92
5-14	703,728	1.94
15-24	266,099	.67
25-34	221,213	.69
35-44	136,373	.59
45-54	149,171	.64
55-64	165,486	.82
65-74	127,825	.90
75+	84,623	1.06
All ages	1,994,536	.94

Note. From "The prevalence of speech and language impairments," by D. J. Fein, 1983/February, Asha, 25, p. 37.
Excludes cleft palate cases and deaf persons who cannot speak.

Problems of Audition

Hearing sensitivity declines commensurate with chronological age within the aging population (Figure 1), although non-aging factors may contribute greatly toward variances in hearing level data among individuals of similar longevity. The National Health Interview Survey reported by Punch (1983) (Table 4) reveals a prevalence rate among noninstitutionalized, civilian persons of 24% between 65 and 74 years and 39% for older age groups. Small sample surveys on the prevalence among nursing home residents reveal much higher figures, ranging upwards to 90% (Chafee, 1967).

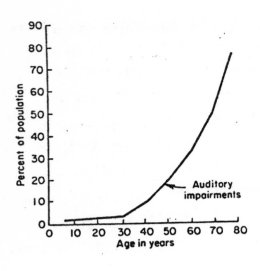

Figure 1. Percentage of persons in U.S. with auditory impairments, ages 6-79 years. From Fact book on aging: A profile of America's older population (p. 100) by C. S. Harris (1978). Washington, DC: The National Council on Aging.

Table 4. Prevalence rates of hearing impairment, per 100 persons, in the civilian, noninstitutionalized population of the U.S.

Age group in years	Number	Prevalence rate %
5	96,034	0.63
5-14	592,595	1.63
15-24	922,012	2.32
25-34	1,380,760	4.29
35-44	1,344,130	5.82
45-54	2,269,974	9.79
55-64	3,095,322	15.35
65-74	3,430,852	24.10
75+	3,087,095	38.55
All	16,218,774	7.64

Note. From "The prevalence of hearing impairment," by J. Punch, 1983/ April, Asha, 25, p. 27. Rates are based on 1977 interview data from the National Center for Health Statistics, 1982.

The decline of hearing sensitivity reported in surveys is only one aspect of the receptive communication problem among older persons. Declines in performance on central auditory processing tasks involving auditory memory storage and retrieval, phonemic analysis and synthesis, message conduction speed, comprehension in noise, and comprehension of degraded messages all suggest central auditory aging effects. The prevalence of these changes is not known, although it seems likely that they are related to increasing neuron depletion accompanying biological aging.

Neurological Disorders

Neurological disorders that may affect the reception, organization, perception, and expression of language include those of sudden onset, such as traumatic cerebrovascular accidents, and progressive neurological impairments such as Alzheimer's and Parkinson's diseases. The prevalence of stroke by age decade is shown in Figure 2. Nearly 75% of all acute stroke attacks in the United States occur in persons 65 years and older. Data from the 1981 national Survey of Stroke conducted by the National Institute of Neurological and Communicative Disorders and Stroke further indicated that at least some degree of speech or language impairment is present in nearly 60% of non-comatose stroke patients and 55% of those who were initially comatose and recovered (Weinfeld, 1981).

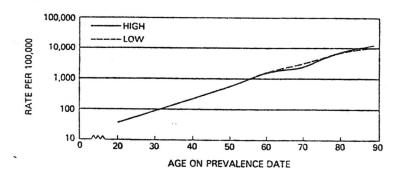

Figure 2. High and low age-specific prevalence rates of stroke per 100,000 population in the United States. From "The 1981 National Survey of Stroke." Stroke, 1(12), 1-67.

The highest incidence of diagnosed aphasia is found in the nursing home population, where 11% have been reported with symbolic language problems (Mueller & Peters, 1981). The incidence of stroke in the general population has been estimated by the National Center for Health Statistics (NCHS). Following a household health interview survey, NCHS indicated that approximately 2.7 million individuals 20 years and older had a history of stroke (Weinfeld, 1981). Mace and Rabins (1983) attribute 20% of the incidence of senile dementia to multiple infarcts, or small, often unnoticed strokes.

17

Surveys on the prevalence of senile dementia indicate that occurrence ranges from 4.2% (Bergmann, 1975) to 15% (Safford, 1980) in the general community of aging, and to 50% to 63% in the institutionalized elderly (Wang & Busse, 1971). Although a major cause of dementia is Alzheimer's disease, which accounts for about 50% of the cases, other factors responsible may include metabolic disorders, structural problems in the brain, infections, toxins, autoimmune diseases, vascular problems, psychiatric diseases, and multiple sclerosis (Mace & Rabins, 1983). Memory loss is the most common characteristic of senile dementia, and one of the earliest signs is inability to judge the passage of time (Mace & Rabins, 1983). Both expressive and receptive communication problems are observed in senile dementia. However, one rarely finds expressive disorders in the early stages of Alzheimer's disease.

Neuromuscular Disorders Affecting Speech Production

The incidence of motor speech disorders among the general aging population is unknown, although many of the progressive conditions such as Alzheimer's and Parkinson's disease, and more traumatic neurological disorders can be held responsible. It has been estimated that in the nursing home community 19% of the communication disorders consist of dysarthrias and other articulation difficulties, while 21% consist of voice disorders, largely consisting of inadequate loudness or quality disturbances (Mueller & Peters, 1981). Although most normal aging persons do not manifest either dyspraxic or dysarthric conditions, transient disturbances of both speech and language have been observed, along with a deterioration in mental functions associated with fluctuations in blood flow (Wilkie, 1980). Finally, this author has observed clinically that unsupervised drug ingestion in a highly medicated group may also account for changes in cognitive functioning including social communication skills.

Head and Neck Pathologies

Laryngeal problems, including vocal nodules, polyps, contact ulcers, and vocal fold paralysis occur among aging persons (Batza, 1977). Vocal fatigue and vocal weakness have also been linked to depression and increased anxiety states (Cooper, 1970; Damste & Lerman, 1975) common to older individuals, this may suggest the need for referral to a speech-language pathologist.

Prevalence and incidence data are best documented among laryngectomized persons, who largely constitute an aging population. The International Association of Laryngectomees indicates that the average age of individuals who have undergone laryngectomy is 55 years. American Cancer Society data suggests that approximately 9,000 cases of cancer of the larynx are discovered each year in the United States (American Cancer Society, 1978). The population of laryngectomees in this country has been estimated to be 30,000 (International Association of Laryngectomees, 1975).

Traumatic injury or falls may be responsible for some head and neck problems which may produce communication disorders. Although the elderly have a relatively low accident rate compared with other age groups (Hogue, 1980), they have a higher incidence of injuries and deaths due to falling (Iskrant & Joliet, 1968). Moreover, physical frailties and reduced calcium in the bony structures, particularly in those over the age of 70, make the elderly especially susceptible to injury.

Problems With Current Intervention Approaches

Many of the tests and measurements of the past, as well as a number of intervention strategies, have tended to "infantalize" the elderly, in the sense that they were normalized or developed for younger age groups. Body systems age and demonstrate performance decrements at different rates, both within the same person and for various individuals of equivalent chronological age. Similarly, a wide disparity may also be observed in communicative skills. Consequently, the development of a profile of performance skills for normal aging persons of various chronologies would appear to be a useful foundation from which to assess disorders (Bloomer, 1980).

Moreover, what constitutes a communicative "handicap" for one older person may lack significance in another, at least insofar as causing a reduction in life satisfaction. Instruments which assess the extent to which various disabilities are actually handicapping in the geriatric environment would permit a more relevant focus in rehabilitation. As indicated by Ventry and Weinstein (1983), the combination of quantifying both the extent of impairment and deriving the perceived handicap from an attitudinal questionnaire seems to be a better method to delineate the needs of the elderly.

Bloomer (1980) cites a number of other limitations with present intervention methods among the aging, which are summarized below:

1. Our profession has given little attention to preventive measures.
2. Speech and hearing specialists should participate more with other disciplines when dealing with geriatric cases.
3. Research should be aimed at adapting evaluative procedures to serve multiple disorders.
4. Members of our profession should promote sociability among the aging and utilize family and community to reduce social neglect.

The point is well-taken that members of the profession must make themselves more accessible to the elderly, many of whom lack the mobility of younger persons. In addition, the dialectics of the aging environment (Windley & Scheidt, 1980) should become as familiar to speech-language pathologists and audiologists as those of school-age clients. Reducing barriers and tailoring clinical settings for optimal intervention is as important in older age groups as it is for children.

Accessibility extends beyond the physical environment. There is a professional responsibility to see that communication problems among the elderly are revealed to others. In recent years, a number of authors have alluded to the continuing responsibility for providing education and guidance within the geriatric support system (Bloomer, 1980; Lubinski & Chapey, 1980; Mueller & Peters, 1981; Safford, 1980). Regional workshops conducted by the American Speech-Language-Hearing Association (ASHA) have focused on this important aspect (Diggs, 1980). However, the responsibility falls to the individual practitioner to see that family members, cohorts, and professionals from other disciplines learn to recognize communication problems, act as knowledgeable referral sources, and participate in intervention. The relevance and need for our services must achieve increased visibility through commitment as a caring profession within a "caring society" (Comfort, 1978).

Purpose of Training

One means by which a "caring society" might be fostered is through a conscious effort at recognizing, understanding, and remembering that communication does not occur as a static isolated event. Rather, the form and content of messages are determined by the individual's present physical and psychological abilities as well as by previous experiences, and the context in which the communication occurs. Thus, changes in physical condition, psychological state, or socialization patterns associated with aging may result in concomitant changes in communication.

With knowledge, understanding, and sensitivity to the characteristics of aging--changes in cognitive development from adulthood to old age, psychological needs, neurological correlates of aging, and socialization patterns of aging persons--comes the ability to provide efficient, effective, and appropriate speech-language and hearing services in an effort to foster the maintenance of independent quality living for the aging person.

Thus, the purpose of this training manual is to enhance speech-language pathologists' and audiologists' awareness of the physical, psychological, and sociological changes associated with aging. The end result is that communication disorders specialists be better prepared to generate more appropriate intervention strategies for communication problems present in the aging population and to interact in closer cooperation with other members of the health care team.

Self Study Questions

1. What evidence contraindicates the aging myths about "educability" and "intelligence?"

2. What key factors tend to draw the older person inward in a social communicative sense?

3. It has been suggested that the aging population is not homogeneous. What significance does this have on our interpretation of what is a communication "disorder" in this age group?

4. In this chapter older persons have been described as the largest multiply handicapped segment of the population. What evidence supports this statement?

5. What are the principle problems in our profession that affect current intervention approaches among the aging?

REFERENCES

Adamowicz, J. (1976). Visual short term memory and aging. <u>Journal of Gerontology</u>, <u>31</u>, 39-46.

American Cancer Society, (1978). <u>Facts on cancer of the larynx</u>. (p. 1). New York.

Batza, E. M. (1977). Adventures in vocal rehabilitation. In M. Cooper & M. H. Cooper (Eds.), <u>Approaches to vocal rehabilitation</u>. Springfield, IL: Charles C. Thomas.

Bergmann, K. (1975). The epidemiology of senile dementia. <u>British Journal of Psychiatry</u>, (Special Publication), <u>9</u>, 100-109.

Berkman, L. F., & Syme, S. L. (1979). Social networks, host resistance, and mortality: A nine year follow up study of Alameda County residents. <u>American Journal of Epidemology</u>, <u>109</u>, 186-204.

Bloomer, H. (1980). Speaking of aging. Guest Editorial, <u>Asha</u>, <u>22</u>, 459.

Botwinick, J. (1977). Aging and intelligence. In J. E. Birren & K. W. Schaie (Eds.), <u>Handbook of the psychology of aging</u>. New York: Van Nostrand.

Butler, R. N. (1975). <u>Why survive? Being old in America</u>. (pp. 9-10). New York: Harper & Row.

Cameron, P. (1970a). The generation gap: Beliefs about sexuality and self-reported sexuality. <u>Developmental Psychology</u>, <u>3</u>, 272.

Cameron, P. (1970b). The generation gap: Which generation is believed powerful versus generational members' self appraisal of power? <u>Developmental Psychology</u>, <u>3</u>, 403-404.

Cameron, P. (1973). Which generation is believed to be intellectually superior and which generation believe itself intellectually superior? <u>International Journal of Aging and Human Development</u>, <u>4</u>, 157-170.

Carmichael, C. W. (1982). In L. A. Samovar & R. E. Porter (Eds.), <u>Intercultural communication: A reader</u>. (p. 155). Belmont, CA.

Cattell, R. B. (1963). The theory of fluid and crystallized intelligence: A critical experiment. <u>Journal of Educational Psychology</u>, <u>54</u>, 1.

Chafee, C. E. (1967). Rehabilitation needs of nursing home patients: A report of a survey. <u>Rehabilitation Literature</u>, <u>28</u>, 377.

Comfort, A. (1978, April). <u>Keynote address</u>. Presented at the 24th annual meeting of the Western Gerontological Society, Tucson, AZ.

Cooper, M. (1970). Voice problems of the geriatric patient. *Geriatrics,* *25,* 107-110.

Curtin, S. (1972). Aging in the land of the young. *Atlantic Monthly,* *230,* 68.

Damste, P. H., & Lerman, J. W. (1975). *An introduction to voice pathology.* Springfield, IL: Charles C. Thomas.

Demming, J. A., & Pressey, S. L. (1957). Tests 'indigenous' to the adult and older years. *Journal of Counseling Psychology,* *4,* 144-148.

Demo, M. P. (1980). Education and the elderly. *Communication Education,* *29,* 78-85.

Diggs, C. C. (1980). ASHA recognized needs of older persons. *Asha,* *22,* 401-403.

Epstein, L. (1976). Symposium on age differentiation in depressive illness: Depression in the elderly. *Journal of Gerontology,* *31,* 278-282.

Fein, D. J. (1983a). Population data from the U.S. Census Bureau. *Asha,* *25,* 37.

Fein, D. J. (1983b). The prevalence of speech and language impairments. *Asha,* *25,* 37.

Harris, C. S. (1978). *Fact book on aging: A people of America's older population.* The National Council on Aging, Washington, DC.

Hirsch, B. J. (1981). Social networks and the coping process: Creating personal communities. In B. H. Gottleib (Ed.), *Social networks and social support.* (pp. 149-170). Beverly Hills, CA.

Hogue, C. C. (1980). Epidemiology of injury in old age. In *Epidemiology of aging: Second conference* (Publication 80-969). (p. 128). U. S. Public Health Service.

International Association of Laryngectomees, (1975). *Laryngectomized speaker's source book.* (p. 9). New York: International Association of Laryngectomees.

Iskrant, A. P., & Joliet, P. V. (1968). *Accident and homocide.* Cambridge: Harvard University Press.

Jernigan, J. (1979, November). *The biologically elite.* Paper presented at the third annual conference on the medical aspects of aging, University of Florida, Gainesville, FL.

Kemp, B. J., & Vash, C. L. (1971). Productivity after injury in a sample of spinal cord injured persons: A pilot study. Journal of Chronic Disease, 24, 259-275.

Lubinski, R., & Chapey, R. (1980). Communication services in home health care agencies: Availability and scope. Asha, 22, 929-934.

Mace, N. L., & Rabins, P. V. (1983). The 36-hour day. (7th ed.). (pp. 36-37). Baltimore: The Johns Hopkins University Press.

McKinlay, J. B. (1981). Social network influences on morbid episodes and the career of help seeking. In L. Eisenberg & A. Kleinman (Eds.), The relevance of social science for medicine. (pp. 77-107). Holland: Dordrecht.

Miller, A. H., Gurin, P., & Gurin, G. (1980). Age consciousness and political mobilization of older Americans. The Gerontologist, 20, 691-700.

Mueller, P. B., & Peters, T. J. (1981). Needs and services in geriatric speech-language pathology and audiology. Asha, 23, 627.

Price, L. J., Fein, G., & Feinberg, I. (1980). Neuropsychological assessment of cognitive function in the elderly. In L. W. Poon, (Ed.), Aging in the 1980's: Psychological issues. (pp. 78-85). Washington, DC: American Psychological Association.

Punch, J. (1983). The prevalence of hearing impairment. Asha, 25, 27.

Rau, M. (1984). Personal communication.

Safford, F. (1980). A program for families of the mentally impaired elderly. The Gerontologist, 20(6), 656.

Schaie, K. W. (1978). External validity in the assessment of intellectual performance in adulthood. Journal of Gerontology, 33, 695-701.

Schuetz, J. (1980). Lifelong learning: Communication education for the elderly. Communication Education, 29, 35-36.

Schulz, R., & Decker, S. (1983, August). Long term adjustment to physical disabilities: The role of social comparison processes, social support, and perceived control. Paper presented at the annual meeting of the American Psychological Association, Anaheim, CA.

Soldo, B. J. (1980). America's elderly in the 1980's. Population Bulletin, 35(4), 11.

Spakes, P. R. (1979). Family, friendship, and community interaction as related to life satisfaction of the elderly. Journal of Gerontological Social Work, 1, 279-294.

Ventry, I. M., & Weinstein, B. E. (1983). Identification of elderly people with hearing problems. Asha, 25(7), 37-45.

Wang, H. S., & Busse, E. W. (1971). Dementia in old age. In C. E. Wells (Ed.), Dementia. Philadelphia: Davis.

Weinfeld, F. D. (1981). The 1981 national survey of stroke. Stroke, 1(12), 1-22.

Wetrogan, S. I. (1983). Provisional projections of the population of states by age and sex: 1980-2000. Bureau of Census, U.S. Dept. Commerce, Population Estimates and Projections, Series P-25, 937.

Wilkie, F. L. (1980). Blood pressure and cognitive functioning. In Epidemiology of aging: Second conference (NIH Publication 80-969, pp. 105-126). U.S. Public Health Service.

Windley, P. G., & Scheidt, R. J. (1980). Person-environment dialectics: Implications for competent functioning in old age. In L. W. Poon (Ed.), Aging in the eighties. Washington, DC: American Psychological Association, 407-423.

Wolfe, L. M. (1963). Lifelong learning and adjustment in the later years. Adult Education, 14, 26-32.

Suggested Readings

Mace, N. L., & Rabins, P. V. (1981). The 36 hour day. Baltimore: Johns Hopkins University Press.

Holland, A. (Ed.). (1984). Language disorders in adults. San Diego: College Hill Press.

Butler, R. N. (1975). Why Survive? Being old in America. New York: Harper & Row.

Beasley, D. S., & Davis, G. A. (Eds.). (1981). Aging communication processes and disorders. New York: Grune & Stratton.

Maurer, J. F., & Rupp, R. R. (1979). Hearing and aging: Tactics for intervention. New York: Grune & Stratton.

Bergman, M. (1980). Aging and the perception of speech. Baltimore: University Park Press.

Schow, R. L., Hutchinson, J. M., & Nerbonne, M. A. (1978). Communication disorders of the aged. Baltimore: University Park Press.

Oyer, J. J., & Oyer, E. J. (Eds.). (1976). Aging and communication. Baltimore: University Park Press.

Physical Changes In Aging

Linda Jacobs-Condit
American Speech-Language-Hearing Association, Rockville, Maryland

and

Mary Louise Ortenzo
George Washington University, Washington, DC

Aging is a universal and natural process which begins at conception and continues throughout the life cycle. Although heredity plays a role in the way in which each of us ages (Comfort, 1979), other determinants include health, degree of physical activity, lifestyle, employment, and exposure to harmful substances. Obviously each of these factors may be so intertwined as to obscure our ability to separate disease entities from normal aging. However, the purpose of this chapter is to provide for the reader general information regarding normal physiological changes which are directly related to the normal process of aging as it affects the nervous system, cardiovascular and respiratory systems, musculoskeletal system, sensory processes, and nutrition in the elderly.

Central Nervous System

The nervous system in man includes the central nervous system, the peripheral nervous system (including pairs of 12 cranial and 31 spinal nerves), and the autonomic nervous system (sympathetic and parasympathetic divisions to maintain internal homeostasis). For the purposes of this chapter, the discussion will address primarily the physiological changes which occur within the central nervous system as a function of the aging process.

Comprised of the brain and spinal cord, the central nervous system is the "primary biological basis for intelligence and personality" (Schaie & Geiwitz, 1982, p. 353). Although significant changes in neurological function occur during the aging process (Wantz & Gay, 1981), the age of onset and rate of decline differs within and between individuals (Ordy, Brizzee, & Beavers, 1980).

One frequently cited change with age is a decrease in weight of the human brain. Arendt (1972) reported that a decrease in brain weight occurs earlier for women (at age 60-70 years) than for men (at age 70-80 years). In a comparison between males aged 20-30 years and those aged 70-80 years, Dekaban and Sadowsky (1978) reported a decrease in mean brain weight from 1,449 grams to 1,344 grams with increasing age. This represents a 7% decrease in brain weight of the elderly males studied.

Although a loss of neurons in the central nervous system is not anatomically uniform, Wisniewski and Terry (1973) suggested that this probably accounted for the decline in brain weight which occurs with age. This would appear to be a plausible hypothesis. "Since cells in the central nervous system do not reproduce themselves, when neurons are lost, they are not replaced" (Wantz & Gay, 1981, p. 134).

Not only have researchers reported a decrease in brain weight, but in brain volume as well. Blinkov and Glezer (1968) reported a decrease in total brain volume from about 1300 cubic centimeters at age 20, to 1100 cubic centimeters at age 80. Davis and Wright (1977) observed a constant relationship between brain volume and cranial cavity volume in normal young adults and middle-aged adults (under 55 years of age), suggesting that any deviation from this value in the elderly would be indicative of altered brain volume.

Given that a reduction in cell numbers with age could be related to a decrease in brain weight and brain volume, then it is also likely that these changes could be correlated with reduced efficiency of the brain's functioning (Wantz & Gay, 1981). For example, Schaie (1982) indicated that remaining neurons might be "less efficient than before, conducting nerve impulses at a slightly slower rate" (p. 354). A change which occurs gradually throughout the life span, this reduced nerve conductivity may easily be reflected in longer reaction time or in changes in the electroencephalogram (EEG) (Hultsch & Deutsch, 1981).

Birren (1965) reported that a decline in reaction time is one of the most consistent changes with aging. A function of the central nervous system, the components of reaction time are sensory transmission time, motor execution time, and a central component including interpretation, decision-making and association (Schaie, 1982). The central processing component accounts for a greater percentage of the total reaction time (almost 80%) than do the sensory input or motor output components (Botwinick, 1978).

Reaction time tasks range from the very simple (i.e., time required to push a button after a buzzer sounds) to the very complex (e.g., speed of typing). Welford (1977) reported significantly lengthened reaction time for older adults--20% increase in the performance of simple tasks and more than 50% for complex tasks. Independent of task and situation (Birren, Riegel, & Morrison, 1962), the alteration (slowing) in reaction time with age apparently reflects a change in the "speed with which the central nervous system processes information" (Birren, 1974, p. 808). The hypothesis that with age the central nervous system becomes sluggish and reaction time slows could account for many differences in memory, perception, learning, and intelligence (Birren, 1974; Birren, Woods, & Williams, 1980).

Botwinick (1978) has suggested that physical exercise can substantially improve reaction times in the elderly. In fact, the average reaction time of the elderly who remain physically active (i.e, jog, walk, play racquetball) has been shown to be much faster than that among nonathletic young people. Spirduso and Clifford (1978) reported "sizable differences" between athletic 60-70-year-old males and nonathletic 20-year-old males. Because exercise increases the flow of blood to the brain, increases oxygen levels in the blood and may affect the quality of neural tissue, these factors may easily be related to typical age differences in reaction time (Birren, Woods, & Williams, 1980).

Slowing of behavior and reaction times in the elderly has also been linked to changes in brain electrical activity (Marsh & Thompson, 1977; Woodruff, 1979) as reflected in EEG recordings. The continuous rhythmic activity displayed in the EEG can be divided into four basic patterns and associated behavior states. The dominant, alpha rhythm, at a frequency of 8-13 cps, is associated with a relaxed, awake state with eyes closed. At a faster frequency of 18-30 cps, the beta rhythm is associated with an attentive alert state. Associated with drowsiness and sleep are the slower frequencies, theta at 5-7 cps and delta (0.5-4 cps) waves, respectively.

It is not until individuals reach their late 50s or early 60s that differences in EEG are easily noticeable (Obrist, 1980), the most reliable being a slowing of the alpha rhythm. The alpha occurs at approximately 10-11 cps in young adults, at about 9 cps in those aged 60 years, and at 8 cps in the elderly over 80 years of age. This slowing of the brain and central nervous system activity with age (Schaie, 1982), as reflected in the EEG, may be due to reduced cerebral blood flow which results in neuronal loss (Obrist, 1972), or may be an index of reduced cortical excitability (Woodruff, 1979).

To summarize to this point, several relatively consistent changes within the central nervous system occur with age. As the number of neuronal cells within the brain and spinal cord diminishes, weight and volume (size) of the brain decreases. The elderly also experience an alteration (slowing) in reaction time, and a slowing of alpha waves as depicted on the electroencephalogram (EEG). It is likely that the overall effects of changes within the central nervous system are widespread, influencing a number of behaviors and motor skills. Regardless of the cause of central nervous system changes with age, any behavior or motoric activity mediated by the central nervous system can be "expected to show the characteristic slowing with advancing age" (Wantz & Gay, 1981, p. 136).

An issue which warrants clarification is that surrounding the notion that senility is common to the elderly. Not a normal aspect of the aging process (Maurer & Rupp, 1979; NIA, 1980), senility is often used to describe a wide variety of conditions, the causes of which are equally as varied (including anxiety, poor nutrition, head injury, or adverse drug reactions) (NIA, 1980; Ronch, 1982). For example, senility may be used to denote forgetfulness, confusion or a change in personality or behavior. However, such infrequent memory lapses or slight confusions may simply indicate an "overload of facts in the brain's storehouse of information" (NIA, 1980).

In actuality, senility is the result of organic brain disease (Maurer & Rupp, 1979), the incidence of which is very low in that less than 10% of the elderly will ever become demented (Svanborg, 1983). In a recent study of the elderly in Sweden, Hagnell, Lanke, Rorsman, and Ojesjo (1980) indicated a decline in the incidence of organic brain disease in that country despite an increase in the population of elderly.

Due to a variety of organic causes, senile dementia involves a group of symptoms which include "decreased cognitive ability (memory loss, poor judgement, attention problems; impaired social, work or peer relationships; disorientation; and reduced learning ability) in the absence of delirium or specific intellectual dysfunction" (Ronch, 1982, p. 197).

Although the majority of cases of dementia are reversible, some are not. The causes of reversible dementia include infections, metabolic disturbances, intercranial tumors, nutritional disorders, circulatory and pulmonary diseases, adverse drug interactions, and psychiatric disorders (NIH, 1980; Ronch, 1982). Irreversible dementia may be categorized as Alzheimer's disease (50-70% of cases), multifarct or vascular dementia (15-25% of cases), or a mixture of the two (Eisdorfer, Cohen, & Veith, 1981).

Alzheimer's disease is a neurological disorder of unknown origin for which there is no cure or treatment. It has been hypothesized that this disease may be caused by "selective cell death provoked by viral or environmental agents, excessive accumulation of aluminum or other toxins, a genetic defect or predisposition, or by an age-related change in the immune system" (NIH, 1980, p. 7). Whatever the cause, it is expected that individuals would eventually exhibit "mental emptiness" (NIH, 1980, p. 2) characterized by complete disorientation and total memory loss.

In the early stages of the disease, individuals with Alzheimer's may be unable to concentrate, anxious, irritable, agitated, or withdrawn. In later stages, individuals may be unable to calculate, may exhibit lack of judgment, disorientation to time and place, and inability to understand cartoons or jokes. Some may wander about lost, whereas others may easily throw temper tantrums, become depressed, or even forget the names of family, friends, and/or neighbors. Although each individual progresses through these stages at different rates and exhibits varied loss of functioning, all in the final stages of Alzheimer's disease exhibit the same traits of apathy, disorientation, and lack of concern about the opinion of others (NIH, 1980).

The impact of dementia upon the individual is not simply a function of the measureable degree of organic brain damage, but also reflects a subjective value of decreased abilities as well as cultural and emotional reactions (Ronch, 1982). For instance, the elderly person with a combination of visual, auditory or motor impairments may become withdrawn, confused or even angry; and some of this emotion may be projected onto others (Ronch, 1982).

The Musculoskeletal System

Independence is a strong cultural value of our society. Dependency is generally viewed as an undesirable state. One of the most stressful aspects of the aging process is that a decrease in mobility may eventually cause dependency. Studies show that older people view dependency as one of their greatest fears related to growing old. A frequently heard concern among the elderly is, "I don't mind growing old as long as I can care for myself." Dependency among the older population which usually results from diminished physical mobility makes coping with the tasks of independent living difficult if not impossible (Saxon & Etten, 1978).

Muscular Changes in Normal-Aged Persons

Muscle changes that occur in the aged may be divided into those which are the natural result of aging and those which result from disease. In the normal aging process, a person becomes progressively less able to adapt to the challenge and stress of daily life. From skin to bone and throughout the body, changes are constantly occurring. No one remains at the height of his or her physical perfection. Maximum muscular strength is usually attained by age 25 or 30 (Saxon & Etten, 1978), after which there is a gradual decrease in the number of muscle fibers and in their individual bulk. The reduction in the size of the muscle is referred to as atrophy or "wasting" (Grob, 1981). Muscle power increases through increased use, whereas a failure to flex skeletal muscles causes their atrophy. Usually, after the sixth decade there is a slow, steady atrophy, the rate of atrophy directly related to the life habits of the individual. Older persons may be expected to have a decreased capacity for sustained muscular contraction. Although the process of regeneration is not active, the atrophied muscles are replaced with an increasing amount of adipose tissue (Cape, 1978).

Changes in body composition with age are well-documented. For example, a 150 lb. 80-year-old male has less muscle and more fat than his 30-year-old counterpart with comparable weight and height (Rowe & Besdine, 1982). Changes are particularly conspicuous in the small muscles of the hands, which become thin and bony, with deep spaces between the bones. The arm and leg muscles become thin and flabby. Some degree of weakness does occur with muscular wasting but not generally in proportion to the amount of atrophy (Grob, 1978). By the ages of 70-80, the total weight of the lean body mass, which includes muscle, liver, brain, and kidney diminishes by 20%-30% (Cape, 1978). In addition, muscles become less elastic and therefore less flexible with age. This, combined with age-related changes in skeletal joints, contributes to stiffness and immobility. However, the more robustly physical life is, the bulkier and stronger the muscles remain. A survey of available research reports on normal aging shows that physical fitness resulting from regular systematic exercise and proper nutrition appear to be two of the best ways to offset many of the aches, pains, and limitations of mobility in older age (Saxon & Etten, 1978).

Specific Muscle Changes

In general, the aged person usually shows a decrease in movements, which are characteristically slow. However, many visible muscular changes result not from atrophy but from a degeneration of nerves which innervate the muscles. This may accelerate or retard muscle contraction. For example, spontaneous flickering or twitching of the muscles (fasciculations) particularly occur in the calves, eyelids, hands, and feet. It should be noted, however, that the incidence of muscular fasciculations is not necessarily a function of age. On the other hand, the overall facial expression of a normal older person is more fixed showing infrequent blinking of the eyes and a decrease of spontaneous movements (Grob, 1978). The following brief descriptions of the most common changes of movement are seen to a minor degree and underscore the effect of the changes in normal older people.

Muscle cramps may occur at any age, but often become more troublesome with advancing age. Frequently occurring at night following periods of extreme physical activity, they are painful and involuntary, and commonly affect the thigh, calf, hip, or hand. They may occur from a variety of chemical imbalances such as sodium deprivation, a decrease in the plasma concentration of calcium, from a presence of toxins or in association with specific muscle diseases. However, in the great majority of instances, the cause of muscle cramps is unknown (Grob, 1978).

Cramps may frequently be terminated by passive stretch. Their incidence may be diminished by a hot bath at bedtime or by orally administered quinine sulfate, which lengthens the refractory period of muscles, presumably by slowing repolarization (Grob, 1978).

Restless legs, or a constant moving of the legs, sometimes occurs in elderly persons who experience a tingling or burning sensation (paresthesia). Although the paresthesias are usually relieved by motion of the legs and reappear only when the legs have been quiet for a while, the person tends to keep the legs in motion (Grob, 1978).

Masticatory and facial muscles are essential to chewing and speech production, and also affect the appearance of aging in the face. Changes in structure as well as in points of attachment to the skull and facial bones may result in malfunctions. Due to a lack of research in this area, the data deal mainly with structural changes (Kahane, 1981).

The significant effect of aging in the masticatory muscles is a reduction in biting force which decreases from approximately 300 lbs./sq. in. in young people to 50 lbs./sq. in. in older individuals (Kaplan, 1971). This may result from weakness of the masticatory musculature because of atrophy (Greenfield, Shy, Alvord, & Berg, 1957) or from a reduction in biochemical efficiency due to changes in muscle attachments (MacMillan, 1936). The muscular changes described by MacMillan are due primarily to alterations in bone structure and only secondarily to muscle changes (Kahane, 1981). Limited information is available on the effects of aging on specific facial muscles (Pitanguy, 1978). However, the alterations of musculature in the jaw and chin region appear to be largely cosmetic and would not likely have any deleterious effect upon speech production (Kahane, 1981).

The tongue plays an important role in chewing, swallowing, and speech production. Therefore, anatomic and physiologic changes are important (Kahane, 1981). Two significant changes are found in the reduced number of taste buds and a thinning of the surface epithelium (Robinson, Boling, & Lisner, 1942) which occur earlier in women than in men (40-45 years vs. 50-60 years) (Harris, 1951). There is a 60% decrease in the number of taste buds in senile persons (Kaplan, 1971). Bucciante and Luria (1934) studied the musculature of the tongue in aged persons and found an increase in muscle fiber size with an increased amount of connective tissue indicating atrophy of the tongue muscles. However, the overall size of the tongue does not change significantly with age (Kaplan, 1971). Despite taste bud loss, no significant losses in sensitivity from salty, sweet, sour, or bitter substances were found until the fifth decade, followed by marked declines through the sixth to eighth decades (Kahane, 1981). Additional discussion follows later in the chapter.

No age-related changes in tongue movement during swallowing have been found. However, impaired rapid alternating movements of the tongue in geriatric persons between 66 and 93 from both sexes were reported by Ptacek, Sander, Maloney, and Jackson (1966). This suggests that the neuromuscular movements required for rapid speech may be different from those used in swallowing. The former may be more susceptible to age-related changes than the latter (Kahane, 1981).

Oral Mucosa, Connective Tissue, Glands

Several age-related changes have been observed in the structure of the oral mucosa; specifically, a thinning of the mucosa with some loss of elasticity and loss from attachment to underlying connective tissue, muscle, and bone (Squier, Johnson, & Hopps, 1976). Squier et al. (1976) indicated that this reduction in structural support makes the oral epithelium susceptible to trauma and slow to heal. Due to decreased amounts of salivary secretions, the oral mucosa dries which exacerbates the condition (Kahane, 1981).

Data from Truex (1940) has shown that aging oral epithelium may also undergo changes in sensory innervation. He found that sensory ganglion cells undergo fatty degeneration after the fourth decade. Truex concluded that the loss of these sensory cells result in a reduction of sensitivity in the orofacial area.

With regard to the effects of aging on laryngeal epithelia, the evidence is inconclusive. Several investigators reported that laryngeal epithelia thicken with age, whereas others suggest that age is not a factor. Ryan, McDonald, and Devine (1956) reported that laryngeal mucosa in men was innately thicker than in women. Segre (1971) reported that after middle age, the laryngeal mucosa acquired a thin, yellowish appearance and often underwent nonpathologic changes. However, changes in surface epithelia of the larynx are not natural results of aging but should be viewed as pathologic changes.

Ruckes and Hohmann (1963) and Hommerich (1972) found that the mucous glands in the larynx degenerate and atrophy in persons over 70. The diminished production of mucous by the laryngeal glands results in drying out of the laryngeal mucosa, which consequently predisposes it to trauma and disease (Kahane, 1981).

Several investigators have reported that aging laryngeal muscles undergo degeneration and atrophy. However, there has been disagreement among investigators as to which muscles are most affected (Kahane, 1981). Atrophy in all the intrinsic muscles of the larynx was reported by Kofler (1932) and Carnevalle-Ricci (1937). However, subsequent research by several other investigators is not in total corroboration.

Aging changes in laryngeal muscles appear to be closely related to disturbances in the vascular supply to the muscles (Kahane, 1981). This was concluded by a series of independent investigations. According to Kahane (1981) cautious interpretation may suggest that increasing age causes reduced metabolic capabilities and consequently reduced biochemical efficiency of laryngeal muscles. "Though age-related changes in laryngeal muscles have been noted, the etiology has not been established. Some characteristics of aging laryngeal muscles have been identified, but they appear to vary slightly from muscle to muscle and a hierarchy of muscle affectedness has not been determined" (Kahane, 1981, p. 26).

The Skeletal System

The human body changes as it ages and the skeletal system is no exception. Bone has three surfaces called envelopes, each of which has differing anatomical features but identical cellular structure. The surface facing the marrow cavity is the endosteal envelope, the outer surface is the periosteal envelope, and the material in between is the intracortical envelope (Notelovitz & Ware, 1982).

"Bone is a dynamic organ that is constantly being remodeled" (Giansiracusa & Kantrowitz, 1982, p. 24). Throughout childhood, new bone is formed on the outer surface, and a lesser amount of breakdown occurs on the inner surface. During adolescence bone formation occurs on both surfaces producing large gains in bone mass.

In early adulthood bone breakdown occurs at the inner surface and osteopenia, the normal reduction in bone mass begins. It is at this point that the rate of bone breakdown, also referred to as resorption, exceeds the rate of bone formation resulting in a progressive loss of bone (Meunier, 1973).

Both men and women lose bone as they age. Males lose 27% of their honey-combed fibrous trabecular bone mass by age 80. By the time a woman reaches the same age, she will have lost 43% of her trabecular bone mass (Meunier, Courpron, Edouard, Bernard, Bringuier, & Vignon, 1973). Loss of cortical, or outer portion of bone, begins by age 45 in women and age 50 in men. In addition to starting earlier in females, cortical bone loss proceeds at a more rapid rate. Women lose 10% of their central bone mass per decade whereas men lose 5% (Newton-John & Morgan, 1970).

"Although the entire skeleton loses mass with aging, the distribution of bone loss is not uniform. The different proportions of trabecular versus cortical bone in various parts of the skeleton contribute to this discrepancy" (Giansiracusa & Kantrowitz, 1982, p. 243). Several generalizations can be made about bone loss associated with aging. Women experience maximum bone loss between the ages of 50 and 65, whereas for men this occurs between 70 and 80 years. Skeletal mass in young adults is greater in males than females and is greater in Blacks than in Whites. For women there is accelerated bone loss after menopause (Raisz, 1977).

Several possible factors contribute to the age-related loss of bone mass. Calcium deficiency is due to impaired calcium absorption, in that the percentage of total daily intake of calcium absorbed in persons under 65 correlates inversely with dietary calcium intake. This inverse correlation does not occur in individuals over 65. When faced with a fall in dietary calcium, the aged intestine loses its capacity to increase calcium absorption (Bullamore, Wilkinson, & Gallagher, 1970). Further, there is evidence to suggest that protein metabolism in the older adult interferes with calcium absorption (Notelovitz & Ware, 1982). In addition, the lack of regular and systematic exercise and decrease in estrogen often associated with the postmenopausal years (Saxon & Etten, 1978) may contribute to reduced bone mass.

Osteoporosis is the pathologic state of osteopenia in which bone mass is so reduced that the skeleton loses its integrity and becomes unable to perform its supportive function. (Avioli, 1977). The most common age-related disorder of the skeleton, with which there is an uncoupling of the tightly balanced bone remodeling process. During this process of accelerated bone loss, excessive amounts of bone tissue are lost and skeleton reduction may reach several inches (Notelovitz & Ware, 1982).

The most common type of osteoporosis found in the elderly population results from a complex interplay of heredity, hormones, and nutrition. Clinically, the persons most often affected with osteoporosis are postmenopausal White women, in that 29% of women and 10% of men between the ages of 45 and 79 have osteoporosis" (Giansiracusa & Kantrowitz, 1982, p. 246). Black women have greater bone masses than White women and are affected less frequently. Women who weigh less than 140 lbs. develop osteoporosis more frequently than do heavier individuals, because the adipose (fat) tissue that stores estrogens protects the bones from physical stresses (Jowsey, 1977).

Several possible causes of osteoporosis have been proposed. Normal bone loss may be accelerated as a function of aging, an abnormally low skeletal mass at skeletal maturity may continue to decrease at a normal rate, or a combination of these may occur (Giansiracusa & Kantrowitz, 1982). Jowsey (1977) further states, "morphologically, the only significant difference between individuals with normal senile osteopenic bone and those with pathologic osteoporotic bone is the quantity of bone" (p. 247). Thus, patients with osteoporosis may simply be at the extreme end of the spectrum of physiologic senile osteopenia. The rate of bone formation in patients with untreated osteoporosis is normal, wheras the rate of resorption is increased (Giansiracusa & Kantrowitz, 1982).

Table 1 illustrates that low bone mass at skeletal maturity and an accelerated rate of bone loss characterize osteoporotic patients as compared to normal individuals.

Table 1. Bone turnover in osteoporosis (X ± SD).*

	Age	N	Formation %	Resorption
Normals	20-44	37	2.3 + 1.3	4.0 + 1.4
Patients with osteoporosis	45-75	58	2.0 + 1.4	3.9 + 1.4
	20-44	12	2.9 + 1.7	8.9 + 3.5
	45-75	143	2.6 + 1.7	10.5 + 5.1

Note. In untreated osteoporotic patients, the rate of bone formation is normal, but the rate of bone resorption is several times greater than normal. Source: From Jowsey J. (1977). Osteoporosis: Idiopathic, post-menopausal, and senile. In C. B. Sledge (Ed.), Metabolic diseases of bone. Philadelphia: Saunders.

Osteoporosis affects not only the amount but also the strength of the bone. As bone begins to erode, the porous trabecular bone becomes even more porous and cortical bone becomes thinner. Thin porous bones, no longer strong enough to withstand the physical stresses of everyday activity, are highly susceptible to fracture.

The incidence of vertebral body (spine), femoral neck (hip), and Colles' (wrist) fractures increases with age as shown in Figure 1 (Jowsey, 1977). Of approximately 1 million fractures per year in the U.S. for women 45 years or older, 70% occur in osteoporotic women (Notelovitz & Ware, 1982). Although vertebral bones are primarily composed of trabecular bone, they usually show the effects of osteoporosis first.

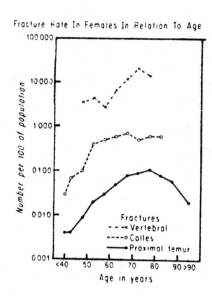

Figure 1. Fracture rate in women in relation to age. From Jowsey, J. (1977). Osteoporosis: Idiopathic, post-menopausal, and senile. In C. B. Sledge (Ed.), Metabolic diseases of bone. Philadelphia: Saunders.

Fractures

Vertebral fractures can occur spontaneously, so that the weakened bones collapse under the weight of the body. Although they generally follow sudden attempts to extend the spine from a flexed position, these fractures can occur from everyday activities. Continued fractures may result in the rib cage tilting downward toward the hips, eventually coming to rest on the hipbones. The result is outward curvature of the upper spine (kyphosis) leading to the dowager's hump; inward curvature of the lower spine (lordosis) and a protruding abdomen, because the downward movement of the ribs forces the internal organs outward (Notelovitz & Ware, 1982).

Pain associated with vertebral osteoporosis takes two forms. Sharp, acute pain varies in intensity from mild to severe, and may be localized at the fracture site or may radiate laterally from the midline to the abdomen. Occasionally, it radiates to the hip and legs. Any movement that increases pain in the abdominal region may exacerbate the pain (Avioli, 1977).

Less localized, chronic pain may be felt up and down both sides of the spine, is often associated with spasming of the muscles or may be aggravated by motion such as coughing, sneezing, straining, and sitting. Treatment of back pains described above consists of strict bed rest from one to several weeks with an emphasis on the need to lie flat in bed. Application of moist heat and muscle relaxants may decrease muscle spasm but should not replace bed rest. Under these conditions, acute pain usually subsides in a few weeks. Persons with severe osteoporosis generally suffer repeated vertebral microfracture that will cause persistent pain (Giansiracusa & Kantrowitz, 1982).

Wrist fractures usually occur when a person extends his or her arm to break a fall. Fractures incurred in this manner are sometimes called Colles' fractures, which usually heal easily and do not lead to complications. However, they may serve as a warning that loss of cortical bone is occurring. The lower part of the radius contains about 25% trabecular and 75% cortical bone, a loss which would thin and weaken the bone. This could account for a dramatic increase in wrist fractures in women over the age of 50, which are 10 times more common in women than in men (Notelovitz & Ware, 1982).

According to Notelovitz & Ware (1982), a hip fracture is actually a fracture of the upper part of the thigh bone (femur). Most fractures occur at the weakest part, the neck, although they can also occur in the shaft or head of the femur.

Hip fractures require immediate medical attention, and the patient is usually hospitalized for 3-6 weeks. Metal pins or screws are generally used to join the broken sections of the bone; severe fractures may require replacement of the femoral head with an artificial device. Recovery from a hip fracture depends on the severity of the fracture, the age and general state of health of the elderly person (Notelovitz & Ware, 1982).

After a hip fracture, serious and even fatal complications may arise. If the femoral neck is severely fractured and fails to heal, the head of the femur can lose its blood supply and die. When this happens, the femoral head must be removed and replaced with an artificial one (Notelovitz & Ware, 1982). The incidence of hip fractures among White women between 80 and 90 years approaches 10%. The average age of patients with femoral neck fractures is 75 years (Tronzo, 1973). These are the most disabling and life-threatening consequences of osteoporosis. The loss of cortical bone is a major factor in hip fractures. Therefore, it is the older woman with advanced osteoporosis who will most likely sustain a hip fracture. Fewer than one-half of all women who suffer a hip fracture regain normal function. Fifteen percent die shortly after and 30% die within 1 year (Notelovitz & Ware, 1982). One of the reasons hip fractures are so dangerous is that they frequently recur. Persons suffering a break in the upper part of the femur are 20 times more likely to develop a hip fracture on the opposite side (Notelovitz & Ware, 1982).

The incidence of hip fractures among White women between 80 and 90 years approaches 10%. The average age of patients with femoral neck fractures is 75 years (Tronzo, 1973). These are the most disabling and life-threatening consequences of osteoporosis. The loss of cortical bone is a major factor in hip fractures. Therefore, it is the older woman with advanced osteoporosis who will most likely sustain a hip fracture. Fewer than one-half of all women who suffer a hip fracture regain normal function. Fifteen percent die shortly after and 30% die within 1 year (Notelovitz & Ware, 1982).

Each year 200,000 osteoporotic American women over the age of 45 fracture one or more of their bones. Of these, over 40,000 die from complications following their injuries. Many others lead significantly altered lives due to chronic pain and disability. As the American population, as well as the populations of other developed nations, continues to age and the life expectancy of women increases, problems related to osteoporosis will also increase (Notelovitz & Ware, 1982).

Cardiovascular System

In the aging process, significant changes occur which affect the function and to some degree the structure of the cardiovascular system. This report examines these anatomic and physiologic changes as well as their effect on the heart and vascular system.

General Structural Changes

Normally, the size of the heart does not change significantly with age. According to Agate (1970), it is not unusual to find the heart of an older person to be anatomically, clinically, and electrically comparable to the heart of a very young person. Contrary to popular belief, an enlarged heart is not necessarily a result of aging, but is more likely to be the result of a pathological condition (Saxon & Etten, 1978).

When cardiac tissue is damaged or destroyed, the body is unable to replace the lost cells. Over time there may be an increase in the collagenous and amyloid deposits (fatty substance) in the heart muscle itself. The heart valves generally become more rigid and thicker, and the walls of the blood vessels, particularly the arteries, lose their elasticity. All of these changes contribute to the loss of the efficiency of the cardiovascular system (Beard, 1983).

The terms used to describe two common vascular changes are arteriosclerosis and atherosclerosis. Arteriosclerosis is a general term to describe vascular changes leading to progressive thickening and loss of resiliency of arterial walls. Atherosclerosis is a form of arteriosclerosis in which fatty deposits accumulate on the inside walls of arteries and may gradually occlude the channel. Even if occlusion does not occur, a rough surface develops on the inner wall which increases the incidence of platelet adhesion. This generally causes the formation of clots, which can either occlude or embolize, the latter causing sudden occlusion. The vessels most often affected are the aorta, coronary arteries, and other major arteries which supply blood to the brain, abdomen, and legs (Saxon & Etten, 1978).

General Functional Changes

The cardiac muscle of an older person requires a slightly longer time period between alternate rhythmic dilations (diastole) and contractions (systole) of the heart musculature (Beard, 1983). This may limit the older person from participating in the type of activity which requires a faster than normal heart beat. At rest, the heart rate of young and old is essentially identical (Saxon & Etten, 1978). According to Beard (1983)

the left and right ventricular filling pressures at rest are normal, are the same in both young and old individuals. During exercise, however, these filling pressures increase significantly more in the aged. These increased filling pressures during exercise in old age are thought to be necessary adjustments to overcome the decreased ventricular compliance and are therefore an essential step in increasing the stroke volume. (p. 66)

Some medical researchers suggest that arrhythmias, such as skipped or extra heart beats, become more common with advancing age. Arrhythmias sometimes produce anxiety in older persons who fail to understand that this is not necessarily indicative of heart disease. In addition, the aging heart is less able to increase its rate in response to stress (Saxon & Etten, 1978). According to Beard, (1978), the aging heart frequently sustains an increase of fibrotic tissue and loss of muscle fiber in the (pacemaker) node responsible for maintaining a regular heart beat. This condition interferes with the automatic functioning of the pacemaker and may account for the high incidence of disturbances in rate and rhythm of the heart beat which accompanies old age (Cape, Coe, & Rossman, 1983).

Cardiac output declines with age thus reducing the amount of oxygen that will be delivered to body tissues and organs. For example, an 80-year-old person receives one-third less oxygen into his/her system than does a 20-year-old. By age 90 the volume of blood which the heart must circulate is estimated to be half the amount it pumped at age 20 (Saxon & Etten, 1978). Cross-sectional studies suggest that cardiac output during exercise in both the sitting and supine positions, or at rest in the supine position, is lower in elderly men than in young men. The decrease in cardiac output at rest and during submaximal exercise is the result of a reduction in stroke volume. Older subjects cannot develop as great an increase in cardiac output during maximal exertion as young subjects (Beard, 1983). These facts may help understand why most older persons tire more quickly or lack the endurance for strenuous work or physical activity. Current research suggests that one way to promote continued adequate cardiac output is through regular systematic exercise (Saxon & Etten, 1978).

Arteries, and to a lesser degree veins, become less elastic with aging. In order to maintain the circulation of blood, the heart must exert a greater effort to overcome the resistance of the less flexible arteries. Blood pressure therefore increases as arterial resistance increases. Such increases in blood pressure are common to the aging population (Saxon & Etten, 1978).

Common Age-related Disorders of the Cardiovascular System

Hypertension

It is estimated that 60 million Americans may suffer from high blood pressure, affecting about 40% of the White population and more than 50% of the Black population over age 65. About 90% of the cases of high blood pressure cannot be cured, but can be controlled by continuous treatment (NIA, 1981).

Many factors can contribute to persistent abnormally high blood pressure. The body systems directly involved are: (a) the cardiovascular because of its tendency towards sclerosis; the endocrine because it acts to retain sodium chloride in the body; (b) the excretory when excess amounts of renin are secreted or when the kidneys do not properly secrete sodium and water is reabsorbed from urinary tubules; and (c) the nervous system because it responds to excessive and prolonged emotional tension by producing an increase in peripheral resistance to blood flow. Long-term untreated hypertension may cause enlargement of the heart, with the possibility of heart failure, as well as further and more widespread arteriosclerosis and possible rupture of blood vessels especially in the brain (stroke) or even kidney dysfunction (Saxon & Etten, 1978).

An 18-year study was conducted to examine the risk associated with hypertension as it relates to cardiovascular mortality. Results of the study suggest that the incidence of cardiovascular mortality of hypertension in men who reached 65 to 74 years of age during the study was 2.4 times greater than in men with normal arterial blood pressure; in women the risk was almost eight times as great in those with hypertension (Lakatta & Gerstenblith, 1982). Given the high incidence of cardiovascular mortality related to blood pressure--two areas remain to be investigated--a mechanism to select candidates for treatment and a determination of the intensity of treatment (Lakatta & Gerstenblith, 1982).

Coronary Artery Disease

"The major cause of death in the 65+ age group worldwide is heart disease, and in a typical Western nation ischemic (narrowing of blood vessels) heart disease accounts for 80 to 90% of all cardiac death" (Lakatta & Gerstenblith, 1982, p. 193).

Coronary heart disease results when the blood supply to the heart muscle itself is reduced or blocked. As described earlier, the coronary arteries are sometimes blocked by clots or the inner walls have accumulated fatty deposits. Both interfere with blood flow to the heart muscle. In addition, if the blood pressure in the coronary arteries is too high the blood vessels may rupture causing a hemorrhage. A rupture which is more likely to occur at a weak spot in the coronary arterial wall is known as an aneurysm (Saxon & Etten, 1978).

When blood flow through the heart is reduced, cardiac tissue becomes oxygen starved and heart rhythm becomes erratic or may cease. Coronary heart disease manifests itself either suddenly in the form of a heart attack or gradually as angina pectoris (Saxon & Etten, 1978).

"Presently we cannot resolve the question of whether the marked prevalence of coronary artery disease in the elderly is related to an effect of age per se or to another effect such as that of risk factors acting over time with no true age-specific component" (Lakatta & Gerstenblith, 1982, p. 194). Most of the evidence concerning the risk factors for acquiring coronary heart disease has been gathered in middle-age populations (Pooling Project Research Group, 1978). Other risk factors that significantly appear to increase the chances of heart disease are elevated cholesterol, smoking, obesity, diabetes, hypertension, inactivity, and a family history of heart problems (Saxon & Etten, 1978). "The complex interaction of risk factors and age must be elucidated before we can test the real significance of risk factors at any age" (Lakatta & Gerstenblith, 1982, p. 194).

Respiratory System

The level of quality and enjoyment of life for the aging person is often dependent in great measure on their ability to remain physically active. This ability is closely linked to the normal functioning of the respiratory system. From the third decade of life and onward, an individual may expect his/her vital lung capacity, maximum breathing capacity, diffusion and absorption of oxygen all to be lowered with a decrease in diaphragm action. Theoretically, the change in diaphragmatic function occurs simultaneously with postural changes (Wantz & Gay, 1981).

Age-Related Changes

Although age-related changes occur in this system, they are difficult to precisely determine. The prevalence of environmental insults, occupational hazards, and smoking complicate, if not prevent, researchers from providing hard data on the changes due strictly to normal aging process.

However, a decrease in normal respiratory efficiency is affected by several factors. First of all, skeletal changes such as calcification of the rib cartilage, osteoporosis, kyphosis, and scoliosis limit rib cage expansion. Muscles used to regulate the size of the thoracic cavity may become weakened or atrophy with age. This directly influences the amount of air actually in the lungs. Several studies conducted over the past half century document the movement of the bronchi and lungs to a lower position in the thoracic cavity. The results suggest that a weakening of the structural support (musculoskeletal system) contributes in large measure to this migration (Kahane, 1981). In addition, elasticity of the lungs decreases with age thus reducing vital capacity. Residual volume increases with age thus leaving less air available for oxygen--carbon dioxide exchange. Structural changes in pleural membranes due to age have been noted by several researchers. The ratios of collagen to elastin content decreases markedly between the young and elderly (Pierce & Ebert, 1965). The pleura of the lungs of the aged are thin, uneven and lack color in comparison to younger persons (McKeown, 1965). The efficiency of pulmonary function due to a stiffer less flexible pleural membrane is reduced with age according to Kahane, (1981). Further, the number of capillaries surrounding alveoli leads to diminished oxygen uptake. An increase in thickness of the alveolar and capillary membranes interfere with normal diffusion (Kahane, 1981).

Attempts have been made to relate the above age-related respiratory changes to intrinsic changes in the lungs that accompany aging. Although data from various studies do not always agree, many pulmonary physiologists believe that a loss of elasticity in the lungs has the most deleterious effect on respiratory functioning (Bates & Christie, 1955; Lynne-Davies, 1977; Mead, Turner, Macklem & Little, 1967; Pierce & Ebert, 1965; Turner, Mead, & Wohl, 1968). Reduced elasticity interferes with the older person's ability to exhale air. This increase in the amount of residual air in the lungs causes an increase in the respiratory rate in order to maintain a sufficient supply of oxygen (Pace, 1970). "It is likely that reduced pulmonary function with increasing age results from a combination of factors, which include decreased elastic recoil pressures of the lungs and conducting airways, smaller vital capacity, and decreased power from the respiratory muscles" (Kahane, 1981, p. 24).

Even though age-related changes occur in the respiratory system, they usually do not unduly handicap older persons in the performance of their daily activities. It is only when strain, stress, or disease is imposed on the system that age-related change becomes significant for adaptive behavior (Saxon & Etten, 1978).

Age-Related Disorders

The cumulative impact of various environments on the aging process, as well as on the respiratory system, often produces irreparable damage. Smoking is the single most significant factor influencing the respiratory system. "The major cause of chronic bronchitis and studies show it (smoking) has been linked to squamous cell carcinomas" (Wantz & Gay, 1981, p. 134). "Habitual smokers have lowered ventilatory performance, often evidenced by reduced air flow rates, although the residual lung volume may be moderately elevated above predicted norms" (Timiras, 1972, p. 135). It is difficult to separate the impact of a lifetime of living from that of lifelong smoking (Wantz & Gay, 1981).

According to most authorities, the respiratory system is affected by the same diseases in both the young and old. However, because symptoms may differ in older people, pathology can be easily overlooked or diagnosed too late for effective treatment (Saxon & Etten, 1978).

In recent years we have witnessed a dramatic decline in the incidence of pulmonary tuberculosis. Generally it appears as a reactivation of a long dormant infection in the older persons whose lowered resistance makes them more susceptible. Due to the gradual development of symptoms, the disease may be far advanced before it is identified. Yet with the advent of modern medicines, treatment is usually successful (Saxon & Etten, 1978).

Lung cancer occurs more frequently among the elderly than among the young and often coexists with chronic lung disease. Factors which influence the development of lung cancers include smoking, occupational hazards such as dust, asbestos, or pollution, and chronic lung tissue damage. Treatment is minimally successful so that prevention should be given high priority (Saxon & Etten, 1978).

A disease responsible for countless deaths prior to the discovery of antibiotics, pneumonia remains a major cause of death among the elderly. Aspiration of foreign materials, decrease in lung functioning, poor circulation, and susceptibility to infection may all lead to pneumonia. Lobar pneumonia (inflammation of one or more lobes of the lungs) is less common in the elderly than bronchopneumonia (more diffuse inflammation of the lung). "Symptoms are not always obvious among the elderly and may go unnoticed or may be misinterpreted until the disease is advanced. Antibiotics and respiratory therapy are used in treatment" (Saxon & Etten, 1978, p. 97).

Diseases of the respiratory system are often progressive and debilitating. Prevention such as avoiding smoking and exposure to pollutants, correcting posture, maintaining an adequate diet, reduction or control of weight are the best prescriptions.

Sensory Changes

Hearing

Most people take for granted the ability to communicate. For the older adults in this country the loss of any aspect of communication can be traumatic, whether related to sight, hearing, or speech. Without communication, the quality of an older person's life is significantly reduced. As Lubinski (1978-1979) indicates

> Communication provides man with a flexible tool
> with which he can share ideas. Perhaps more
> significant than transmission of information,
> spoken communication can be used to fulfill a
> social role... the instrument through which people
> have influence on the environment, impose behavior,
> and demonstrate power (p. 238).

Ruesch (1957) also stressed the psychosocial value of communication in that, "... communication with self and with others and participation in small groups or larger bodies of people are imperative if the individual wishes to survive and remain healthy" (Lubinski, 1978-79, p. 238).

Hearing impairment causes great changes in a person's life. The deterioration of hearing affects the extent to which the elderly can remain in contact with others through social discourse or can stay aware of and in touch with their larger environment through the use of radio, television, films, and theater. Ultimately hearing loss may affect their mental and physical health. They often feel removed from the world and may even lose contact with themselves. Sound is important for self protection and for identification with the environment.

As the older population expands, hearing loss issues can be expected to assume a greater magnitude and demand increased attention. Acknowledgement of this problem is not new. In 1968, Senator Frank Church pointed out to the Senate Special Committee on Aging which dealt with hearing loss, hearing aids, and the elderly that "...the elderly are most in need of trained counsel; they are three times more likely to have significant hearing loss than those younger than they" (p. 1). As a result the Subcommittee directed its attention to three basic areas: (a) the improvement of delivery of services to older people sustaining hearing loss; (b) the sales of hearing aid to older person; and (c) the effects of increasing noise on future generations of Americans (U.S. Senate, 1968). During the past 16 years much has been accomplished, but much more remains to be achieved.

Definitions

In this paper, the elderly population includes those persons 65 years of age and older. Some of the literature distinguishes between the young old (65 to 75) and the old old (75 plus).

Hearing-impaired is a generic term that refers to both hard-of-hearing and deaf persons. Hard-of-hearing refers to an impaired sense of hearing causing difficulty with the comprehension of speech, but which is partially functional. Deafness refers to a degree of hearing loss that is nonfunctional for the ordinary purposes of life (NINDS, 1969).

Hearing loss refers to the measured extent, or severity, to which the hearing is impaired. Hearing acuity is measured in decibels (dB) and the terms generally employed to describe the extent of the acuity loss are normal (0-20 dB), mild loss (20-40 dB), moderate loss (41-55) dB), moderately severe loss (56-70 dB), severe loss (71-90 dB), and profound deafness (90 dB plus) (Knauf, 1978).

In addition to being characterized by a loss of sensitivity (i.e., acuity) for sounds hearing loss can also be characterized by an inability to discriminate or understand speech sounds even when the loss of acuity has been compensated for through amplification. Loss of discrimination is reported in percentages of correctly understood speech (i.e., 100%--all words heard correctly; 0%--no words heard correctly).

Furthermore, hearing impairment can be categorized as unilateral (one ear) or bilateral (both ears); and, the impairment can be temporary, permanent or progressive in nature.

Lastly, tinnitus is a frequent accompanying complaint of those who have hearing loss and is mentioned here simply for clarification. Tinnitus is a ringing or buzzing in the ears or head, the cause of which is unknown. Incidence is greater among those in middle age or later years.

Types and Causes of Hearing Loss Among the Elderly

Types of hearing impairment can be related to the site of structural damage or blockage. These areas are depicted in Figure 2. The common causes of conductive, sensori-neural, mixed, and central hearing impairments follow.

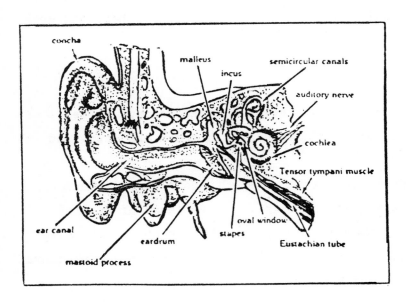

Figure 2. Diagram of the outer, middle, and inner ear. From H. Davis, Benson, Covell, & Fernandez (1983). In Acoustical Society of America, 25, 1180.

A conductive hearing impairment results from involvement of the outer and/or middle ear systems

o External blockage--build-up of wax or foreign object in the ear, which is very common in the population aged 65 years and over.

o Perforated eardrum--a hole or tear in the eardrum which can occur as a result of injury, sudden pressure change, or infection.

o Genetic and congenital abnormalities--malfunction and/or malformation of the outer and/or middle ear which sometimes occur in connection with hereditary diseases.

o Otitis media--middle ear infection and accumulation of fluid.

o Otosclerosis--thought to be hereditary, a disease process affecting the mobility of the ossicular chain, but primarily affecting the stapes.

A sensori-neural hearing impairment is that which stems from damage to the inner ear, the cochlea and/or neural fibers of the VIIIth nerve.

o Presbycusis--literally, the term means "old hearing." Historically, it it has been used to describe hearing impairment that occurs with old age. Presbycusis may be sensory, neural, metabolic, mechanical, or vascular in nature.

o Hereditary hearing loss--includes a great variety of disorders that affect the sensori-neural mechanism and are usually present at birth.

o Trauma-induced--a severe blow to the head, an accident, stroke or brain hemorrhage that affect the ear, auditory pathways, and/or brain centers.

o Tumors--acoustic neuromas and other tumors that invade the VIIIth nerve nucleus and brain stem.

o Noise damage--brief or continued exposure to high intensity sound which irreparably damages the hair cells of the cochlea.

o Vascular incidents--related to hypertension, heart disease, or other vascular problems which may alter blood flow to the inner ear.

o Drug-induced hearing loss--drugs such as aspirin, and some antibiotics, diuretics, and certain powerful anti-cancer drugs can damage the hair cells or other vital structures of the inner ear.

o Viral and bacterial illness--such as mumps, meningitis encephalitis as well as rubella contracted by expectant mothers are some common disease processes which are well-documented as etiologies for hearing impairment.

o Meniere's disease--as a result of endolymphatic hydrops of unknown origin, the syndrome can be characterized by fluctuating hearing loss, vertigo, and tinnitus; symptoms may be exacerbated by or resemble allergy, hypothyroidism, and diabetes.

A _mixed_ hearing impairment, as the term implies, is one which is comprised of both conductive and sensori-neural components.

A central processing disorder is a hearing impairment which influences one's understanding of spoken language, and is related to damage to the auditory pathways in the brain.

Hearing impairments may lead to a reduction in the loudness of sounds, and may also lead to a distortion of sound. Thus the person might complain, "I can hear you, but I can't understand you." This is a common complaint of elderly persons with hearing impairment. Thus, the hearing-impaired elderly person may not be able to tell the difference between many of the sounds of speech either because the sounds cannot be heard or because they are distorted. Another problem often seen in persons with hearing impairments is an inability to tolerate loud sounds or voices. Referred to as "recruitment," this difficulty often creates problems in satisfactory hearing aid fitting.

Finally, a hearing impairment may lead to the inability to capture the meaning of words even though the words are loud enough. In this case, the elderly hearing-impaired person may hear the words but not make any sense out of them. The words are a meaningless jumble of sounds, almost as if the person were listening to a foreign language. This kind of hearing impairment may be caused by certain disorders of the inner ear or to central auditory processing disorders. In the elderly person, the speed of nerve impulses may be considerably slower than normal or the brain itself may lose its ability to interpret words that come at a rapid pace.

Hearing impairment is not a simple matter. The loss of hearing for the elderly has many causes and there are many related problems which may result from hearing inabilities. Further, there are diverse individual differences in reactions to varying degrees of hearing loss.

Vision

The most thoroughly studied sense relative to age (Storandt, 1983), there are several consistent biological changes within the visual system which occur during adulthood (Schaie & Geiwitz, 1982). For example, between the ages of 34 and 45, changes in the lens and other external parts of the eye (see Figure 3) affect the transmission of light waves (Fozard, 1977). In later years, between 55 and 65 years of age, changes within the retina and ocular nervous system

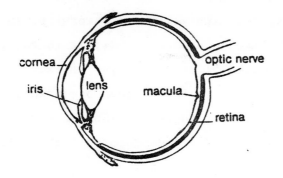

Figure 3. Diagram of the eye. From: NIA (1983). Aging and your eyes. Age Page, U.S. Government Printing Office: 1983-416-519.

affect the sensitivity of the retina (Schaie & Geiwitz, 1982). Thus, since structural changes variously effect visual function, vision is dependent upon structures of the eye as well as the integrity of the nerve pathways from the eye to the brain (Yurick, 1980b). Further, visual perception involves the processes of sensing, interpreting, and responding to visual information (Fozard, et al., 1977).

The lens of the eye yellows and becomes harder and less flexible with age (Fozard, et al., 1977; Schaie & Geiwitz, 1982; Storandt, 1983), reducing and changing the spectral distribution of light which reaches the retina (Yurick, 1980b). Comprised of epithelial tissue (such as is found in skin, hair, nails), the lens grows throughout life. However, unlike the other tissues, because excess cells cannot be shed by the lens, it becomes more compact and less flexible with age (Schaie & Geiwitz, 1982).

The resultant loss of flexibility decreases the ability of the lens to view and focus onto close objects. Strictly defined, accommodation is the "ability of the eye to discriminate detail of near objects" (Storandt, 1983, p. 417). Thus, difficulty with accommodation results in presbyopia, more commonly called "farsightedness". Common in those over 40 years of age, presbyopia is easily corrected by the use of bifocal glasses (NIA, 1983; Porcino, 1983).

Other problems which result from the change in density and flexibility of the lens cannot be so easily remediated. Although the amount of light which reaches the retina is reduced, the elderly require almost twice as much illumination than do younger persons (Cristarella, 1977; Crouch, 1945; Fozard et al., 1977; Schaie & Geiwitz, 1982), yet are highly susceptible to glare (Hatton, 1977). As the lens yellows, it increasingly absorbs the blue-green wavelengths of the color spectrum; thus, reds and yellows are more easily discriminated than blues and violets (Hultsch & Deutsch, 1981; Storandt, 1983).

Somewhat related to a need for increased illumination is the fact that as individuals age the eye's ability to adapt to varying degrees of darkness decreases (Fozard & Popkin, 1978; Hultsch & Deutsch, 1981; Wantz & Gay, 1981). This alteration in dark adaptation is the result of age-related decrements in circulation and metabolism of the retina (Yurick, 1980b).

Within the retina are the rods and cones, sensitive receptors of light (Murch, 1973). The rods are found in the periphery whereas the cones are contained in the central portion of the retina. The rods are sensitive to low intensities of light whereas the cones provide information on detail by analyzing color, brightness, and contour (Murch, 1973). The retina is very sensitive to vascular changes and decreased oxygen supply, which is thought to "affect the efficiency of dark adaptation in the elderly person" (Yurick, 1980b, p. 314). This could easily explain why many persons often experience increasing difficulty with night vision as they grow older.

All too often we hear someone jokingly say, "if only my arms were longer, then I could read this newspaper." Unfortunately, this and other visual changes with age are no joking matter. Farsightedness, the need for greater lighting yet not so much as to cause glare, difficulty in identifying colors, as well as seeing in the dark or semi-dark can have varying effects on individuals as they age. Some of these changes can be easily corrected by the use of glasses or by using higher wattage light bulbs. However, other changes can not be easily corrected and as a result must compensated for. For example, many persons simply choose not to drive at night anymore. Yet, how the person reacts to and accepts each of these age-related changes and the resultant decrease in visual acuity may ultimately affect how he or she copes with the need to alter a long-established lifestyle.

Chemical Senses (Taste and Smell)

Although chemical sensitivity to taste and smell is basic to all organisms, these have often been considered to be the most primitive and elementary of senses (Ordy, Brizzee, & Beavers, 1980). Although often considered to be separate senses, taste and smell have several features in common. For instance, both respond to dissolved substances and are important in the development of attitudes toward food and good nutritional habits (Farber, 1978; Ordy, Brizzee, & Beavers, 1980; Schaie & Geiwitz, 1982). Smell and taste are basic to biological drives, because their role is key in the "reinforcing or reward properties to stimuli" (Ordy, Brizzee, & Beavers, 1980, p. 55). A keen sense of taste and smell can serve as protection from life-threatening situations, such as tainted or spoiled food, smoke or gas fumes (Colavita, 1978; Engen, 1977; Farber, 1978; Schaie & Geiwitz, 1982; Schiffman & Pasternak, 1979). At any rate, individual responses to odors may be affected by age, health, sex, and ethnic background, as well as previous experience with the odor (Yurick, 1980a).

The sense of smell (olfaction) has been the subject of research less often than have the senses of vision, taste, and hearing (Burnside, 1976). Although limited, data indicates several consistent changes with age. Butler & Lewis (1977) indicated that of the elderly aged 80 years, 30% experienced difficulty in identifying common substances by smell. In a comparative study of 100 persons aged 10-90 years, Rous (1969) reported a significant decrease in olfactory sensitivity with age as well as a decline in olfactory adaptation time. Schiffman (1977) reported decline in olfactory sensitivity, discrimination, and recognition with age. A degeneration of the cortical and subcortical olfactory pathway to the brain was reported by Schiffman & Pasternak (1979) who indicated that this could be associated with the aging process.

Although there is general agreement of a decline in sense of smell, Yurick (1980a) as well as Wantz & Gay (1981) attributed this degeneration not only to aging, but also to general decline in the health of individuals. Research has also shown that certain changes in olfactory perception occur throughout a person's life. Colavita (1978) observed that occupational odors, airborne toxic agents, and smoking may cause changes in the sense of smell. Diminished sense of smell may also be associated with respiratory and other diseases common to the elderly (Engen, 1977; Yurick, 1980a). Although the reasons may not be clear, it appears evident that certain degenerative changes are extensive in the elderly. Ruben (1971) found that by the age of 80 approximately 75% of olfactory fibers have degenerated or been lost.

The sense of taste is closely related to the senses of smell and vision. As a matter-of-fact, the "perception of taste can either be enhanced or diminished by the sight and smell of food" (Yurick, 1980a, p. 305).

Sensations of taste for bitter, sweet, salty, and sour are perceived by taste buds (papillae) on the tongue. Sweet tastes are perceived by the anterior (frontal) portion of the tip of the tongue whereas the posterior surface of the tongue perceives bitter tastes, and the lateral edges of the tongue perceive sour tastes. Salty taste is perceived by all of the tongue's surface (Yurick, 1980a).

Schaie & Geiwitz (1982) reported that the elderly experience greater sensitivity for or ability to taste bitter and sour substances than for sweet or salty substances. This would likely be due to the fact that the taste buds which identify the bitter and the sour atrophy. Several researchers have indicated that such a degree of atrophy is unlikely to occur before the ages of 60, 70, or 80 years (Arey, Tremaine, & Monzingo, 1936; Kahane, 1981; Shore, 1976). Despite a loss of taste buds with age, however, the overall size of the tongue does not alter significantly (Corso, 1981; Kaplan, 1971).

Other Senses

Research is scattered, however, there is evidence to suggest that the elderly experience decreased sensitivity to touch and pain, and are less able to detect temperature changes (Schaie & Geiwitz, 1982; Wantz & Gay, 1981; Yurick, 1980a). Although the degree of loss varies among individuals, Kenshalo (1977) has indicated a change of sensitivity to touch in the palm of the hand and the sole of the foot. This decreased acuity for touch could "affect the elderly person's ability to localize stimuli and ...reduce the speed of reaction to tactile stimulation" (Yurick, 1980a, p. 294). The elderly may have difficulty with everyday tasks, such as fastening buttons, identifying coins, or even adjusting a hearing aid. Moreover, this could be related to decreased ability to detect pain and may result in injury from noxious agents, extreme temperatures or even shoes that are too tight. Evidence suggests that the elderly react less quickly to temperature changes, and may be at risk for frostbite or possibly death if accidentally overexposed to the cold (Schaie & Geiwitz, 1982).

Nutrition

Proper nutrition is important for all individuals and can have a profound effect throughout the life cycle (Young, 1983). Nutrition may be conducive to health and fitness, influence quality of life, and may contribute to the development or inhibition of health changes often associated with aging (Young, 1983). For instance, nutritional status is critical for the normal healthy growth and development of infants and children (Weg, 1981). It is important that adults of all ages consume a variety of foods and nutrients to provide sufficient energy to maintain body functions (Wantz & Gay, 1981) and to respond to environmental demands (Henderson, 1983). Moreover, as Young (1983) has indicated, "lifelong patterns of eating are beginning to emerge as fundamental influences of nutritional well-being in later life" (p. 296).

Although data relative to the specific nutrient requirements of the elderly are limited, several researchers have indicated that throughout adulthood nutritional needs are stable (Castor, 1983; Wantz & Gay, 1981), and thus the elderly's requirements are not significantly different from those of younger adults (Foley & Tideiksaar, 1983; Harper, 1978; Katona-Apte & Anderson, 1977; Todhunter & Darby, 1978; Young, 1983). It should be noted, however, that as people age their degree of activity often lessens, metabolic rate declines, and therefore, there is a reduced need for calories (Hickler & Wayne, 1984; Katona-Apte & Anderson, 1977; Wantz & Gay, 1981; Young, 1983). For instance, Lamy (1981) has indicated that energy (caloric) expenditure in men decreases by 21% from 20 to 74 years of age and by an additional 31% by the age of 99.

Nutrients which are essential for maintenance of body functions regardless of age include protein, carbohydrate, fat, vitamins, minerals, and water. Although not a nutrient in the true sense of the word, water is essential to the body's ability to transport nutrients throughout the body to cool down the body and to eliminate wastes (Wantz & Gay, 1981).

According to Wantz & Gay (1981), proteins which should comprise 15% of the dietary intake of calories, are highly complex amino acids and serve three basic functions in the diet: "(1) aid tissue growth and maintenance; (2) aid in the production of enzymes, antibodies and hormones; (3) provide energy" (p. 262). Proteins are readily found in red meats, fish, poultry and dairy products, as well as in a combination of vegetables and grains. Foley (1983) has suggested limited ingestion of red meat in favor of the other sources of protein in order to "reduce intake of saturated fat and increase calcium intake" (p. 361).

Researchers have recommended that simple (sugar) and complex (starch) carbohydrates comprise 55% of daily caloric intake (Foley & Tideiksaar, 1983; Wantz & Gay, 1981) to provide the body with quick energy, regulate fats used for fuel, prevent use of protein for energy, and maintain interrelationship with vitamins. These simple and complex carbohydrates can be found in foods such as bread, cereal, macaroni, fruits, vegetables, dairy products, and refined products. Carbohydrates are converted by the body into glucose for rapid oxidation into energy, heat, water, and carbon dioxide (Wantz & Gay, 1981).

A lasting source of energy is that derived from fats which comprises about 30% of the caloric intake (Foley & Tideiksaar, 1983; Wantz & Gay, 1981; Winick, 1976). Animal fats and some types of vegetables are sources of saturated fats whereas unsaturated fats (mono- and poly-unsaturated) can be found in plants, poultry, and fish. Fats are sources of energy and assist in the body's ability to utilize and transport fat-soluble vitamins (A,D,E,K). When stored, fats insulate the body and protect vital organs. It has been recommended that the daily caloric consumption be equally divided among the fats--10% saturated, 10% mono-unsaturated, 10% poly-unsaturated (U.S. Senate, 1977).

Although they provide no energy and are only required in limited amounts, vitamins are essential for stimulating the function and maintenance of numerous body systems. Vitamins are water-soluble (transported and dissolved in water, see Table 2) or are fat-soluble (transported, dissolved and stored in fat see Table 3). The water-soluble vitamins (B vitamins, niacin, pantothenic acid, folic acid, Vitamin C) stimulate digestion and appetite, metabolism, function of the central nervous, endocrine, integumentary (skin, hair, nails...) and muscular systems, among others. The fat-soluble vitamins (A, D, E, K) influence the digestive and integumentary systems, balance of calcium, mineral metabolism, formation of blood platelets, and blood clotting (Wantz & Gay, 1981).

Table 2. Water-soluble vitamins.

Vitamin	RDA[1]	Result of deficiency	Food source
B_1 (thiamine)	1.0-1.4 mg	Beriberi, loss of appetite, indigestion, fatigue, neuritis, irritability	Pork, beef, liver, legumes, whole grains
B_2 (riboflavin)	1.5-1.7 mg	Dermatitis, eye irritation	Milk, liver, enriched cereals
B_6 (pyridoxine)	2.0 mg	Anemia	Wheat, corn, meat, liver
B_{12} (cobalamin)	3.0 mg	Extrinsic factor in pernicious anemia	Liver, milk, eggs, cheese, meat
Niacin	13-18 mg	Pellagra, neuritis, dermatitis, lassitude, weakness	Meat, peanuts, enriched grains
Pantothenic acid	—[2]	Decreased breakdown of glucose to energy	Liver, eggs, skimmed milk
Folic acid	400 mg	Megaloblastic anemia	Liver, green leafy vegetables, asparagus
Biotin	—[2]	Decreased breakdown of glucose to energy	Egg yolk, liver
Ascorbic acid	55-60 mg	Weakened capillary walls	Citrus fruits, tomatoes, cabbage, potatoes, strawberries, broccoli, brussels sprouts

[1] U.S. recommended daily allowance for females ages 18-35 (first number) and males ages 18-35 (second number).
[2] No current recommendation for dietary intake.
Source: Wantz & Gay (1981). The aging process: A health perspective. Cambridge, MA: Winthrop Publishers.

Table 3. Fat-soluble vitamins.

Vitamin	RDA[1]	Result of deficiency	Food source
A	5000 IU	Reduced ability to adapt from bright light to darkness, decreased appetite, physical weakness, retardation of growth and development	Liver, kidney, cream, butter, egg yolk, yellow and green vegetables, fortified foods
D	400 IU	Reduced ability of body to utilize calcium	Sunlight, yeast, fish oil, fortified foods
E	12-15 IU	Less integrity in red blood cell, anemia	Vegetable oil, milk, eggs, muscle meats, fish, cereal, green leafy vegetables
K	—[2]	Reduced blood clotting ability	Green leafy vegetables, cheese, egg yolk, liver

[1]U.S. recommended daily allowance for females ages 18-35 (first number) and males ages 18-35 (second number).
[2]No current recommendation for dietary intake.
Source: Wantz & Gay (1981). The aging process: A health perspective. Cambridge, MA: Winthrop Publishers.

The ability to ingest the recommended daily allowance of major minerals (calcium, chlorine, magnesium, phosphorus, potassium, sodium, sulphur) and trace minerals (copper, fluorine, iron, manganese, zinc) is fairly easy if a balanced diet is eaten every day (Wantz & Gay, 1981).

Table 4. Major minerals.

Mineral	RDA[1]	Result of deficiency	Food source
Calcium	800-1200 mg	Affects bone and tooth formation, normal clotting of bold, muscle contraction and relaxation; rickets	Milk, cheese, egg yolk, nuts, whole grains, green leafy vegetables
Chlorine	—[2]	Affects fluid balance maintenance and proper stomach acidity	Abundant in most foods
Magnesium	300-400 mg	Affects protein metabolism, growth, and maintenance processes	Abundant in most foods
Phosphorus	800-1200 mg	Affects acid-base balance in body	Same as calcium
Potassium	—[2]	Affects cellular fluid balance, muscle excitability, metabolism of carbohydrate and protein	Abundant in many foods
Sodium	—[2]	Affects normal fluid balance betweeen inside of cell and its surroundings; affects cell permeability and muscle excitability	Table salt, some foods
Sulfur	—[2]	Affects energy metabolism	Abundant in many foods

[1]U.S. recommended daily allowance for females ages 18-35 (first number) and males ages 18-35 (second number).
[2]No current recommendation for dietary intake.
Source: Wantz & Gay (1981). The aging process: A health perspective.
Cambridge, MA: Winthrop Publishers.

Table 5. Trace minerals.

Vitamin	RDA[1]	Result of deficiency	Food source
Copper	—[2]	Affects iron utilization, bone formation, and brain tisssue maintenance	Liver, meat, seafood, nuts, whole grains
Fluorine	1 PPM[3]	Affects teeth and bones	Water
Iodine	100-150 mg	Development of a goiter	Seafood, iodized salt
Iron	18 mg	Affects hemoglobin formation	Liver, meat, egg yolk, whole grains enriched bread, nuts, green vegetables
Manganese	300-400 mg	Affects protein metabolism, synthesis of fatty acids, and blood sugar oxidation	Cereal, tea, nuts, soybeans
Zinc	15 mg	Liver disease	Liver, seafood

[1]U.S. recommended daily allowance for females ages 18-35 (first number) and males ages 18-35 (second number).
[2]No current recommendation for dietary intake.
[3]One part per million per gallon of water.
Source: Wantz & Gay (1981). The aging process: A health perspective.
Cambridge, MA: Winthrop Publishers.

Thus, nutritional requirements for the elderly closely parallel those for younger age groups. However, there are several factors which may influence the ability of the elderly to meet these needs, including drug-diet interactions, change in body functions or activity levels, restricted funds, dental problems and social or personal factors (Foley & Tideiksaar, 1983; Henderson, 1983; Hickler & Wayne, 1984; Katona-Apte & Anderson, 1977; Wantz & Gay, 1981; Weg, 1973, 1981; Young, 1983.

As the largest consumers of drugs (Hickler & Wayne, 1984), the elderly often take several medications simultaneously for long periods of time (Rivlin, 1982). Thus, the elderly are highly susceptible to adverse drug-drug and/or drug-diet interactions, which may include increased excretion of nutrients, increased nutrient utilization, or competition between drug and nutrient at the site of action (Rozovski, 1984).

The ability to ingest the recommended daily allowance of major minerals (calcium, chlorine, magnesium, phosphorus, potassium, sodium, sulphur) and trace minerals (copper, fluorine, iron, manganese, zinc) is fairly easy if a balanced diet is eaten every day (Wantz & Gay, 1981).

Dental problems (i.e., decayed or missing teeth) may present nutritional difficulties for individuals of age. Since 50% of Americans have lost their teeth by age 65 (McBean & Speckmann, 1974; Nizel, 1967, 1981), untold numbers of elderly ay be faced with difficulties in eating. May elderly do have dentures, however, over time they may become loose and ill-fitting. This, too, may make it difficult for the elderly to consume a proper diet which should include meats, fish, raw fruits and vegetables. The end result might be insufficient intake of daily required nutrients.

Personal/social factors, such as reduced income, mobility or transportation, attitude or motivation, have the potential to become significant barriers to proper eating and nutrition for the elderly (Henderson, 1983; Richmond, 1979; Wantz & Gay, 1981; Young, 1983). The elderly person whose income is relatively fixed is often presented with the problem of meeting needs for daily living, including food, the price of which increases yearly (Wattenberg, 1978). Similarly, the elderly who have poor mobility such as occurs with arthritis, or who lack adequate transportation may not be able to shop for groceries, prepare meals or feed themselves (Young, 1983). These factors, as well as the problem of eating alone, may directly affect attitude ad motivation for eating and may ultimately result in poor nutrition.

Adequate diet and nutrition are critical to the health and well being of the elderly. According to several researchers (Beauchene & Davis, 1979; Weg, 1980b, 1981; Yearick, Wang & Pisias, 1980) the nutrients most frequently deficient among the elderly--calcium, iron, magnesium and vitamins A, C, B complex (thiamin, niacin, folic acid)--are highly correlated to the incidence of nervous, circulatory, respiratory and skeletal disorders (Weg, 1980a). Of increasing prevalence among the middle-aged and elderly (Exton-Smith, 1968, 1973; Mayer, 1974; Weg, 1979, 1980ab), borderline or subclinical malnutrition may result in a variety of symptoms, including listlessness, fatigue, headache, insomnia, confusion, poor memory, anxiety, or irratibility (Clements, 1875; Weg, 1980ab). Frequently viewed by health professionals as related to normal aging, these signs may often be neglected. Thus, "malnutrition may be intensified and leave the cells, tissues, and organ systems less able to respond to injury, infection, or emotional stress" (Weg, 1981).

Summary

The chapter described in varying detail a number of the physical and physiological alterations which occur with advancing age. Not a disease, the process of aging results in decreased ability to withstand and counteract the stresses of daily living which can be intertwined with and compounded by disease processes as well as environmental insults. If the quality of life of the elderly is to be improved and insured the environment should be structured in a way that will reduce the incidence and magnitude of stressors as well as be responsive to the physiological capabilities of the normal healthy elderly person.

Self-Study Questions

1. It has been stated that there is a decrease in brain weight and brain volume with advancing age. How is this related to changes in cognitive processing skills?

2. It has been suggested that the elderly are less able to detect changes in temperature and experience decreased sensitivity to touch and pain. What impact can this have on the lifestyle and safety for the elderly?

3. A variety of factors determine the way each of us ages. What are they and what can we do to achieve healthful old age?

4. What are the symptoms typically present in senile dementia?

5. As we age, the lens of the eye becomes less clear and more rigid. What effect do these changes have on vision and on the mobility of the elderly?

6. There is decreased absorption of calcium by the body as we age. What consequence can this have?

REFERENCES

Agate, J. (1970). The practice of geriatrics (2nd ed.). Springfield, IL: Charles C. Thomas.

Arendt, A. (1972). Altern des zentralnerven-systems. In G. Holle (Ed), Handbuk der allegemeinen pathologie. New York: Springer-Verlag.

Arey, L. B., Tremaine, M. J., & Monzingo, F. R., (1936). The numerical and topographical relations of taste buds to human circumvallate papillae throughout the life span. Anatomical Record, 64, 9.

Avioli, L. V. (1977). Osteoporosis: Pathogenesis and therapy. In J. W. Rowe and R. W. Besdine (Eds.), Health and disease in old age. Boston: Little, Brown.

Bates, D. & Christie, R. V. (1955). Effects of aging on respiratory function in man. In G. F. Wolstenholme & M. P. Cameron (Eds.). Ciba foundation colloquia on aging Vol. 1. Boston: Little, Brown.

Beard, Owen W. (1983). Age-related physiological changes in the cardiovascular system. In R. Cape, R. Coe, & I. Rossman (Eds.), Fundamentals of geriatric medicine. New York: Raven Press.

Beauchene, R. E., Davis, T. A. (1979). The nutritional status of aged in the USA. Age, 2(1), 23-28.

Birren, J. E. (1965). Age changes in speed of behavior: Its central nature and physiological correlates. In A. T. Welford & J. E. Birren (Eds.), Behavior, aging, and the nervous system. Springfield, IL: Charles C. Thomas.

Birren, J. E. (1974). Translations in gerontology-from lab to life. Psychophysiology and speed of response. American Psychologist, 29, 808-815.

Birren, J. E., Riegel, K. F. & Morrison, D. F. (1962). Age differences in response speed as a function of controlled variations of stimulus conditions: Evidence of a general speed factor. Gerontologia, 6, 1-18.

Birren, J. E., Woods, A. M., & Williams, M. V. (1980). Behavioral slowing with age: Causes, organizations and consequences. In L. W. Poon (Ed.), Aging in the 1980s. American Psychological Association.

Blinker, S. M., Glezer, I. I. (1968). Techniques of quantitative measurement of morphological structures of the central nervous system. In S. M. Blinker, I. I. Glezer (Eds.), The human brain in figures and tables. New York: Basic Books.

Botwinich, J. (1978). Aging and behavior. New York: Springer-Verlag.

Bucciante, L., & Luria, S. (1934). Trasformazioni nella struttura dei muscoli voluntari dell uoma nella senescenza. Archivio Italiano di anatomia e di embriologia.

Bullamore, J. R., Wilkinson, R., & Gallagher, J. C. (1970). Effect of age on calcium absorption. Lancet, 2, 535.

Burnside, I. M. (Ed.). (1976). Nursing and the aged. New York: McGraw-Hill.

Butler, R. N., & Lewis, M. I. (1977). Aging and mental health: Positive psychosocial approaches. St. Louis: C.V. Mosby.

Cape, R. (1978). Aging: Its complex management. Hagerstown, MD: Harper & Row.

Caper, R., Coe, R. M., & Rossman, I. (1983). Fundamentals of geriatric medicine. New York: Raven Press.

Castor, W. O. (1983). The role of nutrition in human aging. In D. Platt (Ed.), Geriatrics 2. New York: Springer-Verlag.

Clements, F. W. (1975). Nutrition 7: Vitamins and mineral supplementation. Medical Journal of Australia, 1(19), 595-599.

Colavita, F. B. (1978). Sensory changes in the elderly. Springfield, IL: Charles C. Thomas.

Comfort, A. (1979). The biology of senescence (3rd ed.). New York: Elsevier.

Corso, J. F. (1981). Aging sensory systems and perception. New York: Praeger.

Cristarella, M. C. (1977). Visual function of the elderly. American Journal of Occupational Therapy, 31, 432.

Crouch, C. L. (1945). The relation between illumination and vision. Illuminating Engineering, 40, 747.

Carnevalle-Ricci, F. (1937). Osservazioni isopathologiche sulla laringe nells senescenza. Archivo Italiano di Otologia, Rinologia e Laringologia, 49, 1.

Davis, H., Benson, R. W., Covell, W. P., & Fernandex, C. (1953). Anatomy and physiology of the auditory mechanism." _Acoustical Society of America_, _25_, 1180.

Davis, P. J. M., & Wright, E. A. (1977). A new method for measuring cranial cavity volume and its application to the assessment of cerebral atrophy at autopsy. _Neuropathology in Applied Neurobiology_, _3_, 341-358.

Dekaban, A. S., & Sadowsky, D. (1978). Changes in brain weights during the span of human life: Relation of brain weights to body heights and body weights. _Annals Neurology_, _4_, 345-356.

Eisdorfer, C., Cohen, D., & Veith, R. (1981). The psychopathology of aging. _Current Concepts_. Kalamazoo, MI: Upjohn.

Engen, T. (1977). Taste and smell. In J. E. Birren & K. W. Schaie (Eds.), _Handbook of the psychology of aging_. New York: Van Nostrand Reinhold.

Exton-Smith, A. N. (1973). Nutritional deficiencies in the elderly. In A. N. Howard & I. McLean (Eds.), _Nutritional deficiencies in modern society_, London: Baird Newman.

Exton-Smith, A. N. (1968). The problem of subclinical malnutrition in the elderly. In A. N. Exton-Smith, & D. L. Scott (Eds.), _Vitamins in the elderly_. Bristol: Wright & Sons Ltd.

Farber, S. D. (1978). Olfaction in health and disease. _Journal of Occupational Therapy_, _32_, 155.

Foley, C. J., Tideiksaar, R. (1983). Nutritional problems in the elderly. In S. R. Gambert (Ed.), _Contemporary geriatric medicine_. Vol. 1. New York: Plenum.

Fozard, J. L. (1977). Visual perception and communication. In J. E. Birren & K. W. Schaie (Eds.), _Handbook of the psychology of aging_. New York: Van Nostrand Reinhold.

Fozard, J. L., & Popkin, S. J. (1978). Optimizing adult developement: Ends and means of an applied psychology of aging. _American Psychologist_, _33_, 975-989.

Giansiracusa, D. F., & Kantrowitz, F. G. (1982). Metabolic bone disease. In J. W. Rowe & R. W. Besdine (Eds.), _Health and disease in old age_. Boston: Little, Brown.

Greenfield, J. C., Shy, G. M., Alverd, E. C., & Berg, L. (1957). _Atlas of muscle pathology in neuromuscular diseases_. Edinburgh: Livingstone.

Grob, D. (1978). Common disorders of muscles in the aged. In W. Reichel (Ed.), _Clinical aspects of aging_. Baltimore: Williams & Wilkins.

Hagnell, O., Lanke, J., Rorsman, B., Ojesjo, L. (1980). The Lundby project. _Socialstyrelsen Redovisar_, _7_, 49.

Harper, A. E. (1978). Recommended dietary allowances for the elderly. Geriatrics, 33, 73-80.

Harris, W. (1951). The fifth and seventh cranial nerves in relation to the nervous mechanism of taste sensation. British Medical Journal, 1, 831-836.

Hatton, J. (1977). Aging and the glare problem. Journal of Gerontological Nursing, 3(5), 38.

Henderson, J. (1983). Nutritional advice for the elderly. In F. I. Caird & J. G. Evans (Eds.), Advanced geriatric medicine. Vol. 3. (pp. 29-35). Baltimore, MD: Urban & Schwarzenberg.

Hickler, R. B., & Wayne, K. S. (1984, March). Nutrition and the elderly. American Family Physician, 29(3), 137-145.

Hommerich, K. W., (1972). Der alternde larynz: Morphologische aspekte. Hals Nasen Ohrenaerzte, 20, 115-120.

Hultsch, D. F., Deutsch, F. (1981). Adult development & aging: A life-span perspective. New York: McGraw-Hill.

Jowsey, J. (1977). Osteoporosis: Idiopathic, post-menopausal, and senile. In C. B. Sledge (Ed.), Metabolic diseases of bone. Philadelphia: Saunders.

Kahane, J. C. (1981). Anatomic and physiologic changes in the aging peripheral speech mechanism. In D. S. Beasley & G. A. Davis (Eds.), Aging: Communication processes and disorders. New York: Grune & Stratton.

Kaplan, H. (1971). The oral cavity in geriatrics. Geriatrics, 26, 96-102.

Katona-Apte, J., & Anderson, J. B. (1977). Nutrition, physical activity and aging. Chapel Hill, NC: Health Sciences Consortium.

Kenshalo, D. R. (1977). Age changes in touch, vibration, temperature, kinesthesis, and pain sensitivity. In J. E. Birren & K. W. Schaie (Eds.), Handbook of the psychology of aging. New York: Van Nostrand Reinhold.

Knauf, V. H. (1978). (2nd ed.). Communication training. In J. Katz (Ed.), Handbook of clinical audiology. Baltimore: Williams & Wilkins.

Kofler, K. (1932). Die altersveranderungen in larynx. Monatsschrift fuer Ohrenheilkunde und Laryngo-Rhinologie (Wein), 66, 1468.

Lakatta, E. G., & Gerstenblith, G. (1982). Cardiovascular system. In J. W. Rowe & R. W. Besdine (Eds.), Health and disease in old age. Boston: Little, Brown.

Lamy, P. P. (1981). Nutrition & the elderly. Drug Intell Clinical Pharmacology, 15, 887-891.

Lubinski, R. B. (1978-1979). Why so little interest in whether or not old people talk: A review of recent research on verbal communication among the elderly. International Journal on Aging and Human Development, 9, 238.

Lynn-Davies, P. (1977). Influence of age on the respiratory system. Geriatrics, 32, 57-60.

Macmillan, H. W. (1936). Anatomy of the throat, mylohyoid region and mandible in relation to retention of mandibular artificial dentures. Journal of the American Dental Association, 23, 1435-1442.

Marsh, G. R., & Thompson, L. W. (1977). Psychophysiology of aging. In J. E. Birren & K. W. Schaie (Eds.), Handbook of the psychology of aging. New York: Van Nostrand Reinhold.

Maurer, J. F., & Rupp, R. R. (1979). Hearing and aging: Tactics for intervention, New York: Grune & Stratton.

Mayer, J. (1974). Aging & nutrition. Geriatrics, 29(5), 57-59.

Mead, J., Turner, J. M., Macklem, P. T., C. Little, J. B. (1967). Significance of the relationship between lung recoil and maximum expiratory flow. Journal of Applied Physiology, 22, 95-108.

Meunier, P., Courpron, P., Edouard, C., Bernard, J., Bringuier, J., & Vignon, G. (1973). Physiological senile involution and pathological rarefaction of bone. Clinical Endocrinology & Metabolic, 2, 239.

Murch, G. M. (1973). Visual and auditory perception, New York: Bobbs-Merrill.

McBean, L. D., & Speckman, E. W. (1974). A review: The importance of nutrition in oral health. Journal of the American Dental Association, 89, 109-114.

McKeown, F. (1965). Pathology of the aged. London: Butterworths.

National Institute of Aging, (1980, October). Senility: Myth or madness? Age Page, NIH U.S. Government Printing Office: #1981-0-354-635.

National Institute of Aging (1981, May). High blood pressure: A common but controllable disorder, Age Page, NIH SDHHS.

National Institute of Aging (1983, September). Aging and your eyes. Age Page, NIH, U.S. Government Printing Office #1983-416-519.

National Institute of Health (1980). Alzheimer's disease, A scientific guide for health practitioners, NINDS; Office of Scientific and Health Reports.

National Institute of Neurological Disease and Stroke (NINDS). (1969). National Institutes of Health, U.S. Department of Health, Education, and Welfare. Human communication and its disorders: An overview. Bethesda, MD: NINDS Monograph No. 10, p. 16.

Newton-John, H. F., & Morgan, D. B. (1970). The loss of bone with age, osteoporosis, and fractures. Clinical Orthopedics, 71, 229.

Nizel, A. E. (1967). Food and nutrition for the new denture wearer, particularly the geriatric patient. In The science of nutrition & its application in clinical dentistry. Philadelphia: W. B. Saunders.

Nizel, A. E. (1981). Nutritional management of the elderly, especially those with dentures. In Nutrition in preventive dentistry: Science & practice. Philadelphia, PA: W. B. Saunders.

Notelovitz, M., & Ware, M. (1982). Stand tall: The Informal Woman's Guide to preventing osteoporosis. Gainesville, FL: Triad Publishing.

Obrist, W. D. (1972). Cerebral physiology of the aged: Influence of circulatory disorder. In C. M. Gaitz (Ed.), Aging and the brain. New York: Prenum Press.

Obrist, W. D. (1980). Cerebral blood flow and EEG changes associated with aging and dementia. In E. W. Busse & D. G. Blazer (Eds.), Handbook of geriatric psychiatry, New York: Van Nostrand Reinhold.

Ordy, J. M., Brizzee, K. R., & Beavers, T. L. (1980). Sensory function and short-term memory in aging. In G. J. Maletta & F. J. Pirozzolo (Eds.), The aging nervous system. New York: Praeger Publishers.

Pace, W. R. (1970). Pulmonary physiology in clinical practice (2nd ed.). Philadelphia: F. A. Davis.

Pierce, J. A., & Ebert, R. V. (1965). Fibrous network of the lung and its change with age. Thorax, 20, 469-476.

Pitanguy, I. (1978). Ancillary procedures in face lifting. Clinics in Plastic Surgery, 5, 51-70.

Pooling Project Research Group (1978). Journal of Chronic Disease, 31, 201.

Porcino, J. (1983). Growing older, getting better. Reading, MA: Addison-Wesley.

Ptacek, P. H., Sander, E. K., Maloney, W. H. & Jackson, C. C. R. (1966). Phonatory and related changes with advanced age. Journal of Speech and Hearing Research, 9, 353-360.

Raisz, L. G. (1977). Bone metabolism and calcium regulation. In L. V. Avioli & S. M. Krane (Eds.), Metabolic bone disease. New York: Academic Press.

Richmond, J. B. (1979, May-June). Health promotion & disease prevention in old age. Aging, 11-15.

Rivlin, R. S. (1982). Summary & concluding statements: Evidence relating selected vitamins & minerals to health & disease in the elderly population in the U.S. American Journal of Clinical Nutrition, 36(5): 1083-1086.

Robinson, H. B., Boling, L. R., & Lisher, B. E. (1942). Teeth and jaws. In E. V. Cowdry (Ed.), Problems of aging (2nd ed.). Baltimore: Williams & Wilkins.

Ronch, J. L. (1982). Who are these aging persons? In R. H. Hull (Ed.), Rehabilitative audiology. New York: Grune & Stratton.

Rous, J. (1969). The effect of age on the functional capacity of smell analysis. Ceskoslovenska Otolaryngologic, 18, 248-256.

Rowe, J. W., & Besdine, W. (Eds.). (1982). Health and disease in old age. Boston: Little, Brown.

Rozovski, S. J. (1984, April/May). Nutrition for older Americans. Aging, 344, 49-63.

Ruben, R. (1971). Aging and hearing. In I. Rossman (Ed.), Clinical Geriatrics. Philadelphia: Lippincott.

Ruckes, J., & Hohmann, M. (1963). On the topography and presence of fatty tissue in the human superior vocal cord in relation to age, weight, and disease. Anatomischer Anzieger, 112, 405-425.

Ruesch, J. (1957). Disturbed communication, the clinical assessment of normal and pathological communication behavior, New York: Worton.

Ryan, R. F., McDonald, J. R., & Devine, K. D. (1956). Changes in laryngeal epithelium: Relation to age, sex, and certain other factors. Mayo Clinic Proceedings, 31, 47-52.

Saxon, S. V., & Etten, M. J. (1978). Physical change and aging: A guide for the helping professions. New York: Tiresias Press.

Schaie, W. K. (1982). The Seattle longitudinal study: A 21-year explosion of psychometric intelligence in adulthood. In K. W. Schaie (Ed.), Longitudinal studies of adult psychological development. Guilford Press.

Schaie, W. K., & Geiwitz, J. (1982). Adult development & aging. Boston: Little, Brown.

Schiffman, S. (1977). Food recognition by the elderly. Journal of Gerontology, 32, 586-592.

Schiffman, S., & Pasternak M, (1979). Decreased discrimination of food odors in the elderly. Journal of Gerontology, 34, 73.

Segre, R. (1971). Senescence of the voice. Eye, Ear, Nose and Throat Monthly, 50, 62-68.

Shore, H. (1976). Designing a training program for understanding sensory loss in aging. The Gerontologist, 16, 157.

Spirduso, W. W., & Clifford, P. (1978). Replication of age and physical activity effects on reaction and movement time. Journal of Gerontology, 33, 26-30.

Squier, C. A., Johnson, N. W., & Hopps, R. M. (1976). Human oral mucosa. London: Blackwell Scientific Publications.

Storandt, M. (1983). Psychologic aspects. In F. V. Steinberg, (Ed.), Care of the geriatric patient. St. Louis: C. V. Mosby.

Svanborg, A. (1983). The physiology of aging in man - diagnostic and therapeutic aspects. In F. I. Caird & J. G. Evans (Eds.), Advanced geriatric medicine 3, Baltimore, MD: Urban & Schwarzenberg.

Timiras, P. S. (1972). Cardiovascular alterations with age: atherosclerosis. In F. S. Timiras (Ed.), Developmental physiology and aging. New York: Macmillan.

Todhunter, E. N., & Darby, W. J. (1978). Guidelines for maintaining adequate nutrition in old ages. Geriatrics, 33, 49-56.

Truex, R. (1940). Morphological alterations in the Gasserian ganglion cells and their association with senescence in man. American Journal of Pathology, 16, 255-268.

Turner, J. M., Mead, J., & Wohl, M. E. (1968). Elasticity of human lungs in relation to age. Journal of Applied Physiology, 25, 664-671.

U.S. Senate (1968, July). Hearing loss, hearing aids and the elderly. Report 98-912, Washington, DC: U.S. Government Printing Office.

U.S. Senate (1977, December). Select committee in nutrition & human needs, (2nd ed.). Dietary goals for the U.S. Washington, DC: U.S. Government Printing Office.

Wantz, M. S., & Gay, J. E. (1981). The aging process: A health perspective. Cambridge, MA: Winthrop Publishers.

Wattenberg, B. (1978). The U.S. fact book. New York: Grosset & Dunlop.

Weg, R. B. (1973). Drug interaction with the changing physiology of the aged: Practice & potential. In R. David (Ed.), Drugs & the elderly. Los Angeles: Andrus Gerontology Center.

Weg, R. B. (1979). Nutrition & the later years. Los Angeles: USC Press.

Weg, R. B. (1980a). Changing physiology and nutrition in aging. In H. C. Slavkin (Ed.), Proceeding new horizons in nutrition for the health professions. Los Angeles: USC Press.

Weg, R. B. (1980b). Prolonged mild nutritional deficiencies: Significance for health maintenance. Journal of Nutrition for the Elderly, 1(1), 3-22.

Weg, R. B. (1981). The changing physiology of aging. In R. H. Davis (Ed.), Aging: Prospects & issues. Los Angeles: USC Press.

Welford, A. T. (1977). Motor performance. In J. E. Birren & K. W. Schaie (Eds.), Handbook of the psychology of aging. New York: Van Nostrand Reinhold.

Winick, M. (Ed.) (1976). Nutrition & aging. New York: John Wiley.

Wisniewski, H. M., & Terry, R. D. (1973). Morphology of the aging brain, human, and animal. Progress Brain Research, 40, 167-187.

Woodruff, D. S. (1979). Brain electrical activity and behavior relationships over the life span. In P. B. Baltes (Ed.), Life-span development and behavior. Vol. 1. New York: Academic Press.

Yearick, E. S.; Wang, M. S. L., & Pisias, S. J. (1980). Nutritional status of the elderly: Dietary and biochemical findings. Journal of Gerontology, 3(5), 663-671.

Young, E. A. (1983, March). Nutrition, aging and the aged. Medical Clinics of North America, 67(2), 295-313.

Yurick, A. G. (1980a). The nursing process as applied to the adaptive experience of the aged. In A. G. Yurick, S. S. Robb, B. E. Spier, & N. J. Ebert (Eds.), The aged person & the nursing process. Englewood Cliffs, NJ: Prentice-Hall.

Yurick, A. G. (1980b). Vision in the elderly person and the nursing process. In A. G. Yurick, S. S. Robb, B. E. Spier, & N. J. Ebert (Eds.), The aged person and the nursing process. Englewood Cliffs, NJ: Prentice-Hall.

Psychological Changes With Aging

Elizabeth Robertson-Tchabo
University of Maryland, College Park, Maryland

The purpose of this chapter is to review the normal and abnormal age-related changes in mental functioning and to consider the psychological resources potentially needed to cope with the losses frequently associated with advancing age. One limitation of gerontological training is that few professionals who are contributing to the scientific aging literature or to the delivery of services to the elderly have experienced the process of becoming "seasoned citizens." Cowley (1980) wrote:

> To enter the country of age is a new experience, different from what you supposed it to be. Nobody, man or woman, knows the country until he has lived in it and taken out his citizenship papers. "Put cotton in your ears and pebbles in you shoes," said a gerontologist, a member of that new profession dedicated to alleviating all maladies of old people except the passage of years. "Pull on rubber gloves. Smear Vaseline over your glasses, and there you have it: instant aging." Not quite. His formula omits the messages from the social world, which are louder, in most cases, than those from within. We start by growing old in other people's eyes, then slowly we come to share their judgment. (p. 2, 5)

One theme running through the various sections of this paper is that gerontological training requires joint consideration of the objective behavioral facts of human aging and of the subjective psychological impact of these changes.

The psychology of aging is part of the field of developmental psychology which is concerned with behavioral changes within individuals across the entire life span and with differences between and similarities among people in the nature of these changes. The objectives of life span developmental psychology include describing within-individual changes and between-individual differences, explaining how such changes and differences come about, and

modifying behavior in an optimal way (Baltes, Reese, & Nesselroade, 1977).
Because changes within an individual occur gradually, it is helpful to know
about the past as well as the present to explain current behavior and to
predict future behavior. A focus on age-related changes within an individual
requires a longitudinal study design which seems compatible with the way
in which information is gathered in many clinical contexts. Unfortunately,
studies in the gerontological literature consist almost entirely of
cross-sectional research. In such designs, two or more age groups of different
people born at different times are compared on some measurable performance at
one point in time. However, representative groups of subjects differing in
chronological age are also likely to differ in other attributes, such as
educational level and health status, that co-vary both with chronological age
and with performance on a particular task. A cross-sectional approach provides
measures of age/cohort differences, whereas a longitudinal approach provides
direct measures of age changes.

This does not mean that a longitudinal approach solves all of the problems
in describing what happens to individuals as they mature (see Nesselroade &
Baltes, 1979). For example, repeating measures (practice) can affect
performance. Moreover, subjects who continue to participate in a study may
not be representative of the initial study group; that is, "survivors" tend
to perform better on the initial performance measures than subjects who do not
return for further tests (Arenberg, 1974).

A General Conceptual Framework: Person-Environment Transactions

In developmental theories, there is at least tacit recognition of the
fact that an individual changes in a changing world, and that the context
of development can affect the nature of individual change. Nevertheless,
gerontological research frequently has described psychobiological functions
isolated from social context and has presented aging as a process characterized
by declines in health, strength, and mental functioning. This decremental
model of aging precludes intervention and modification of behavior since
decline is considered to be inevitable. More recently, investigatorsstimulated
by public concern for the problems of housing the elderly and of improving
the quality of institutional environments have examined the effects

74

of various environmental factors on the behavior of older persons (Altman, Wohlwill, & Lawton, 1984; Atchley & Byerts, 1975; Byerts, Howell, & Pastalan, 1979; Golant, 1979; Lawton, 1980; Rowles & Ohta, 1983; Windley, Byerts, & Ernst, 1975). The studies showed that many behaviors considered to be less than optimal were, in part, a consequence of a specific social environment rather than of chronological age per se. Moreover, the behavioral competence of elderly people could be increased by changing environmental conditions so that there was a better "match" between environmental demands and the older persons' abilities. The importance of understanding how environmental features interact with personal characteristics to influence behavioral competence and psychological well-being has been recognized, and gradually ecological models have replaced decremental views of the aging process.

Rapid expansion of the aging-environment field led to a proliferation of theoretical models. Pastalan (1975) proposed an "age-loss continuum" in which aging was viewed in terms of progressive lifespan contraction associated with a series of role losses. Lawton and Simon (1968) proposed an "environmental docility hypothesis" which posited that, with increasing age, personal competence declines and external and environmental influences become progressively more pervasive in limiting activity and in determining an older person's life-style and level of environmental participation. This view was elaborated in Lawton and Nahemow's (1973) ecological model of adaptation and aging. An additional level of complexity was provided by Kahana (1975) with her "environmental congruence model." This model addressed the highly individualistic sets of need and preferences that ideally are consonant with facilitating or supportive characteristics of an environmental context. When a balance between individual needs and environmental characteristics is achieved, a state of congruence is said to exist. Kahana's model incorporated several social and psychological dimensions (including privacy, autonomy or control, and potential for individual expression) which provide a more elaborate analysis of the old person-environment interaction. Subsequently, Rowles (1978) proposed a "hypothesis of changing emphasis" which describes changes with advanced age in four domains of the old person-environment transaction - action, orientation, feeling, and fantasy.

Investigators have moved gradually to more complex analyses of the person-environment transaction as it became apparent that studies which explored single aspects of the relationship, such as the design of a residence or the architectural barriers to mobility, lacked a sense of the total context. In a recent evaluation of the state of the art in the aging-environment literature, Rowles and Ohta (1983) concluded that it is becoming increasingly apparent that to fully appreciate the older person-environment transaction, it is necessary to adopt a holistic stance, utilizing a broader view of milieu and incorporating into the older person's environmental context consideration of societally determined norms of "appropriate activity," changing sex role expectations, and other social, cultural, and political components. They also pointed out that the preference for more holistic interpretation risks the development of fuzzy conceptual frameworks that are so complex and inclusive that they could not be studied empirically even with the most sophisticated multivariate techniques.

In contrast to the earlier studies of aging-environment transactions which were concerned primarily with institutionalized populations and tended to focus on themes of "losses" or "decrements" with advanced old age, future research can be expected to shift attention to the more able, community-dwelling, elderly individual. The focus has shifted to ways in which old people actively mold not only their physical environment but also the psychological and social milieu in which they reside. With the shift in emphasis, mediators of the person-environment interaction have become more important (Parr, 1980). Mediation involves intellectual processes of cognitive appraisal, and mediating variables include how people perceive the environment, the importance to them of environmental characteristics, what they expect to receive from an environment, and how they expect to be able to change it. By definition, mediators are influenced by both personal and environmental characteristics, but they should not be considered as end products. Rather, the outcome of a person-environment interaction should be judged by behavioral measures that are collected in specific environmental contexts.

It is interesting to note that ecological models have also been employed for some time in the speech and hearing field. Goetzinger (1967) suggested that the impact of hearing impairment is manifested by a change in the interaction between a person and his environment. Maurer and Rupp (1979) have emphasized that "...loss of hearing sensitivity should be considered in terms of the geriatric environment" (p. 191).

Two other methodological issues related to ecological validity will be addressed here. The first concerns the external validity of measures collected in the controlled environment of the experimental laboratory; that is, age differences in performance measured in the laboratory should be capable of being generalized to other settings especially everyday, "real-life" environments. Frequently, the laboratory and usual, everyday environments are different. Everyday settings may provide compensatory, support systems for proficient performance that have no counterparts in laboratory settings.

The second issue related to ecological validity is the degree to which test materials are relevant to the everyday environments of elderly individuals. Typically, tests used to assess the performance of older people have not been developed specifically for use with older populations. Consequently, a test developed and standardized upon behavior sampled in young adults may be inappropriate to test similar facets in older individuals, either in terms of content or instructional set (Schaie, 1977, 1978). McNair (1979) has suggested guidelines for assessment tools for the elderly: (a) they should be brief to prevent fatigue; (b) easily read with respect to legibility of print and level of reading difficulty; (c) provide age-relevant items; and (d) provide age-relevant norms.

Defining Old Age

The problem of defining what is meant by the term, "older people," becomes apparent from even a cursory inspection of the literature. One investigator's "old" group is another investigator's "middle-aged" group. In addition to the age range of the subjects sampled, the task selected for study also determines whether significant age differences or changes appear. Clearly, aging affects various physiological functions and perhaps mental abilities at vastly different rates. The terms, "older person" and "late in life," will be used to refer to individuals aged 70 years or older, a position consistent with the age at which significant age-related changes in mental functioning have been found (Arenberg, 1974, 1978, 1982a, 1982b, 1983).

It is also important to distinguish "normal" or "primary" aging from "pathological" or "secondary" aging (Busse, 1969). Aging is not synonymous with disease. Normal or primary aging refers to the biological processes which are time-related and not a function of stress, trauma, or disease. Secondary or pathological aging refers to decrements in functioning attributable to trauma or to chronic disease. Secondary aging processes are not attributable to maturational effects although they are correlated with chronological age since the prevalence of chronic diseases increases with age.

The preceding points have implications for selection and description of subjects in aging studies. The elderly are not a homogeneous group. For many measures, there is greater variability in the old group than in any other age group. The strategy of looking for subjects where people of a given age are likely to be found, such as college classrooms, senior citizens' centers, or audiology centers is efficient from a practical point of view, but unquestionably non-random sampling biases the samples in known and unknown ways (e.g., see Humphrey, Gilhome-Herbst, & Faurqi, 1981). Samples of people drawn from a single site undoubtedly do not constitute a representative sample of the total population. In conducting correlational research, correlations are necessarily low when the variance of a variable is attenuated. Moreover, differences in sample selection contribute to differences in obtained results.

Cognitive Functioning

Intelligence

Because cognition plays a central role in adaptation to aging, we will start by reviewing age changes in cognitive performance. Longitudinal studies of intelligence which did not extend to late life typically found little or no decline in performance. In 1949, Owens (1953) retested individuals who were first given the Army Alpha test of intelligence when they entered college in 1919. The mean performance for seven of the eight subtests of the Army Alpha improved from the time when the subjects were in their late teens to the retest when they were in their late forties. In 1960, these subjects were tested a third time, when in their early sixties; no decline was found over this 11-year interval (Owens, 1966). Similar results were reported in a study by Cunningham and Birren (1976), wherein the Army Alpha was administered to college students. Twenty-eight years later when in their late forties, those who could be retested showed no decline. Several other studies, using a variety of tests with subjects in their forties at the last time of measurement, also reported small if any decline (Bayley & Oden, 1955; Nisbet, 1957; Tuddenham, Blumenkrantz, & Wilkins, 1968).

In more recent longitudinal studies, older subjects were included and age changes were found late in life. Eisdorfer and Wilkie (1973) described declines in performance on the Wechsler Adult Intelligence Scale over a 10-year period. Mean decrements were moderate for the subjects who were in their sixties at the time of the first test and who completed four test sessions during this 10-year period. For the subjects initially in their seventies who completed all four test series, mean declines were somewhat greater. Blum, Fosshage, and Jarvik (1972) used several subtests from the Wechsler-Bellevue Intelligence Scale and obtained measures from subjects who were initially in their mid-sixties and followed until they were in their mid-eighties. Declines were found in all subtests over the 20-year interval.

The most extensive and systematic longitudinal study of intelligence and aging has been conducted by Schaie and his colleagues (Schaie, Labouvie, & Buech, 1973; Schaie & Lobouvie-Vief, 1974; Schaie & Strother, 1968a, 1968b) using the Primary Mental Abilities Test (PMA). Subjects, all volunteers obtained from the membership of a prepaid medical plan, were tested in 1956, 1963, and 1970. In 1956, men and women aged 20-70 years were tested. Some of these subjects were retested in 1963 and the "survivors" were tested a third time in 1970. Additional subjects were added in 1963 and some of them were retested in 1970. Additional subjects were added in 1963 and some of them were retested in 1970. In addition to the direct measures of change based on repeated testing of the same individual, estimates of age change were based on comparisons of independent samples of the same birth cohort tested 7 or 14 years apart. For example, each of three groups of subjects all born in 1889 were tested at one of the three times of measurement. The group tested in 1956 was 67; the group tested in 1963 was 74 years; and the group tested in 1970 was 81 years. The mean difference in performance among these groups are estimates of age changes late in life for this birth cohort.

For every age group initially 60 years or older, mean declines were found for almost every 7-year and 14-year measure of change and estimate of change on each of the five subtests of the PMA, although the consistent mean declines were not large even for the 14-year test interval. Performances of the groups initially under 60 typically improved or remained stable over the 14-year testing period. Although sex differences were found to be significant for several variables (space, reasoning, and psychomotor speed), these differences

primarily affect the level of performance rather than the slope of the age
change functions (Schaie & Strother, 1968b).

In summary, the results of the studies of intelligence and aging are
consistent. In cross-sectional studies, age differences are found across the
entire adult life span. In longitudinal studies, age changes in intelligence
test performance are not found until late in life.

Memory and Learning

Although few longitudinal studies of memory and learning have been
published, the results are similar to those found in the longitudinal studies
of intelligence. Arenberg (1978) reported cross-sectional age differences
and longitudinal age changes on the Benton Revised Visual Retention Test
(BVRT). The pattern of findings in both the cross-sectional and longitudinal
analyses were very similar: (a) small if any age differences and changes in
early adulthood, (b) moderate differences and changes for subjects initially
in their fifties and sixties, and (c) substantial declines late in life.

The BVRT is a memory-for-designs task. Ten designs of geometric figures,
each displayed for 10 seconds, are drawn immediately from memory with no
time limit. The dependent measure is the total number of errors made in the
reproduction of all 10 designs. In this study, three cross-sectional and
two longitudinal analyses were reported for men in the Baltimore Longitudinal
Study of Aging (BLSA). The first cross-sectional analysis of men aged 20-102
years found a correlation of .47 between age and total errors. Two subsequent
samples of men aged 17-83 years and 21-90 years found correlations of .47
and .51, respectively. These are among the highest correlations between
chronological age and cognitive performance reported in the literature.

Some of the men in the first sample, returned six (or more) years later
for retesting. The groups initially in their thirties and forties declined
very little; those initially in their fifties and sixties declined little
more; but the group initially in their seventies declined substantially. Some
of the men in the second sample also were retested at least six years later.
Again, errors increased substantially only for the men initially in their
seventies. In both longitudinal analyses, the magnitudes of the age changes
were consistent with the age differences in the cross-sectional analyses.

It should be noted that the age-related declines in performance cited
above were found for a group of men who were more highly educated, more

economically secure, and healthier than the general population. With these biases operating, the age-related decrements that were found for these men undoubtedly underestimate the magnitude of change in the general population. It is of note that the longitudinal and cross-sectional results were more similar than longitudinal and cross-sectional results in the studies of intelligence. One likely possibility is that memory-for-designs performance is affected less by the social and cultural changes which have substantial effects on measures of intelligence. Cross-sectional comparisons, which confound aging with birth cohort (generation) differences, are less likely to match longitudinal changes when nonmaturational factors are important predictors of performance.

Performance on most psychological tasks is affected by several variables. Kausler (1982) distinguished primary factors, proficiency in processes that are involved in performance of a particular task, from secondary factors, general processes that may affect performance level on a wide range of tasks varying considerably in their underlying abilities or primary factors. In general primary and secondary factors interact to determine a level of performance. Common secondary factors include a subject's motivational level, general health, degree of recent practice of skills relevant to a particular task performed in the laboratory, formal educational level, or socioeconomic status. Socioeconomic status is correlated highly with level of formal education, which in representative samples of the general population is frequently a more powerful predictor of performance than chronological age.

Studies of verbal learning also are included in the BLSA although the sample sizes in each study were not large and only preliminary results have been published (Arenberg, 1983; Arenberg & Robertson-Tchabo, 1977). Both serial and paired-associate learning performance were measured; and in each paradigm, two pacing conditions were included. Subjects were randomly assigned to either a short anticipation interval, which allowed little time to respond to each item, or to a longer interval. The primary measure in both learning procedures was the number of errors to reach the criterion of an errorless trial. The men ranged in age from 20 to 87 years at the time of the first test.

Mean differences for the younger men who participated in the paired-associate learning task at the fast pace were small. Mean errors for the group in their mid-sixties, however, were high; and for the group in their late sixties or early seventies, mean errors were higher still. Six years after the first measure, some of these men were retested. For the younger groups, mean changes were small, but for the groups who reached their late sixties or early seventies, mean declines were substantial, and for the oldest group who had reached their late seventies, declines were even more dramatic. The pattern of results for paired-associate learning at the fast pace was very similar to that for the Benton data. Furthermore, the pattern of results for the paired-associated learning at the slower pace was not markedly different although mean errors were fewer than at the fast pace.

The results of the serial learning studies were somewhat less systematic, but the pattern at both pace conditions was similar. In general, small age differences and changes were found for the youngest groups, and the largest age differences and changes were found for the oldest groups.

Problem Solving and Aging

Two studies of problem solving were included in the BLSA. The first (Arenberg, 1974) is a completed study of logical problem solving, while the second (Arenberg, 1982a) is a progress report of a continuing study of conceptual problem-solving.

Substantial age differences had been reported in two cross-sectional studies using similar logical problems (Jerome, 1962; Young, 1966). Arenberg (1974) confirmed these findings and showed age differences both in the proportions of men who solved each problem and in measures of effectiveness in reaching a solution.

An interesting effect of attrition emerged from the longitudinal follow-up. Of the original sample of 300 men, 263 solved the first problem; and of these, 193 returned and solved that problem six years later. In the first session, substantial age differences in mean effectiveness were found using the data for the 263 men who sowed the problem. However, when the first-time measures were analyzed only for the 193 men who returned and again solved the problem, the age differences disappeared. For all age groups under 70 years when first tested, performance improved on the second measure; but for the group over 70 years at the time of the first test, performance declined substantially at the second measure. Despite the positive bias due to attrition (better initial performers in the older groups who returned and solved the problem six years later), the oldest group declined significantly.

There was a relationship between successfully solving the problem the first time and subsequent mortality. Twelve of the 49 men aged 70 years and over when first tested died during the 6-year retest interval. Six nonsurvivors were among the 36 men who had solved the first problem, and 6 were among the 13 who had not solved the problem. In other words, 17% of the solvers died, but 46% of those who failed died. Interestingly, survivors and nonsurvivors did not differ on the Vocabulary subtest of the Wechsler Adult Intelligence Scale.

Substantial age differences also are emerging from cross-sectional analyses of the concept-problem solving study (Arenberg, 1982a). Using the number of problems solved, the means declined monotonically from the twenties to the eighties. As in the logical problem-solving study, dropouts plus nonsolvers resulted in the better performers in the older groups returning and attempting all 12 problems 6 or 7 years later. The four youngest age groups had small mean improvements in number of problems solved the second time, but means for the groups in their sixties and seventies when measured initially declined somewhat. All of these findings are consistent with a decline in reasoning performance late in life.

The conclusion that there are age changes in several aspects of cognitive performance is based on the group mean change. However, in every age group, including the oldest, there were some men who did not decline. Further research is needed on individual differences in cognitive change (Denney, 1982). The relationship between cognitive change and level and change of other important variables, such as personality traits (Robertson-Tchabo, Arenberg, & Costa, 1979) and health status (Hertzog, Schaie, & Gribbin, 1978) may help to explain why some people decline and others maintain performance levels. Moreover, the BLSA data that have been discussed here were for samples of men. In 1978, the BLSA was expanded to include women. Whether the longitudinal findings for women will parallel those of the men, particularly with respect to the age at which one begins to find a significant decline (given the longer average life expectancy for women) remains to be seen. Although sex-related differences in cognition have been reviewed recently (Cohen & Wilkie, 1979; Kramer & Jarvik, 1979; Turner, 1982), the literature on sex-related differences in cognitive performance of the elderly is extremely limited and the findings are not consistent.

Explanations of Age Differences and Age Changes

A primary goal of longitudinal studies is to describe maturational changes. However, documentation of a significant age change on a particular performance task typically does not provide information concerning which structure or process is altered by maturational change. Considerable information has been gathered from cross-sectional studies with respect to the nature of age-related performance differences. The experimental questions usually include: (a) Are there age differences in performance, (b) Are there treatment effects; and (c) Are there significant age x treatment interactions; that is, are the age differences smaller under one condition than under another.

Kausler (1982) emphasized that the presence or absence of interaction effects is one way to gain insight into what processes are affected by aging and what processes are not. Once a specific process or condition of learning has been identified as age sensitive, there is then a possibility of finding ways to circumvent or to overcome the deleterious effects. We will review briefly selected cross-sectional studies with an emphasis on age sensitive aspects of performance.

Secondary Memory. Information processing models, which have dominated the analysis of age differences in performance, view the sequences of operations and transformations involved in cognitive activity as a complex system with many interacting stages. A basic assumption in information processing models of cognition is that the output is not an immediate consequence of stimulation but rather it is the product of a number of decision processes at successive levels of recoding. Primary and secondary memory are terms used by Craik (1977) to describe a dual stage memory model. Primary memory denotes a limited capacity store and secondary memory denotes a much larger, more stable store limited only by the rate at which it can accept information. Generally, age differences in primary memory capacity are minimal with undemanding conditions; that is, when a task does not require manipulation of information or division of attention during registration (Craik, 1977; Hartley, Harker, & Walsh, 1980). When the number of items to be remembered exceeds the primary memory span, however, older people do not recall as much information as young adults. Research has attempted to identify the nature of the age-related deficit in secondary memory (Smith, 1980) by differentiating registration, storage, and retrieval stages of memory. Earlier studies (e.g., Laurence, 1967; Schonfield

& Robertson, 1966) implicated retrieval as an age-sensitive process. Although older subjects could not access stored information at the time of recall, under conditions that minimized the search and retrieval requirement (recognition or cued recall conditions), there were not age differences. Subsequent studies have shown small age differences in recognition, but recall differences typically have been substantial. More recently, experimenters have been aware of the interdependence of registration and retrieval stages. Evidence is accumulating that older and younger individuals do not organize information in the same way at the time of registration which necessarily is reflected in age differences in the number and type of retrieval cues available at a subsequent time of recall (Burke & Light, 1981; Canestrari, 1968; Craik & Simon, 1980, Hulicka & Grossman, 1967).

In addition to studies that have found substantial age differences and age changes for information presented in the visual modality, results of several studies have indicated that older persons generally process auditory information (including spoken communications) less efficiently than younger individuals (e.g., Cohen, 1979; Rabbitt, 1982).

Pacing and Rate of Presentation. Because slowing is one of the most pervasive behavioral effects of aging, it is not surprising that pacing variables have been investigated extensively. Several studies investigated age differences in performance on rote learning tasks (Arenberg, 1965; Canestrari, 1963). Paired-associate learning is a rote procedure in which the task is to learn to respond with the response component that has been paired with a stimulus. Time to respond is called the anticipation interval. During this interval, a subject attempts to voice the correct response. The time that a stimulus together with its response is displayed is termed the inspection interval. During the inspection interval, a subject can study the stimulus-response word pair. Monge and Hultsch (1971) varied both the duration of the anticipation interval and the inspection interval. They found that either a longer inspection interval or a longer anticipation interval reduced the number of trials required by the older individuals to reach the criterion of one errorless trial. Longer inspection intervals equally benefitted both the young and the old groups, but increasing the duration of the anticipation interval was particularly beneficial for the older individuals. Additional time to respond has been found consistently to result in more effective learning for elderly individuals.

It is valuable to remember that the problem of speed stress is not restricted to experimental studies of cognitive functioning (see Welford, 1977). Schonfield (1980) has cautioned that anyone conversing with an elderly person should attempt to cultivate an unhurried tempo, and that the advice applies especially to professional consultations. Moreover, sensitivity to pacing variables appears in middle age (Monge & Hultsch, 1971). Pacing would undoubtedly be a factor in the acquisition by older persons of speechreading or signing skills.

Aids to Cognitive Performance. Older people frequently express concern about memory impairment (Zelinski, Gilewski, & Thompson, 1980). Although self-assessment of mental status is not always a reliable index of objective memory performance (Kahn, Zarit, Hilbert, & Niederehe, 1975), community surveys have indicated that one half of persons aged 60 years or older report serious memory problems (Lowenthal, Berkman, Beuhler, Pierce, Robinson, & Tier, 1967). In response to this need, psychologists have begun to develop practical memory remediation techniques for the elderly and to investigate the efficacy of such procedures. It should also be noted that it is not necessary that a deficit in cognitive performance exist in order to improve one's level of functioning.

Zarit, Cole, & Guider (1981) reported two studies of elderly community residents that investigated the effects of teaching four memory training strategies on subsequent recall performance. In the first study, subjects were randomly assigned to either the memory training group or to a current events discussion (control) group. Participants in the memory training group attended four, 90-minute sessions and at each session were instructed in an encoding strategy appropriate to enhance performance on a particular task. In the first session, subjects were instructed to cluster items in a categorized list of 10 items. In the second session, subjects were instructed to construct a meaningful connection between 10 pairs of individual pictures and corresponding names. In the third session, subjects were given lists of 10 unrelated items and instructed to visualize mental images to connect successive words. In the fourth session, subjects were read a long paragraph and told to use categories, images, and personal associations to the material to remember fractual information. Significant treatment effects were found for two of the tasks: (a) recall of related items and (b) recall of unrelated items.

Another important finding was that subjects in both the training and the control groups reported fewer subjective memory complaints at the completion of the study. The authors noted that training on tasks may be less important than changing expectations to help older adults view episodes of forgetfulness in a more balanced way. Forgetting does not usually represent a barrier to competent functioning in normal elderly adults. As Rabbitt (1977) commented, "In view of the deterioration of memory and perceptual motor performance with advanced age the right kind of question may well be not 'why are old people so bad at cognitive tasks' but rather 'how in spite of growing disabilities, do old people preserve such relatively good performance?'" (p. 623).

Imagery or Visual Mnemonics

One specific encoding strategy that has frequently been shown to enhance the performance of elderly individuals is visual imagery (see Poon, Walsh-Sweeney, & Fozard, 1980). Robertson-Tchabo, Hausman, and Arenberg (1976) employed a mnemonic procedure, the method of loci, to facilitate the recall performance of elderly community residents. Using this method, a subject is instructed to take a mental trip through his residence stopping in order at 16 places. When he learns a list of unrelated words, he retraces the trip visualizing one of the items in association with each stopping place. This method capitalizes on familiar (more automatic) stopping places and their natural-order attributes that provide effective retrieval cues. Using familiar spatial locations profits from self-generated mediators, reduces the interference from dividing attention between encoding and storage, and may reduce search failure as a subject knows where to resume a "trip."

Yesavage, Rose, and Bower (1983) investigated the relative effectiveness of three training conditions for elderly subjects. The image group was taught the standard mnemonic technique (McCarty, 1980) to learn name-to-face associations for each of a series of 12 face-name pairs. The image-plus-judgment group received identical mnemonic instructions and were also asked to judge the pleasantness of the image. The no-image group was treated like the image group except that they were not instructed to form an image when applying the mnemonic. The image group and the image-plus-judgment group showed higher recall than the no-image control group, and the image-plus-judgment group maintained their recall performance even after 48 hours. Additional elaboration of visual image associations is a technique which undoubtedly will be added to cognitive skill training programs for aged persons.

Two other points should be made. The first is that the time invested in training is not trivial. For example, Yesavage, Rose, and Bower (1983) instructed their subjects over five consecutive days with each session lasting 2 hours, and other investigators have needed comparable amounts of time. A second point is that such a substantial investment in training does not guarantee that subjects will transfer the training to day-to-day tasks. It is not clear why this happens. Perhaps psychologists need to gain a better understanding of the nature of the cognitive demands placed upon elderly individuals in their daily lives. Hulicka's (1982) report of an elderly participant's comment to the director of a cognitive training program, "Lady, your training program deals with your problems rather than mine" (p. 350) suggests that we might profit by attending more to the concerns of the elderly individuals whom we purport to serve.

Environmental Manipulation

In addition to changing an individual's behavior to enhance cognitive performance, manipulation of the environment also has been demonstrated to improve performance (Lawton, 1977). Ideally, of course, one might consider simultaneous manipulations of both the individual and the context to achieve optimal performance. Langer, Rodin, Beck, Weinman, & Spitzer (1979) conducted two studies with nursing home residents to enhance memory performance by increasing the cognitive demands. In the first study, motivation to practice cognitive activities was manipulated by varying the degree of reciprocal self-disclosure (i.e., mutual sharing of experiences) offered by student interviewers in a series of dyadic interactions. In the second study, motivation was manipulated by varying whether a subsequent reward was contingent upon attending to and remembering recommended cognitive activities (names of nurses and other residents). In both studies, the experimental treatments designed to elicit high cognitive activity resulted in improved performance on recall tasks.

Practice

In addition to these specific procedures which have been demonstrated to improve performance on a variety of cognitive tasks, it is important to note that practice alone (in the absence of specific instruction to process information in a particular manner) sometimes results in significant improvement in the performance of older individuals (e.g., Labouvie-Vief & Gonda, 1976). Exposure to a variety of cognitive tasks also results in improved performance on targeted behaviors (Baltes & Willis, 1982).

Implications

An index of an individual's level of cognitive functioning is useful to the extent that such a measure is related to behaviors of practical and social consequence. Assessment and evaluation of an individual's cognitive performance may influence decisions regarding when to retire, maintenance of independence, assessment of educability, and recommendation for rehabilitation training. Assessment of cognitive functioning should be part of a routine checkup especially since self-reported memory complaints have been identified as a symptom of depression in the elderly (see Kahn, Zarit, Hilbert, & Niederhe, 1975). However, a simple question such as, "Would you say you have memory problems?" is not sufficient to examine this complex problem. Three factors that have been identified as important are the frequency of cognitive failures, the importance to the individual of the memory failures, and the amount of effort made by the individual to avoid failures (see Zelinski, Gilewski, & Thompson, 1980). Others factors which could be included and might be helpful in examining a cognitive complaint include the familiarity of the task to the person and the context and circumstances in which a task was performed.

Cognitive Style and a Conservative Approach to Tasks

Studies of aging and cognitive functioning have been concerned primarily with quantitative differences; that is, with age differences in the level of performance, but the previously cited studies of age-related differences in encoding processes raise the question of qualitative differences in performance. Cognitive styles refer to individual variations in typical modes of perceiving, remembering, thinking, and problem solving; or to distinctive ways of apprehending, storing, transforming, and utilizing information (Kogan,

1973). Although abilities also involve the foregoing operations, there is a difference in emphasis. Abilities are concerned with the level of skill (better or poorer performance) whereas cognitive styles are related to the manner and form of cognition.

Field Dependence/Field Independence

One measure of cognitive style that has received considerable attention in the aging literature is field dependence-field independence. This dimension refers to individual differences in sensitivity to contextual and irrelevant stimuli. People considered to be field-dependent are said to rely largely on external stimuli in making perceptual judgments and to experience their environments in a global, relatively undifferentiated way. People classified as being field independent are believed to rely largely on internal stimuli in making perceptual judgments and to experience their environments in a relatively differentiated way (Witkin, Dyk, Faterson, Goodenough, & Karp, 1962). Field-dependent people, therefore, are more likely to be distracted by irrelevant stimuli and to suffer attentional problems when confronted by multiple stimulus sources. The popular notion is that people become more field dependent as they become older.

The two tests generally employed in the assessment of field dependence-field independence are the Rod-and-Frame test and the Embedded Figures test. Limitation of any construct to one or two tests poses a problem, particularly when the test materials do not have intrinsic interest and inadequate time is allowed for subjects to become familiar with the tasks. The Rod-and-Frame tests involves trying to adjust a rod in a darkened room so that it is vertical to the ground. Because the laboratory is dark, the person must rely on an internal sense of vertical rather than on environmental cues. In the Embedded Figures test, subjects attempt to find simple geometric figures hidden within more complex geometric designs. Accuracy is aging-contingent upon a subject's ability to ignore contextual information. For both tasks, the time required to make a response is the dependent measure used most frequently, and we have already noted that older persons are particularly disadvantaged on performance of paced tasks. Results of cross-sectional studies using the Rod-and-Frame and Embedded Figures tests generally have supported the hypothesis that field dependence increases from early to late adulthood

(Comalli, Wapner, & Werner, 1959; Eisner, 1972; Kogan, 1973; Lee & Pollack, 1978; Markus, 1971; Panek, Barrett, Sterns, & Alexander, 1978; Schwartz & Karp, 1967). However, we cannot rule out cohort differences as an explanation of this difference in field dependence. Moreover, other individual differences that are related to both field dependence-field independence and to age such as sensory acuity, educational level, and health status are usually not controlled.

Although the external validity of the Rod-and-Frame test and the Embedded Figures test may be challenged, field independence is related to one important, extra-laboratory task, driving an automobile. Independent of age, automobile accident rates are higher for field dependent than for field independent individuals (Mihal & Barrett, 1976). While we have noted that speed of response may contribute to age differences in field independence, speed of response is a necessary component of many everyday tasks including driving an automobile.

Cautiousness. Another dimension of cognitive style that has special importance in the evaluation of cognitive performance of the elderly is that of cautiousness. Again, the popular belief is that elderly people are more cautious and less willing to take risks than younger people. However, as with many other stereotypes, behavioral evidence in support of increasing cautiousness with increasing age is equivocal, and other explanations of the obtained age differences are also possible.

Signal detection methodology has been used to separate the two components of sensitivity (capacity) and response criterion (the response bias). In continuous recognition tasks, for example, there is the possibility that lower accuracy scores found for older subjects reflect a more stringent response criterion. However, if this were the case, it would be expected that there would also be a lower false alarm rate for older subjects compared to younger subjects. In fact, this is not the case. If anything, elderly subjects have been found to exhibit higher false alarm rates than younger persons (see Rankin & Kausler, 1979).

Other paradigms for the assessment of age differences in cautiousness and risk-taking have produced similarly equivocal results. Wallach and Kogan (1961) examined age differences in response to the Choice Dilemmas Questionnaire. On this test, subjects are given discriptions of life situations involving a person who is faced with a decision. They reported that their elderly subjects were more cautious than younger subjects in making decisions. Unfortunately, the usefulness of this paradigm is compromised considerably by its apparent low reliability (Okun, Stock, & Ceurvorst, 1980).

Although older individuals as a group cannot be characterized as being overly cautious, it is important to note that cautiousness could affect the task performance of some individuals. Varying the incentive conditions within a testing situation is one way to determine the range of response possible for an individual. Moreover, the separation of sensitivity and criterion aspects of performance by use of signal detection procedures might be useful in the assessment of hearing loss (see Corso, 1981).

Stress and Coping

Personality

The shift from a focus on stressors frequently encountered in advanced age to a consideration of individual differences in coping resources was mentioned previously in the discussion of a conceptual framework for this paper. In other words, given a particular objective stressor such as mild hearing impairment, how can we account for the wide range in self-reported impact of a common threat? One step in an ecological analysis of adjustment to life events and changes in life style is consideration of personal characteristics that are likely to affect adaptation to change. Lieberman (1978) and Costa & McCrae (1980b) have pointed out the importance of personality characteristics in explanations of adaptation to the expected and unexpected stressors of life. Fortunately, the literature concerning age differences in personality has been reviewed frequently (see Bromley, 1978; Chown, 1968; Lawton, Whelihan, & Belsky, 1980; McCrae & Costa, 1984; Moss & Susman, 1980; Neugarten, 1963, 1973, 1977; Riegel, 1959; & Thomae, 1980) and extensive consideration of theoretical and methodological issues in personality assessment is beyond the scope of this paper.

One of the most controversial issues in the psychology of aging is the question of the relative stability of adult personality; that is, are there consistent age changes in personality? An unequivocal answer is complicated by the multiple theoretical and methodological approaches to the study of personality and aging and by the fact that almost all of literally hundreds of studies have been cross-sectional (Neugarten, 1977). Typically, those studies focused on age differences in a single trait or dimension of personality, and the findings have been inconsistent with respect to age differences in personality traits. A trait is a generalized tendency toward thoughts, feelings, and behaviors and can be viewed as a structure of personality that accounts for relatively enduring dispositions and consistencies in an individual's behavior over time. Sociability is one example of a trait. Trait measurement generally relies on a standardized, self-report psychometric inventory or questionnaire, and usually the test items have been identified through factor analysis.

More recently, longitudinal studies of age changes in temperamental traits have been conducted (e.g., Costa & McCrae, 1977, 1978; Costa, McCrae & Arenberg, 1980; Douglas & Arenberg, 1978; Siegler, George, & Okun, 1979). In contrast to the cross-sectional data, evidence for long-term stability of personality traits in normal adults was consistently found using differentpersonality inventories and different dependent measures of stability (e.g., a retest correlation taken over a period of years, mean levels of a trait, or factor structure invariance). Rather than continuing to use personality as a dependent measure and to ask how does personality change as individuals grow older, it would be more appropriate to view personality as an important independent variable and to ask how individuals with different personality profiles differ in their adaptation to the aging process (McCrae & Costa, 1982).

Using a trait model of personality, Costa and McCrae (1980b) identified a limited set of three dimensions of personality which they have found useful to predict psychologically important, global characteristics of individuals. The three basic, but not necessarily exhaustive, trait domains which have been identified using a variety of self-report personality scales include Neuroticism, Extraversion, and Openness to Experience (NEO). Neuroticism refers to a dimension of adjustment-maladjustment and appears to be an index of the vulnerability of the individual to stress of all kinds. Extraversion characterizes an interpersonal style dimension, and Openness to Experience refers to an experiential style dimension which contrasts alternative adaptive strategies. An open style maximizes the input of new information to find the best solution whereas a closed type minimizes new information and disruption of existing order. Within each of these broad personality domains, Costa and McCrae (1980a) have identified six well-established traits. Their six facets of Neuroticism include Anxiety, Hostility, Depression, Self-consciousness, Impulsiveness, and Vulnerability. In the interpersonal cluster of Extraversion, the six components include Attachment and Gregariousness (both aspects of sociability), Assertiveness, Activity, Excitement-seeking, and Positive Emotions. The six facets of Openness to Experience include the content areas of Esthetics, Feelings, Phantasy, Ideas, Actions, and Values.

Individual differences in these trait domains have predicted self-reported, subjective levels of adjustment. In the gerontological literature, adjustment is usually defined operationally by scores on a test of general well-being measuring morale, life satisfaction, or happiness. In a large sample of adult men, Costa and McCrae (1980b) have found that happiness was related to both Extraversion and to Neuroticism. Adjusted and extraverted men were happier than neurotic and introverted men.

The independence of positive affect and negative affect has been appreciated for some time (see Bradburn, 1969); Costa and McCrae (1976) have made an important contribution with their explanation of this phenomenon. They suggested that positive affect or satisfaction with life is related strongly to Extraversion. Negative affect or dissatisfaction with life is predicted by Neuroticism. Because Extraversion and Neuroticism are independent (uncorrelated), general satisfaction and dissatisfaction also are independent. Moreover, self-reported health status is influenced strongly by Neuroticism. The important implication of these results is that stable personality characteristics are more important predictors of general well-being than objective life circumstances. Costa and McCrae (1980a) concluded that ". . . adjusted extraverts will tend to find satisfaction in almost any life situation, whereas the neurotic will never be pleased" (p. 85).

Thus, the validity of a global measure of subjective well-being as an index of either adjustment of a major life event or of the effectiveness of a program for the elderly must be considered in the context of individual differences in Neuroticism and Extraversion. Stable personality characteristics also were shown to have important implications for the study of coping with expected and unexpected stressors associated with male mid-life crisis (Costa & McCrae, 1978).

Life Events

Adaptation, adjustment, and coping have remained central themes in gerontological research. The question of how the dynamics of stress and coping change with the processes of aging and the circumstances of living is answered best by a longitudinal perspective. Again, not surprisingly, most of the research has been cross-sectional and has addressed the somewhat different question of whether adults of various ages use different coping strategies and face different stressors. Most of these studies have used measures of general well-being as an index of adjustment (see Larson, 1978; Lohmann, 1980), and we have discussed the problems associated with the interpretation of such indices in the previous section. With the exception of self-reported health, which is moderately and frequently correlated with life satisfaction (r = .40), no other variables appear to be important and consistent correlates of general well-being. Rather, variability is typical--many people manage well, but some manage poorly.

Two different approaches to stress and coping research are found in the current literature. The more common model defines stressors as major life events that involve role change and require adaptation. Life events became ofinterest when Holmes and Rahe (1967) proposed that adaptation required by major life changes substantially increased the risk of physical illness. Their major life events approach to the study of stress (the Social Readjustment Rating Scale) has dominated research despite the fact that cumulated life events correlate only weakly with health outcomes and that extensive methodological criticisms have been noted (see Rabkin & Streuning, 1976). In addition, lists of life events omit many events of importance to aging adults, such as disability due to chronic health problems, loneliness, and an unresponsive environment. Moreover, mediating processes of cognitive appraisal such as the personal significance of an event are not considered. It is not the event, but the significance of the event at a particular time in a person's life, that should be taken into account (Lazarus & Delongis, 1983). Throughout life, people struggle to make sense out of what happens to them and to provide themselves with a sense of order and continuity (Butler, 1975).

In a thoughtful theoretical examination of life events from a developmental perspective, several researchers (Brim, 1980; Brim & Ryff, 1980) have suggested that life events can be classified by three properties of events: (a) the probability that an event will take place for a particular person, "Will it happen to me?"; (b) the correlation of the event with chronological age, "If so, when will it happen?"; and (c) the social distribution of the event, "If it happens, will there be other people like me or will I be the only one?" The probability that a particular event will take place as assessed by an individual is especially significant because it is likely that people selectively attend to only those events that are likely to happen to them. Age-relatedness is important because it influences whether or not a person is prepared for or is caught unexpected by a life event. Neugarten (1977) has referred to "on-time" and "off-time" transitions and has suggested that "off-time" events are more disruptive. Social distribution is important because it determines whether or not an individual is likely to have a support system to help buffer a crisis and whether a role model is likely to be available.

When life events are cross-classified by the three properties, eight types of events are identified. When an event is shared by many individuals in a society, the probability of occurrence is high, and the event is related to age, anticipatory socialization is possible. Retirement is one example of these so-called Type 1 events. Educational interventions can be designed so that values, attitudes and overt behaviors required by the change in status can be learned prior to the event and potentially necessary resources can also be identified.

Recently, Schlossberg (1984) has reviewed the extensive literature on adjustment to major transitional life events, and has developed a model to assess the process of adjustment to such changes. However, unlike the adjustments required by abrupt changes in status, such as retirement or widowhood, to which the majority of adults eventually experience positive outcomes, the stressors implicit in advanced old age are the lower-level, chronic stresses or daily hassles of everyday existence. The range of coping mechanisms in the latter case has not been well-studied.

Daily Hassles

The second approach to stress and coping research supplements the life events strategy and focuses on daily hassles (DeLongis, Coyne, Dakof, Folkman, & Lazarus, 1982; Kanner, Coyne, Schaefer, & Lazarus, 1981; Lazarus & DeLongis, 1983). Daily hassles refer to the irritating, frustrating, and distressing demands and troubled relationships that to some degree characterize everyday transactions with the environment. Some of these hassles are transient, others are recurrent or even chronic, but they should be distinguished from dramatic, change-centered, major life events. The Hassles Scale (Kanner, Coyne, Schaefer, & Lazarus, 1981) assesses both the frequency and severity of these stressors, and includes items such as misplacing or losing things, concern about weight, rising prices, and not having enough time for one's family. DeLongis et al. (1982) found that scores on the Hassles Scale were better predictors than major life events of health outcomes. In addition to measuring hassles, positive experiences or daily uplifts are measured concurrently (Kanner et al., 1981).

An integral component of the daily hassles and uplifts model is a person's cognitive appraisal of the significance of a stressor. Coping is a second key mediating process that accounts for individual differences in perceived strain given similar environmental conditions. Folkman and Lazarus (1980) assessed coping in a middle-aged sample using the Ways of Coping Checklist and distinguished two basic functions of coping--problem solving and the regulation of emotion. They found that most stressful situations generated both sorts of coping activities. McCrae (1982) used a greatly expanded version of the Ways of Coping Checklist, and found that older people generally use the same coping processes as younger people although certain stressors are more common among older people.

Aging and Adjustment to Communication Problems

The problem of acquired hearing loss and communication disorders in the elderly is a topic that recently has received considerable attention (Beasley & Davis, 1981; Corso, 1981; Glendenning, 1982; Henoch, 1979; Hinchcliffe, 1983; Hull, 1981; Maurer & Rupp, 1979; Obler & Albert, 1980; Schow, Christensen, Hutchinson, & Nerbonne, 1978; Wilder & Weinstein, 1984). There is a concensus that adequate rehabilitative management of a hearing-impaired person depends not only on the level of objective hearing loss as measured by standardized audiometric measures but also on a person's subjective, self-assessment of the effect of hearing impairment (hearing handicap) on everyday function (Alpiner, 1979; Gilhome-Herbst, 1983; Harless & McConnell, 1982; Milne, 1976; Rosen, 1979; Rousey, 1971). Several studies (Berkowitz & Hochberg, 1971; McCartney, Maurer, & Sorenson, 1976; Weinstein & Ventry, 1983a) using a variety of self-assessment scales have investigated the magnitude of hearing handicap in a geriatric sample. However, none of these scales were developed exclusively for use with elderly people. It is possible that some of the items in these inventories are inappropriate because the demands of environments on younger and older persons may be different. Fortunately, a self-report inventory to quantitatively measure hearing handicap specifically for elderly clients has been developed recently (Ventry & Weinstein, 1982; Weinstein & Ventry, 1983b). The Hearing Handicap Inventory for the Elderly (HHIE) uses a 3-point scale and includes 12 items that tap social/situational effects of hearing handicap and 13 items that tap emotional response to an auditory deficit. Moreover, considerable attention has been paid to the psychometric adequacy of the inventory. As expected, objective hearing loss measured by pure-tone threshold accounted for only 37% of the variance in hearing handicap, and the authors stated that other individual differences such as personality characteristics probably contribute to the subjective assessment of hearing loss.

In light of Costa and McCrae's (1980a) NEO model, we might speculate that both Neuroticism and Extraversion might contribute to the self-evaluation of hearing handicap. That is, with equivalent levels of hearing loss, individuals with high levels of Neuroticism would evaluate their handicap more negatively than those with low levels of Neuroticism as measured by the Emotional subscale of the HHIE. On the other hand, Extraversion would be expected to be related to the Social/situational subscale because more extraverted individuals perfer group social interaction and stimulation, social situations which may be less than optimal for hearing-impaired individuals. Furthermore, because a change in the HHIE scores as an index of the effectiveness of rehabilitative management might be affected by the inherent bias attributable to different cognitive appraisals of persons high in Neuroticism versus Extraversion. Other dependent measures should be used concurrently.

The prevalence of hearing handicap among samples of elderly suggests that it is appropriate to view hearing impairment as a stressor. Because it is frequently difficult to precisely identify the onset of hearing impairment, it may be that adjustment to communication difficulties may be better understood within the stress and coping framework of daily hassles and uplifts (Folkman & Lazarus, 1980). Moreover, the significance of the hearing loss (cognitive appraisal) to a particular individual may determine the motivational level for participation in anticipatory socialization interventions, such as learning to sign. Finally, longitudinal studies of adjustment to hearing handicap are necessary to improve our understanding of the complex and dynamic person-environment interactions involved.

Severe Maladjustment and Psychopathology

Wells (1980) in a presentation to the American Psychopathological Association stated that even now little can be added to an article published by Sir Martin Roth in 1955 on the natural history of mental disorders in old age. However, Roth (1980) himself was impressed by the expansion of the field of geriatric psychiatry in the last 30 years from discussions of presenile and arteriosclerotic dementia to a much wider range of topics including the differential diagnosis of psychiatric disorders in the elderly, the epidemiology of senile dementia and depression, and the pharmacotherapy of these disorders. The burgeoning interest in the psychiatric problems of the aged reflects growing recognition of the fact that these conditions constitute the most formidable challenge posed by the aging populations of the developed world. Extensive summaries of the literature on the psychopathology of aging are available elsewhere (see Birren & Sloane, 1980; Blazer, 1977; Busse & Blazer, 1980; Busse & Pfeiffer, 1973; Cole & Barrett, 1980; Howells, 1975; Isaacs & Post, 1978; Levy & Post, 1982; Pitt, 1982; Post, 1966; Raskin & Jarvik, 1979; Storandt, Siegler, & Elias, 1978; Verwoedt, 1976; & Zarit, 1980).

Prevalence of mental illness in the elderly. Epidemiology of psychological orders in late life has provided valuable information over the past 2 decades. Although important and unsolved problems still remain in regard to standardization of case finding techniques and of measuring the severity of disturbance with reliability, it is clear from community studies that the prevalence of psychopathology in the elderly is substantial (Bremer, 1951; Essen-Moller, Larsson, Uddenberg & White, 1956; Kay, Beamish, & Roth, 1964; Leighton, Harding, Macklin, Hughes, & Leighton, 1963; Lowenthal et al., 1967).

Studies of psychological disturbance in the later years fall essentially into three categories: (a) those seeking to measure the existence of any, even mild, psychiatric disorders; (b) those measuring only the prevalence of "significant" degrees of psychiatric disturbance; and (c) those studies assessing only the prevalence of mental disorder in which a patient is being seen in a diagnostic or treatment facility.

Leighton et al. (1963) using a criterion of even "mild" emotional disturbance found that between 50% and 60% of their elderly subjects experiences some degree of distress. Although the prevalence is substantial, it does not indicate a remarkable increase with advancing age of the total number of persons with any degree of emotional disorder (Pfeiffer, 1977).

Among studies concerned with the prevalence of psychopathology of at least moderate severity in an elderly population are those of Pasamanick (1962), Lowenthal et al. (1967); and Kay, Beamish, and Roth (1964). The prevalence of moderate to severe psychopathology from these studies falls between 12% and 26%.

Redick, Kramer, and Taube (1973) and Kramer, Taube, and Redick (1973) focus primarily on elderly persons actually receiving mental health services. At the time of the 1970 Census, about 125,000 persons aged 65 years or more were hospitalized in psychiatric hospitals. It was estimated that 70% to 80% of the 700,000 individuals residing in nursing homes suffer from moderate to severe mental disorders. Advanced age may be associated with a high prevalence of psychopathology, and may be particularly noticeable beyond age 75 years.

In the next three sections of this paper, we will consider specific forms of psychopathology. Psychiatric classification systems distinguish functional disorders from organic disorders. Functional disorders include disturbances in adaptation despite intact brain functioning, whereas organic disorders refer to disturbances in behavior occurring because of impaired brain function.

Depression. Affective disturbances, particularly depression, are the most frequent functional disorders in old age. Depressions vary considerably in duration and in degree. Many elderly persons experience fleeting episodes of saddened affect, loss of energy, and short-lived lack of interest frequently in response to some adverse life situation or loss. More severe and more lasting depressive reactions are experienced by substantially fewer elderly persons, usually in response to significant losses or more rarely without recognizable precipitating factors.

It is easy to speculate why there would be a high incidence of transient depressive attacks in older persons and also why these individuals might present somewhat different symptoms than young depressed patients. First, there are significant sensory losses and health problems associated with aging. The consequences of these losses may be more isolation and withdrawal among the elderly than among younger individuals. The elderly are more likely to encounter a variety of adverse psychosocial factors that can precipitate depressions. Advancing age may lead to mandatory retirement, decreased financial resources, and loss of emotional support of an informal support system by the death of spouse, relatives, and friends. One empirical study by Beckman and Brody (1973) confirmed the relationship between role loss and depression in the elderly. They found a statistically significant correlation between a Role Loss Index derived from Dean's Powerless Scale and scores on the Beck Depression Inventory in 167 older men and women with an unspecified age range.

Two issues concerning depression and the elderly will be highlighted here. The first concerns age differences in the presenting symptoms between young and old depressed patients. The second issue is related to the first in that both pharmacological and behavioral treatment approaches to depression in old age have been extremely successful, providing of course that a depressive episode is recognized.

It has been suggested that the elderly are more likely to mask their depression than younger individuals (Goldfarb, 1974; Salzman & Shader, 1978). Many researchers and clinicians are likely to overlook mild depression or even severe depressive illness that involves a predominance of somatic complaints or even cognitive impairment. In contrast, such scales as the Zung Self-Rating Depression Scale (Zung, 1965) may weigh physical symptoms heavily in the identification of depressive disorder. Elderly people with actual physicalillness may then be falsely identified as depressed. Blumenthal (1975) stated that the somatic items on the Zung SDS, such as constipation, weight loss, fatigue, and heart racing, contributed to spuriously high total scores for those aged 65 years and over. On the other hand, Raskin (1979) cautions that not all somatic concerns, complaints of body slowness, and expressions of fatigue and apathy should be considered normal for the elderly. Gurland, Fleiss, Goldberg, Sharpe, Copeland, Kelleher, & Kellett (1976) extracted a large depression factor from the Geriatric Mental State Schedule which included complaints of memory impairment, a loss of interest in social activities, a lack of energy and listlessness, and sleep and vegetative disturbances. Clearly, there is a fine line that separates behaviors than can legitimately be ascribed to the aging process from those associated with depression. Presumably mental health workers skilled in the use of clinical interview techniques can probe for mood disturbances in those instances in which an elderly individual seems primarily concerned with somatic complaints. It may be that individuals from older cohorts are less comfortable talking about mental problems than about physical complaints. Blazer and Williams (1980) reported that in a community survey of 997 elderly people which identified 14.7% of the sample with significant dysphoric symptomatology of whom 3.7% had symptoms of a major depressive disorder, only 1% of the subjects were receiving therapy from a trained counselor.

The typically low utilization rate of mental health services by elderly individuals contrasts with the impressive recovery rate for those individuals who do seek assistance. Stotsky (1975) summarized studies concerned with the efficacy of antidepressant medications for elderly individuals. More recently, Gallagher and Thompson (1981) compared the relative merits of three types of psychosocial treatment, behavioral psychotherapy, cognitive therapy, and brief psychotherapy (which is short-term and psychodynamically oriented). The subjects were diagnosed as experiencing "major depressive disorders," were free of significant cognitive impairment, and were not taking psychotropic medications during the course of treatment. Follow-ups indicated that both behavioral and cognitive treatment were superior to brief psychotherapy at 3 months, 6 months, and 1 year, although all three techniques had been regarded as equally effective immediately after termination of treatment.

Paraphrenia: Paranoid states of late life and deafness. Our concern ith this group of elderly patients is that an association between deafness and paranoid psychosis has been frequently reported that these patients constitute a significant proportion of the elderly mentally ill population, and that most importantly, audiologists are the health professionals most likely to have contact with these individuals prior to their hospitalization. Paranoia can be regarded as a disturbance of perception, intellect, and thinking with has no understandable relationship to a person's life. The term paraphrenia was reintroduced by Roth (1955) to describe schizophrenia with onset after age 60 years, a condition in which paranoid delusions and hallucinations are prominent but signs of organic dementia or sustained confusion are absent. Moreover, from the content of the delusional and hallucinatory symptoms, the condition is judged not to be due to a primary affective disorder. European studies consistently have shown that 10% of elderly psychiatric patients' first admissions to a hospital are for paranoid psychoses. The controversy in psychiatry concerning paranoid states is related to differential diagnosis and subtyping within this group of patients (Post, 1966; Retterstol, 1966). American psychiatry typically has viewed late-life paranoid states either as rare or not part of the schizophrenic syndrome (see Bridge & Wyatt, 1980a, and few American studies have been conducted with this group of psychiatric patients (Berger & Zarit, 1978). Bridge and Wyatt (1980b) urged that an American epidemiologic study be carried out to assess the incidence and prevalence of late-life paranoid states. It should be noted in this regard that the factors most commonly responsible for unreliability in diagnosis between research and hospital staffs were the patients' symptoms of belligerence and paranoid delusions. When these were present, the hospital staff most frequently diagnosed the state as <u>organic</u> whereas the research staff diagnosed the state as <u>functional</u> (Gurland et al., 1976)

The aforementioned association between hearing impairment and paranoid psychosis has been reported frequently (see Kay & Roth, 1961; Post, 1966). However, in these studies of hospitalized psychiatric patients hearing loss was not measured objectively, the duration of the hearing loss was not always known, and no otological diagnoses were made. Subsequently, Cooper, Kay, Curry, Garside, and Roth (1974) interviewed and otologically examined 54 patients with paranoid psychoses and 57 patients with affective psychoses. Members of both groups had become psychotic for the first time after the age of 50 years. In addition, a relative or close friend of the patient was seen in all but five cases. The minimum criterion of social deafness was "difficulty in hearing speech in any part of church/theatre or in group conversation but able to hear speech at close range without aid." After recovery from the acute phase of the illness, pure-tone audiometry was performed and evaluated by researchers who were unaware of the psychiatric diagnosis. Normal hearing was defined as hearing loss within the limit of social adequacy (30 db) over the speech frequency range (512-2048 Hz) and not greater than 40 at the higher frequencies in the better ear, because hearing in the better ear may be presumed largely to determine the degree of social handicap in everyday life. They found that patients with paranoid psychosis had a more severe degree of hearing loss and were more often socially deaf than patients with affective illness. The differences seem to be due to a significantly higher proportion of paranoid patients having longstanding, usually severe, bilateral deafness, which was most commonly caused by chronic middle-ear disease.

Kay, Cooper, Garside, and Roth (1976) examined various premorbid characteristics of the two groups of patients studied by Cooper et al. (1974) to assess the roles of intrinsic and extrinsic factors in the etiology of the late onset paranoid states. Low social class, having few or no surviving children, and social deafness were associated with a diagnosis of paranoid illness. Moreover, patients suffering from paranoid psychosis were rated both by themselves and by a significant other as having greater difficulty in establishing and maintaining satisfactory interpersonal relationships before the onset of the illness and as being more solitary, shy, and reserved, touchy and suspicious, and less able to display sympathy or emotion. The authors concluded that these traits of solitariness, emotional coldness, and hostility described an abnormal premorbid schizoid personality, but the origin of such traits remains unknown.

Cooper and Curry (1976) using an enlarged sample of 27 paranoid and 18 affective patients who had been deaf prior to the onset of their psychosis replicated their earlier findings (Cooper et al., 1974). The long interval between the onset of deafness and the onset of psychosis seems to suggest opportunities for intervention especially because conductive deafness is often surgically remediable. Further research is needed to explore the path from social deafness to paranoid states and it may be that systematic observation (by informed audiologists and speech-language pathologists) of those individuals at risk for paraphrenia may provide further clues to clarify the nature of the relationship.

It should also be noted that Post (1966) reported that with adequate initial phenothiazine therapy plus maintenance, paraphrenic patients were responsive (that is, no longer psychotic), although there was little effect upon social relationships or general adjustment.

Organic Brain Syndromes: Dementia. Dementing illnesses are a group of organic, insidious, irreversible, and progressive cognitive disorders of the middle-aged and the aged characterized by a progressive decline in mental functioning, self-care, and adaptation to the environment culminating in premature death. Concern with and new information about dementia and other pathological conditions that affect cognitive functioning has stimulated extensive research which has been summarized elsewhere (Corkin, Davis, Growdon, Usdin, & Wurtman, 1982; Katzman, Terry, & Bick, 1978; Miller, 1977; Miller & Cohen, 1981).

Folstein and McHugh (1978) outlined three defining characteristics of dementia which include: (a) a history of deterioration in intellectual capacity from a previously higher level as reported by the patient, his family and friends; (b) evidence of a global intellectual disturbance based on a mental status examination; and (c) no disturbance in the state of consciousness such as occurs in coma or delirium. These defining features are all behavioral markers and do not specify a particular neuropathology.

It is important to note that dementia in the aged can be secondary to a wide range of physical conditions which are potentially treatable. Early detection and intervention are imperative because the combination of compromised cerebral function produced by systemic or metabolic disease and subthreshold degenerative change could result in irreversible brain damage (Roth, 1978). The more common etiological factors in secondary dementia include chronic intoxication by drugs, potassium loss from self-purgation, and nutritional deficiencies, especially vitamin B12.

Primary Degenerative Dementia: Senile dementia of the Alzheimer's type. The most common form of dementing illness occurring in 50-70% of affected persons is senile dementia of the Alzheimer's type due to primary neuronal degeneration. A clinical diagnosis is presumptive and is made by the elimination of all other known and testable causes of intellectual impairment, including malnutrition, drug intoxication, alcoholism, depression, and cardiovascular disease. A confirmatory diagnosis is pathological and is made when a large concentration of neurofibrillary tangles and senile plaques is observed in the neocortex and hippocampus at autopsy.

Multi-infarct dementia. Neuropathologic observations indicate that cerebrovascular alterations may be responsible for another 15-25% of dementing illnesses (Terry & Wisniewski, 1977; Tomlinson, Blessed, & Roth, 1970). Cognitive dysfunction resulting from vascular compromise is related to the occurrence of multiple cerebral infarcts. Despite the fact that anecdotally multi-infarct dementia is said to follow a stepwise deterioration in contrast to the progressive, gradual decline observed in senile dementia of the Alzheimer's type, on a case by case basis the cognitive disturbances are difficult to distinguish. Hachinski, Iliff, Zilhka, Dubonlay, McAllister, Marshall, Russell, & Symon (1975) and Hachinski (1978) has devised a clinical ischemic questionnaire which appears to be useful to distinguish nonoverlapping groups. However, Liston and La Rue (1983a, 1983b) have questioned the validity of the criteria used to make a differential diagnosis antemortem. The most salient shortcoming of studies of dementia is the lack of autopsy confirmation of diagnoses, particularly in light of the small sample sizes employed, the incomplete description of sample characteristics, and the nonblind assessment and rating procedures.

The most important issue with respect to the dementing illnesses remains the early and valid diagnosis of the condition. The most serious mistake is the erroneous judgment of dementia in the presence of a depressive illness. Effective treatment of dementia is likely to be optimized only if it is begun early in the course of the illness. One strategy that may be effective is to use the information derived from studies of normal aging to pursue processes which appear to be maintained into old age; for example, tasks of recognition memory and some aspects of language function.

Summary

As Kastenbaum (1971) stated in his popular article, old age has a terrible reputation. However, chronological age is often blamed for losses that would be more accurately attributed to chronic diseases (for which the elderly do not have a monopoly), to environmental deprivation associated with living arrangements, or to a lack of opportunity to maintain a satisfactory life style. In other words, the reputation of old age, good and bad, should be shared with other predictors of behavior. Moreover, the good news is that many of the factors associated with pathological or secondary aging are potentially preventable or medicable for current and future generations of elderly people if adequate resources and services are available.

Aging is the product of a bio-psycho-social process which is constrained by genetic and by physical-environmental factors. There is now a fairly extensive data base concerning age differences and age changes in functional, psychological, and social status which is beginning to provide a clearer understanding of the adaptational difficulties as well as the coping resources involved in successful aging. As health care providers, we have a professional obligation to prepare to meet the needs of this rapidly growing segment of our population, but concern is not enough. More research on individual differences on which we can more appropriately base that concern and care is extremely important.

The elderly are not a homogeneous group, and people do not become more similar as they become older. The statistically significant age changes observed in the performance of standardized, experimental laboratory measures of cognitive functioning can be compensated for by avoiding learning conditions that penalize performance of older individuals (e.g., paced tasks where speed of response is a premium). A more significant problem is related to the appraisal of cognitive abilities by elderly individuals. To the extent that an older person expects cognitive performance to decline with increasing age, he will be more sensitive to and more accepting of instances of memory failure that are common to individuals of all ages. The studies of the interaction of personality characteristics and adjustment to the aging process further suggest that some individuals typically judge themselves and their life circumstances more harshly than other individuals even when these individuals are equated from the level of objective strain. It was suggested that individual differences in Neuroticism, Extraversion, and Openness to Experience as well as in environmental preferences would contribute to the unexplained variance in the adjustment of hearing-impaired elderly individuals.

One more point should be made, and that is that we are kidding ourselves if we choose to believe that aging is merely a timely and perhaps interesting external problem. We too are aging. Since most of us will one day join this distinguished group of "seasoned citizens," we should be motivated by self-interest (if nothing more) to work for our future selves.

Self-Study Questions

Review Questions: Fill in the blanks.

1. An ecological view of aging considers the _____

2. Mediators of the older person-environment interaction include:

    (a) _____

    (b) _____

    (c) _____

    (d) _____

3. Tests that have not been developed specifically for use with older
    populations may not be appropriate to assess the performance of older
    people. Criteria to evaluate assessment tools for the elderly include:

    (a) _____

    (b) _____

    (c) _____

    (d) _____

4. "Normal" or "primary" aging is _____
    _____.

5. In longitudinal studies of intelligence test performance, visual memory,
    verbal learning, and problem solving task performance age changes are found
    _____.

6. Performance on most psychological tasks is affected by several variables.
    In addition to primary ability factors, secondary factors that may affect
    performance on a wide range of tasks include:

    (a) _____

    (b) _____

    (c) _____

    (d) _____

7. Pacing and speed of response are important instructional variables. Rate
    of presentation of information affects the rate of acquisition new
    information for people of all ages. Older people benefit more than younger
    people when the time to make a response is _____.

8. Older individuals can improve their cognitive performance using a variety of strategies that include:

    (a) _____

    (b) _____

    (c) _____

    (d) _____

9. Conclusions about age-related qualitative differences in performance have been tentative and the studies have been cross-sectional. Field dependence is _____

    _____.

10. Older individuals as a group _____ be characterized as being overly cautious.

11. A personality trait is _____

    _____.

12. Costa and McCraie's NEO model includes three trait dimensions of personality which are:

    (a) _____

    (b) _____

    (c) _____

    (d) _____

13. In what way do personality traits contribute to adjustment to aging?

14. Two approaches to the study of stress and coping include

    (a) _____

    (b) _____

15. Advanced age is associated with a high prevalence of psychopathology. The most frequent functional psychiatric disorder in old age is

16. Dementia is characterized by _____

    _____

17. The most common form of dementing illness is _____

    _____.

REFERENCES

Alpiner, J. G. (1979). Psychological and social aspects of aging as related to hearing rehabilitation of elderly clients. In M. A. Henock (Ed.), Aural rehabilitation for the elderly. New York: Grune & Stratton.

Altman, I., Wohlwill, J., & Lawton, M. P. (Eds.). (1984). Human behavior and environment: The elderly and the physical environment. New York: Plenum.

Arenbert, D. (1965). Anticipation interval and age differences in verbal learning. Journal of Abnormal Psychology, 70, 419-425.

Arenberg, D. (1974). A longitudinal study of problem solving in adults. Journal of Gerontology, 29, 650-658.

Arenberg, D. (1978). Differences and changes with age in the Benton Visual Retention Test. Journal of Gerontology, 33, 534-540.

Arenberg, D. (1982a). Changes with age in problem solving. In F. I. M. Craik & S. Trehub (Eds.), Aging and cognitive processes (pp. 221-235). New York: Plenum Press.

Arenberg, D. (1982b). Estimates of age changes on the Benton Visual Retention Test. Journal of Gerontology, 37, 87-90.

Arenberg, D. (1983). Memory and learning do decline late in life. In J. E. Birren, J. M. A. Munnichs, H. Thomae, & M. Marois (Eds.), Aging: A challenge for science and social policy. (Vol. 3). New York: Oxford University Press.

Arenberg, D., & Robertson-Tchabo, E. A. (1977). Learning and aging. In J. E. Birren & K. W. Schaie (Eds.), Handbook of the psychology of aging (pp. 421-449). New York: Van Nostrand Reinhold.

Atchley, R. C., & Byerts, T. O. (Eds.). (1975). Rural environments and aging. Washington, DC: Gerontological Society.

Baltes, P. B., Reese, H. W., & Nesselroade, J. R. (1977). Life-span developmental psychology: Introduction to research methods. Monterey: Brooks/Cole.

Baltes, P. B., & Willis, S. L. (1982). Plasticity and enhancement of intellectual functioning in old age: Penn State's adult development and enrichment project (ADEPT). In F. I. M. Craik & S. Trehub (Eds.), Aging and cognitive processes (pp. 353-389). New York: Plenum Press.

Bayley N., & Oden, M. H., (1955). The maintenance of intellectual ability in gifted adults. Journal of Gerontology, 10, 91-107.

Beasley, D. S., & Davis, G. A. (1981). Aging: Communication processes and disorders. New York: Grune & Stratton.

Beckman, A. C., & Brody, G. F. (1973). Role loss, powerlessness, and depression among older men and women. The Gerontologist, 13, 100.

Berger, K. S., & Zarit, S. H. (1978). Late life paranoid states. American Journal of Orthopsychiatry, 48, 528.

Berkowitz, A. O., & Hochberg, I. (1971). Self assessment of hearing handicap in the aged. Archives of Otolaryngology, 93, 25-28.

Birren, J. E., & Sloane, R. B. (Eds.). (1980). Handbook of mental health and aging. Englewood Cliffs, NJ: Prentice-Hall.

Blazer, D. G. (1977). Psychopathology of aging. Kansas City, MO: American Family Physician.

Blazer, D., & Williams, C. D. (1980). Epidemiology of dysphoria and depression in an elderly population. American Journal of Psychiatry, 137, 439-444.

Blum, J. E., Fosshage, J. L., & Jarvik, L. F. (1972). Intellectual changes and sex differences in octogenarians: A twenty-year longitudinal study of aging. Developmental Psychology, 7, 178-187.

Blumenthal, M. D. (1975). Measuring depressive symptomatology in a general population. Archives of General Psychiatry, 32, 971-978.

Bradburn, N. M. (1969). The structure of psychological well-being. Chicago: Aldine.

Bremer, J. (1951). A social psychiatric investigation of a small community in northern Norway. Acta Psychiatrica et Neurologica Scandinavica (Supplement No. 62).

Bridge, T. P., & Wyatt, R. J. (1980b). Paraphrenia: Paranoid states of late life. II. American European research. Journal of the American Geriatrics Society, 28, 193-200.

Bridge, T. P., & Wyatt, R. J. (1980). Paraphrenia: Paranoid states of late life. I. European research. Journal of the American Geriatrics Society, 28, 201-205.

Brim, O. G., Jr. (1980). Types of life events. Journal of Social Issues, 36(1), 148-157.

Brim, O. G., Jr., & Ryff, C. D. (1980). On the properties of life events. In P. B. Baltes & O. G. Brim, Jr. (Eds.), Life-span development and behavior. (Vol. 3) (pp. 367-388). New York: Academic Press.

Bromley, D. B. (1978). Approaches to the study of personality changes in adult life and old age. In A. D. Isaacs & F. Post (Eds.), Studies in geriatric psychiatry (pp. 17-40). New York: John Wiley.

Burke, D. M., & Light, L. L. (1981). Memory and aging: The role of retrieval processes. Psychological Bulletin, 90, 513-546.

Busse, E. W. (1969). Theories of aging. In E. W. Busse & E. Pfeiffer (Eds.), Behavior and adaptation in late life (pp. 11-32). Boston: Little, Brown.

Busse, E. W., & Blazer, D. G. (1980). Handbook of geriatric psychiatry. New York: Van Nostrand Reinhold.

Busse, E. W., & Pfeiffer, E. (Eds.). (1973). Mental illness in later life. Washington, DC: American Psychiatric Association.

Butler, R. N. (1975). The facade of chronological age: An interpretative summary. In B. L. Neugarten (Ed.), Middle age and aging (pp. 235-242). Chicago: University of Chicago Press.

Byerts, T. O., Howell, S. C., & Pastalan, L. A. (Eds.). (1979). Environmental context of aging: Lifestyles, environmental quality and living arrangements. New York: Garland STPM Press.

Canestrari, R. E., Jr. (1963). Paced and self-paced learning in young and elderly adults. Journal of Gerontology, 18, 165-168.

Canestrari, R. E., Jr. (1968). Age changes in acquisition. In G. A. Talland (Ed.), Human aging and behavior (pp. 169-188). New York: Academic Press.

Chown, S. M. (1968). Personality and aging. In K. W. Schaie (Ed.), Theory and methods of research on aging. Morgantown: West Virginia University Press.

Cohen, D., & Wilkie, F. (1979). Sex-related differences in cognition among the elderly. In M. A. Wittig & A. C. Petersen (Eds.), Sex-related differences in cognitive functioning. New York: Academic Press.

Cohen, G. (1979). Language comprehension in old age. Cognitive Psychology, 11, 412-429.

Cole, J. O., & Barrett, J. E. (Eds.). (1980). Psychopathology in the aged. New York: Raven Press.

Comalli, P. E., Jr., Wapner, S., & Werner, H. (1959). Perception of verticality in middle and old age. Journal of Psychology, 42, 252-266.

Cooper, A. F., & Curry, A. R. (1976). The pathology of deafness in the paranoid and affective psychoses of later life. Journal of Psychosomatic Research, 20, 97-105.

Cooper, A. F., Kay, D. W. K., Curry, A. R., Garside, R. F., & Roth, M. (1974). Hearing loss in paranoid and affective psychoses of the elderly. Lancet, ii, 851-854.

Corkin, S., Davis, K. L., Growdon, J. H., Usdin, E., & Wurtman, R. J. (Eds.). (1982). Alzheimer's disease : A report of progress in research. New York: Raven Press.

Corso, J. F. (1981). Aging, sensory systems and perception. New York: Praeger.

Costa, P. T., Jr., & McCrae, R. R. (1977). Age differences in personality structure revisited: Studies in validity, stability, and change. Aging and Human Development, 8, 261-275.

Costa, P. T., Jr., & McCrae, R. R. (1978). Objective personality assessment. In M. Storandt, I. C. Siegler, & M. F. Elias (Eds.), The clinical psychology of aging (pp. 119-143). New York: Academic Press.

Costa, P. T., Jr., & McCrae, R. R. (1980a). The influence of extraversion and neuroticism on subjective well-being: Happy and unhappy people. Journal of Personality and Social Psychology, 38, 668-678.

Costa, P. T., Jr., & McCrae, R. R. (1980b). Still stable after all these years: Personality as a key to some issues in adulthood and old age. In P. B. Baltes & O. G. Brim, Jr. (Eds.), Life span development and behavior. Vol. 3. (pp. 65-103). New York: Academic Press.

Costa, P. T., Jr., & McCrae, R. R, & Arenberg, D. (1980). Enduring dispositions in adult males. Journal of Personality and Social Psychology, 38, 793-800.

Cowley, M. (1980). The view from 80. New York: Penguin.

Craik, F. I. M. (1977). Age differences in human memory. In J. E. Birren & K. W. Schaie (Eds.), Handbook of the psychology of aging (pp. 384-420). New York: Van Nostrand Reinhold.

Craik, F. I. M., & Simon, E. (1980). Age differences in memory: The roles of attention and depth of processing. In L. W. Poon, J. L. Fozard, L. S. Cermak, D. Arenberg, & L. W. Thompson (Eds.), New directions in memory and aging (pp. 95-112). Hillsdale, NJ: Lawrence Erlbaum.

Cunningham, W. R., & Birren, J. E. (1976). Age changes in human abilities: A 28-year-old longitudinal study. Developmental Psychology, 12, 81-82.

DeLongis, A., Coyne, J. C., Dakof, G., Folkamn, S., & Lazarus, R. S. (1982). Relationship of daily hassles, uplifts, and major life events to health status. Health Psychology, 1(2), 119-136.

Denney, N. W. (1982). Aging and cognitive changes. In B. B. Wolman (Ed.), Handbook of developmental psychology (pp. 807-827). Englewood Cliffs, NJ: Prentice-Hall.

Douglas, K., & Arenberg, D. (1978). Age changes, cohort differences, and cultural change on the Guilford-Zimmerman Temperament Survey. Journal of Gerontology, 33, 737-747.

Eisdorfer, C., & Wilkie, F. (1973). Intellectual changes with advancing age. In L. F. Jarvik, C. Eisdorfer, & J. E. Blum (Eds.), Intellectual functioning in adults (pp. 21-30). New York: Springer.

Eisner, D. A. (1972). Developmental relationships between field independence and fixity-mobility. Perceptual and Motor Skills, 34, 767-770.

Essen-Moller, E., Larsson, H., Uddenberg, C. E., & White, G. (1956). Individual traits and morbidity in a Swedish rural population. Acta Psychiatrica et Neurologica Scandinavica (Supplement No. 100).

Folkman, S., & Lazarus, R. S. (1980). An analysis of coping in a middle-aged community sample. Journal of Health and Social Behavior, 21, 219-239.

Folstein, M., & McHugh, P. (1978). Dementia syndrome of depression. In R. Katzman, R. D. Terry, & K. L. Bick (Eds.), Alzheimer's disease: Senile dementia and related disorders (pp. 87-93). New York: Raven Press.

Gallagher, D., & Thompson, L. W. (1983). Depression in the elderly: A behavioral treatment manual. Los Angeles: University of Southern California Press.

Glendenning, F. (1982). Acquired hearing loss and elderly people. Stoke-on-Trent: J. H. Brookes.

Goetzinger, C. P. (1967). Factors associated with counseling the hearing impaired adult. Journal of Rehabilitation of the Deaf, 1, 32-48.

Golant, S. M. (Ed.). (1979). Location and environment of elderly population. Washington, DC: V. H. Winston & Sons.

Goldfarb, A. I. (1974). Masked depression in the elderly. In S. Lesse (Ed.), Masked depression. New York: Jason Aronson.

Gurland, B. J., Fleiss, J. L., Goldberg, K., Sharpe, L., Copeland, J. R. M., Kelleher, M. J., & Kellett, J. M. (1976). A semi-structured clinical interview for the assessment of diagnosis and mental state in the elderly: The Geriatric Mental State Schedule. II. A factor analysis. Psychological Medicine, 6, 451-460.

Hachinski, V. (1978). Cerebral blood flow: Differentiation of Alzheimer's disease from multi-infarct dementia. In R. Katzman, R. D. Terry, & K. L. Bick (Eds.), Alzheimer's disease: Senile dementia and related disorders (pp. 97-103). New York: Raven Press.

Hachinski, V. C., Iliff, L. D., Zilhka, E., Duboulay, G. H., McAllister, V. L., Marshall, J., Russell, R. W. R., & Symon, L. (1975). Cerebral blood flow in dementia. Archives of Neurology, 32, 632-637.

Harless, E. L., & McConnell, F. (1982). Effects of hearing aid use on self concept in older persons. Journal of Speech and Hearing Disorders, 47, 305-309.

Hartley, J. T., Harker, J. O., & Walsh, D. A. (1980). Contemporary issues and new directions in adult development of learning and memory. In L. W. Poon (Ed.), Aging in the 1980s: Psychological issues (pp. 239-252). Washington, DC: American Psychological Association.

Henoch, M. A., (Ed.). (1979). Aural rehabilitation for the elderly. New York: Grune & Stratton.

Hertzog, C., Schaie, K. W., & Gribbin, K. (1978). Cardiovascular disease and changes in intellectual functioning from middle to old age. Journal of Gerontology, 33, 872-883.

Hinchcliffe, R. (Ed.). (1983). Hearing and balance in the elderly. London: Churchill Livingstone.

Holmes, T. H,, & Rahe, R. H. (1967). The Social Readjustment Rating Scale. Journal of Psychosomatic Research, 11, 213-218.

Howells, J. G. (Ed.). (1975). Modern perspectives in the psychiatry of old age. New York: Brunner Mazel.

Hulicka, I. M. (1982). Memory functioning in late adulthood. In F. I. M. Craik & S. Trehub (Eds.), Aging and cognitive processes (pp. 331-351). New York: Plenum Press.

Hulicka, I. M., & Grossman, J. L. (1967). Age group comparisons for the use of mediators in paired-associate learning. Journal of Gerontology, 22, 46-51.

Hull, R. H. (Ed.). (1981). The communicatively disordered elderly. (Special issue). Seminars in Speech, Language, and Hearing, 2(3).

Humphrey, C., Gilhome-Herbst, K., & Faurqi, S. (1981). Some characteristics of the hearing-impaired elderly who do not present themselves for rehabilitation. British Journal of Audiology, 15, 25-30.

Issacs, A. D., & Post, F. (Eds.). (1978). Studies in geriatric psychiatry. New York: John Wiley.

Jerome, E. A. (1962). Decay of heuristic processes in the aged. In C. Tibbits & W. Donajue (Eds.), Social and psychological aspects of aging. New York: Columbia University Press.

Kahana, E. (1975). A congruence model of person-environment interaction. In P. G. Windley, T. O. Byerts, & F. G. Ernst, F. G. (Eds.), Theory development in environment and aging. Washington, DC: Gerontological Society.

Kahn, R. L., Zarit, S. H., Hilbert, N. M., & Niederehe, G. (1975). Memory complaint and impairment in the aged. Archives of General Psychiatry, 32, 1569-1573.

Kanner, A. D., Coyne, J. C., Schaefer, C., & Lazarus, R. S. (1981). Comparison of two modes of stress measurement: Daily hassles and uplifts versus major life events. Journal of Behavioral Medicine, 4, 1-39.

Kastenbaum, R. (1971). Getting there ahead of time. Psychology Today, 5, 52-58.

Katzman, R., Terry, R. D., & Bick, K. L. (Eds.). (1978). Alzheimer's disease: Senile dementia and related disorders. New York: Raven Press.

Kausler, D. H. (1982). Experimental psychology and human aging. New York: John Wiley.

Kay, D. W. K., Beamish, P., & Roth, M. (1964). Old age mental disorders in Newcastle-upon-Tyne: I. A study of prevalence. British Journal of Psychiatry, 110, 146-158.

Kay, D. W. K., Cooper, A. F., Garside, R. F., & Roth, M. (1976). The differentiation of paranoid from affective psychoses by patient's premorbid characteristics. British Journal of Psychiatry, 129, 207-215.

Kay, D. W. K., & Roth, M. (1961). Environmental and hereditary factors in the schizophrenias of old age ("late paraphrenia") and their bearing on the general problem of causation of schizophrenia. Journal of Mental Science, 107, 649-686.

Kogan, N. (1973). Creativity and cognitive style: A life-span perspective. In P. B. Baltes & K. W. Schaie (Eds.), Life span developmental psychology: Personality and socialization (pp. 145-178). New York: Academic Press.

Kramer, M., Taube, C. A., & Redick, R. W. (1973). Patterns of use of psychiatric facilities by the aged: Past, present, and future. In C. Eisdorfer & M. P. Lawton (Eds.), The psychology of adult developmental and aging (pp. 428-528). Washington, DC: American Psychological Association.

Kramer, N. A., & Jarvik, L. F. (1979). Assessment of intellectual changes in the elderly. In A. Raskin & L. F. Jarvik (Eds.), Psychiatric symptoms and cognitive loss in the elderly (pp. 221-271). Washington, DC: Hemisphere Publishing.

Labouvie-Vief, G., & Gonda, J. N. (1976). Cognitive strategy training and intellectual performance in the elderly. Journal of Gerontology, 31, 327-332.

Langer, E. J., Rodin, J., Beck, P., Weinman, C., & Spitzer, L. (1979). Environmental determinants of memory improvement in late adulthood. Journal of Personality and Social Psychology, 37, 2003-2013.

Larson, R. (1978). Thirty years of research on the subjective well-being of older Americans. Journal of Gerontology, 33, 109-125.

Laurence, M. W. (1967). A developmental look at the usefulness of list categorization as an aid to free recall. Canadian Journal of Psychology, 221, 153-165.

Lawton, M. P. (1977). The impact of the environment of aging. In J. E. Birren & K. W. Schaie (Eds.), Handbook of the psychology of aging (pp. 276-301). New York: Van Nostrand Reinhold.

Lawton, M. P. (1980). Environment and aging. Monterey: Brooks/Cole.

Lawton, M. P., & Nahemow, L. (1973). Ecology and the aging process. In C. Eisdorfer & M. P. Lawton (Eds.), The psychology of adult development and aging (pp. 619-674). Washington, DC: American Psychological Association.

Lawton, M. P., & Simon, B. (1977). The ecology of social relationships in housing for the elderly. The Gerontologist, 8, 108-115.

Lawton, M. P., Whelihan, W. M., & Belsky, J. K. (1980). Personality tests and their uses with older adults. In J. E. Birren & R. B. Sloane (Eds.), Handbook of mental health an aging (pp. 537-553). Englewood Cliffs, NJ: Prentice-Hall.

Lazarus, R. S., & DeLongis, A. (1983). Psychological stress and coping in aging. American Psychologist, 38, 245-254.

Lee, J. A., & Pollack, R. H. (1978). The effect of age on perceptual problem-solving stategies. Experimental Aging Research, 4, 37-54.

Lieberman, M. A. (1978). Social and psychological determinants of adaptation. Aging and Human Development, 9, 115-126.

Leighton, D. C., Harding, J. S., Macklin, D. B., MacMillan, A. M., Leighton, A. N. (1963). The character of danger: Psychiatric symptoms in selected communities: Stirling County study of psychiatric disorder and sociocultural environment. (Vol. 3). New York: Basic Books.

Leighton, D. C., Harding, J. S., Macklin, D. B., MacMillan, A. M., & Leighton, A. H. (1983). Psychiatric findings of the Stirling county study. American Journal of Psychiatry, 119, 1021-1026.

Levy, R., & Post, F. (1982). The psychiatry of late life. Oxford: Blackwell Scientific Publications.

Liston, E. H., & La Rue, A. (1983a). Clinical differentiation of primary degenerative and multi-infarct dementia: A critical review of the evidence. Part I: Clinical studies. Biological Psychiatry, 18, 1451-1465.

Liston, E. H., & La Rue, A. (1983b). Clinical differentiation of primary degenerative and multi-infarct dementia: A critical review of the evidence. Part II: Pathological studies. Biological Psychiatry, 18, 1467-1484.

Lohmann, N. (1980). Life satisfaction research in aging: Implications for policy development. In N. Datan & N. Lohmann (Eds.), Transitions of aging (pp. 27-40). New York: Academic Press.

Lowenthal, M. F., Berkman, P. L., Beuhler, J. A., Pierce, R. C., Robinson, B. C., & Trier, M. L. (1967). Aging and mental disorder in San Francisco. San Francisco: Jossey-Bass.

Markus, E. J. (1971). Perceptual field dependence among aged persons. Perceptual and Motor Skills, 33, 763-768.

Maurer, J. F., & Rupp, R. R. (1979). Hearing and aging: Tactics for intervention. New York: Grune & Stratton.

McCartney, J. H., Maurer, J. F., & Sorenson, F. D. (1976). A comparison of the hearing handicap scale and the hearing measurement scale with standard audiometric measures on a geriatric population. Journal of Auditory Research, 16, 51-58.

McCarty, D. L. (1980). Investigation of a visual imagery mnemonic device for acquiring face-name associations. Journal of Experimental Psychology: Human Learning and Memory, 6, 145-155.

McCrae, R. R. (1982). Age differences in the use of coping mechanisms. Journal of Gerontology, 37, 454-460.

McCrae, R. R., & Costa, P. T., Jr. (1982). Aging, the life course, and models of personality. In T. Field (Ed.), Review of human development. New York: Wiley.

McCrae, R. R., & Costa, P. T., Jr. (1984). Emerging lives, enduring dispositions: The stability of personality in adulthood. Boston: Little, Brown.

McNair, D. M. (1979). Self-rating scales for assessing psychopathology in the elderly. In A. Raskin & L. Jarvik (Eds.), Psychiatric symptoms and cognitive loss in the elderly (pp. 157-168). Washington, DC: Hemisphere.

Mihal, W. L., & Barrett, G. V. (1976). Individual differences in perceptual information processing and their relation to automobile accident involvements. Journal of Applied Psychology, 61, 229-233.

Miller, E. (1977). Abnormal aging. New York: John Wiley.

Miller, N. E., & Cohen, G. D. (1981). Clinical aspects of Alzheimer's disease and senile dementia. New York: Raven Press.

Milne, J. S. (1976). Hearing loss related to some signs and symptoms in older people. British Journal of Audiology, 10, 65-73.

Monge, R., & Hultsch, D. (1971). Paired-associate learning as a function of adult age and the length of the anticipation and inspection intervals. Journal of Gerontology, 26, 157-162.

Moss, H. A., & Susman, E. J. (1980). Constancy and change in personality development. In O. G. Brim, Jr., & J. Kagan (Eds.), Constancy and change in human development. Cambridge, MA: Harvard University Press.

Nesselroade, J. R., & Baltes, P. B. (1979). Longitudinal research in the study of behavior and development. New York: Academic Press.

Neugarten, B. L. (1963). Personality changes during the adult years. In R. G. Kuhlen (Ed.), Psychological backgrounds of adult education. Chicago: Center for the Study of Liberal Education for Adults.

Neugarten, B. L. (1973). Personality change in late life: A developmental perspective. In C. Eisdorfer & M. P. Lawton (Eds.), The psychology of adults and aging. (pp. 311-335). Washington, DC: American Psychological Association.

Neugarten, B. L. (1977). Personality and aging. In J. E. Birren & K. W. Schaie (Eds.), Handbook of the psychology of aging (pp. 626-649). New York: Van Nostrand Reinhold.

Nisbet, J. D. (1957). Intelligence and age: Retesting with twenty-four years' interval. British Journal of Educational Psychology, 27, 190-198.

Obler L. K., & Albert, M. L. (1980). Language and communication in the elderly: Clinical, therapeutic, and experimental issues. Lexington, MA: Lexington Books.

Okun, M. A., Stock, W. A., & Ceurvorst, R. W. (1980). Risk taking through the adult life span. Experimental Aging Research, 6, 463-474.

Owens, W. A., Jr. (1953). Age and mental abilities: A longitudinal study. Genetic Psychology Monographs, 48, 3-54.

Owens, W. A., Jr. (1966). Age and mental abilities: A second adult follow-up. Journal of Educational Psychology, 51, 311-325.

Panek, P. E., Barrett, G. V., Sterns, G. V., & Alexander, R. A. (1978). Age differences in perceptual style, selective attention, and perceptual-motor reaction time. Experimental Aging Research, 4, 377-387.

Parr, J. (1980). The interaction of persons and living environments. In L. W. Poon (Ed.), Aging in the 1980s: Psychological issues (pp. 393-406). Washington, DC: American Psychological Association.

Pasamanick, B. (1962). A survey of mental disease in an urban population. VI. An approach to total prevalence by age. Mental Hygiene, 46, 567-572.

Pastalan, L. A. (1975). Research in environment and aging: An alternative to theory. In P. G. Windley, T. O. Byerts, & F. G., Ernst (Eds.), Theory development in environment and aging. Washington, DC: Gerontological Society.

Pfeiffer, E. (1977). Psychopathology and social pathology. In J. E. Birren & K. W. Schaie (Eds.), Handbook of the psychology of aging (pp. 650-671). New York: Van Nostrand Reinhold.

Pitt, B. (1982). Psychogeriatrics (2nd ed.). London: Churchill Livingstone.

Poon, L. W., Walsh-Sweeney, L., & Fozard, J. L. (1980). Memory skill training for the elderly: Salient issues on the use of imagery mnemonics. In L. W. Poon, J. L. Fozard, L. S. Cermak, D. Arenberg, & L. W. Thompson (Eds.), New directions in memory and aging (pp. 461-484). Hillsdale, NJ: Lawrence Erlbaum.

Post, F. (1966). *Persistent persecutory states of the elderly.* London: Pergamon.

Rabkin, J. G., & Sheuning, E. L. (1976). Life events, stress, and illness. *Science, 194,* 1013-1020.

Rabbitt, P. M. (1977). Changes in problem solving ability in old age. In J. E. Birren & K. W. Schaie (Eds.), *Handbook of the psychology of aging* (pp. 606-625). New York: Van Nostrand Reinhold.

Rabbitt, P. M. (1982). Development of methods to measure changes in activities of daily living in the elderly. In S. Corkin, K. L. Davis, J. H. Growdon, E. Usdin, & R. J. Wurtman (Eds.), *Alzheimer's disease: A report of progress in research* (pp. 127-131). New York: Raven Press.

Rankin, J. L., & Kausler, D. H. (1979). Adult age differences in false recognitions. *Journal of Gerontology, 34,* 58-65.

Raskin, A. (1979). Signs and symptoms of psychopathology in the elderly. In A. Raskin & L. F. Jarvik (Eds.), *Psychiatric symptoms and cognitive loss in the elderly* (pp. 3-18). Washington, DC: Hemisphere.

Raskin, A., & Jarvik, L. F. (1979). *Psychiatric symptoms and cognitive loss in the elderly: Evaluation and assessment techniques.* Washington, DC: Hemisphere.

Redick, R. W., Kramer, M., & Taube, C. A. (1973). Epidemiology of mental illness and utilization of psychiatric facilities among older persons. In E. W., Bussee & E. Pfeiffer (Eds.), *Mental illness in later life.* Washington, DC: American Psychiatric Association.

Retterstol, N. (1966). *Paranoid and paranoic psychoses.* Springfield, IL: Charles C. Thomas.

Riegel, K. F. (1959). Personality theory and aging. In J. E. Birren (Ed.), *Handbook of aging and the individual* (pp. 187-851). Chicago: University of Chicago Press.

Robertson-Tchabo, E. A., Arenberg, D., & Costa, P. T., Jr. (1979). Temperamental predictors of longitudinal change in performance on the Benton Revised Visual Retention Test among seventy year old men: An exploratory study. In F. Hoffmeister & C. Muller (Eds.), *Brain function in old age* (pp. 151-159). New York: Springer-Verlag.

Robertson-Tchabo, E. A., Hausman, C. P., & Arenberg, D. (1976). A classical mnemonic for older learners. *Educational Gerontology, 1,* 215-226.

Rosen, J. K. (1979). Psychological and social aspects of the evaluation of acquired hearing impairment. *Audiology, 18,* 238-252.

Roth, M. (1955). The natural history of mental disorder in old age. *Journal of Mental Science, 101,* 281-301.

Roth, M. (1980). Senile dementia and its borderlands. In J. O. Cole & J. E. Barrett (Eds.), Psychopathology in the aged (pp. 205-232). New York: Raven Press.

Rousey, C. L. (1971). Psychological reactions to hearing loss. Journal of Speech and Hearing Disorders, 36, 382-389.

Rowles, G. D. (1978). Prisoners of space? Exploring the geographical experience of older people. Boulder, CO: Westview Press.

Rowles, G. D., & Ohta, R. J. (1983). Aging and milieu: Environmental perspectives on growing old. New York: Academic Press.

Salzman, C., & Shader, R. I. (1978). Depression in the elderly: I. relationships between depression, psychologic defense mechanisms, and physical illness. Journal of the American Geriatrics Society, 36, 253-260.

Schaie, K. W. (1977). Quasi-experimental research designs in the psychology of aging. In J. E. Birren & K. W. Schaie (Eds.), Handbook of the psychology of aging (pp. 39-58). New York: Van Nostrand Reinhold.

Schaie, K. W. (1978). External validity in the assessment of intellectual development in adulthood. Journal of Gerontology, 33, 695-701.

Schaie, K. W., Labouvie-Vief, G. (1974). Generational versus ontogenetic components of change in adult cognitive behavior: A fourteen-year cross-sequential study. Developmental Psychology, 10, 305-320.

Schaie, K. W., Labouvie-G. V., & Buech, B. U. (1973). Generational and cohort-specific differences in adult cognitive functioning: A fourteen-year study of independent samples. Developmental Psychology, 9, 151-166.

Schaie, K. W., & Strother, C. R. (1968a). A cross-sequential study of age changes in cognitive behavior. Psychological Bulletin, 70, 671-680.

Schaie, K. W., & Strother, C. R. (1968b). The effects of time and cohort differences on the interpretation of age changes in cognitive behavior. Multivariate Behavioral Research, 3, 259-294.

Schlossberg, N. K. (1984). Counseling adults in transition: Linking practice with theory. New York: Springer.

Schonfield, D. (1980). Learning, memory, and aging. In J. E. Birren & R. B. Sloane (Eds.), Handbook of mental health and aging (pp. 214-244). Englewood Cliffs, NJ: Prentice-Hall.

Schow, R. L., Christensen, J. M., Hutchinson, J. M., & Nerbonne, M. A. (1978). Communication disorders of the aged: A guide for health professionals. Baltimore: University Park Press.

Schwartz, D. W., & Karp, S. A. (1967). Field dependence in a geriatric population. Perceptual and Motor Skills, 24, 495-504.

Siegler, I. C., George, L. K., & Okun, M. A. (1979). Cross-sequential analysis of personality. Developmental Psychology, 15, 350-351.

Smith, A. D. (1980). Age differences in encoding, storage, and retrieval. In L. W. Poon, J. L. Fozard, L. S. Cermak, D. Arenberg, & L. W. Thompson (Eds.), New directions in memory and aging (pp. 23-45). Hillsdale, NJ: Lawrence Erlbaum.

Storandt, M., Siegler, I. C., & Elias, M. F. (Eds.). (1978). The clinical psychology of aging. New York: Plenum.

Stotsky, B. (1975). Psychoactive drugs for geriatric patients with psychiatric disorders. In S. Gershon & A Raskin (Eds.), Genesis and treatment of psychologic disorders in the elderly (pp. 229-258). New York: Raven Press.

Terry, R. D., & Wisniewski, H. (1977). The ultrastructure of the neuro-fibrillary tangle and the senile plaque. In G. E. W. Wolstenholme & M. O'Connor (Eds.), Ciba Foundation Symposium on Alzheimer's Disease and Related Conditions (pp. 145-168). London: Churchill.

Thomae, H. (1980). Personality and adjustment to aging. In J. E. Birren & R. B. Sloane (Eds.), Handbook of mental health and aging (pp. 285-309). Englewood Cliffs, NJ: Prentice-Hall.

Tomlinson, B. E., Blessed, G., & Roth, M. (1970). Observations of the brains of demented old people. Journal of Neurological Science, 11, 205-242.

Tuddenham, R. D., Blumnekrantz, J., & Wilkin, W. R. (1968). Age changes on AGCT: A longitudinal study of average adults. Journal of Consulting and Clinical Psychology, 32, 659-663.

Turner, B. F. (1982). Sex-related differences in aging. In B. B. Wolman (Ed.), Handbook of developmental psychology (pp. 912-936). Englewood Cliffs, NJ: Prentice-Hall.

Ventry, I. M., & Weinstein, B. E. (1982). The Hearing Handicap Inventory for the Elderly: A new tool. Ear and Hearing, 3, 128-134.

Verwoerdt, A. (1976). Clinical geropsychiatry. Baltimore: Williams & Wilkins.

Wallach, M. A., & Kogan, N. (1961). Aspects of judgement and decision making: Interrelationships and changes with age. Behavioral Sciences, 6, 23-26.

Weinstein, B. E., & Ventry, I. M. (1982). Hearing impairment and social isolation in the elderly. Journal of Speech and Hearing Research, 25, 593-599.

Weinstein, B. E., & Ventry, I. M. (1983a). Audiologic correlates of the Hearing Handicap Inventory for the Elderly. _Journal of Speech and Hearing Disorders, 26_, 148-151.

Weinstein, B. E., & Ventry, I. M. (1983b). Audiometric correlates of the Hearing Handicap Inventory for the Elderly. _Journal of Speech and Hearing Disorders, 48_, 379-384.

Welford, A. T. (1977). Motor performance. In J. E. Birren & K. W. Schaie (Eds.), _Handbook of the psychology of aging_ (pp. 450-496). New York: Van Nostrand Reinhold.

Wells, C. E. (1980). The differential diagnosis of psychiatric disorders in the elderly. In J. O. Cole & J. E. Barrett (Eds.), _Psychopathology in the aged_ (pp. 19-31). New York: Raven Press.

Wilder, C. N., & Weinstein, B. E. (1984). _Aging and communication: Problems in management._ New York: Haworth.

Windley, P. G., Byerts, T. O., & Ernst, F. G. (Eds.). (1975). _Theory development in environment and aging._ Washington, DC: Gerontological Society.

Witkin, H. A., Dyk, R. B., Faterson, H. F., Goodenough, D. R., & Karom S. A. (1962). _Psychological differentiation._ New York: Wiley.

Yesavage, J. A., Rose, T. L., & Bower, G. H. (1983). Interactive imagery and affective judgements improve face-name learning in the elderly. _Journal of Gerontology, 38_, 197-203.

Young, M. L. (1966). Problem-solving performance in two age groups. _Journal of Gerontology, 21_, 505-509.

Zarit, S. H. (1980). _Aging and mental disorders: Psychological approaches to assessment and treatment._ New York: The Free Press.

Zarit, S. H., Cole, K. D., & Guider, R. L. (1981). Memory training stategies and subjective complaints of memory in the aged. _The Gerontologist, 21_, 158-164.

Zelinski, E. M., Gilewski, M. J., & Thompson, L. W. (1980). Do laboratory memory tests relate to self-assessment of memory ability in the young and old? In L. W. Poon, J. L. Fozard, L. S. Cermak, D. Arenberg, & L. W. Thompson (Eds.), _New directions in memory and aging_ (pp. 519-544). Hillsdale, NJ: Lawrence Erlbaum.

Zung, W. W. K. (1965). A self-rating depression scale. _Archives of General Psychiatry, 12_, 63-70.

Suggested Readings

Albert, M. S. (1981). Geriatric neuropsychology. Journal of Consulting and Clinical Psychology, 49, 835-850.

Atchley, R. C. (1980). The social forces in later life: An introduction to social gerontology (3rd ed.). Belmont: Wadsworth.

Ban, T. A. (1980). Psychopharmacology for the aged. New York: Karger.

Belmore, S. M. (1981). Age-related changes in processing explicit and implicit language. Journal of Gerontology, 36, 316-322.

Bergman, M. (1980). Aging and the perception of speech. Baltimore: University University Park Press.

Botwinick, J. (1967). Cognitive processes in maturity and old age. New York: Springer.

Botwinick, J. (1977). Intellectual abilities. In J. E. Birren & K. W. Schaie (Eds.), Handbook of the psychology of aging (pp. 580-605). New York: Van Nostrand Reinhold.

Botwinick, J. (1987). Aging and behavior (2nd ed.). New York: Springer.

Botwinick, J., & Storandt, M. (1974). Memory, related functions, and age. Springfield, IL: Charles C. Thomas.

Burish, T. G., & Bradley, L. A. (1983). Coping with chronic disease: Research and applications. New York: Academic Press.

Costa, P. T., Jr., & McCrae, R. R. (1976). Age differences in personality structure: A cluster analytic approach. Journal of Gerontology, 31, 564-570.

Crook, R. Ferris, S., & Bartus, R. (Eds.). (1983). Assessment in geriatric psychopharmacology. New Canaan, CT: Mark Powley Associates.

Dixon, R. A., & Hultsch, D. F. (1983). Structure and development of metamemory in adulthood. Journal of Gerontology, 38, 682-688.

Eisdorfer, C., & Friedel, R. O. (Eds.). (1977). Cognitive and emotional disturbance in the elderly. Chicago: Year Book Medical Publishers.

Elias, M. F., & Streeten, D. H. P. (Eds.). (1980). Hypertension and cognitive processes. Mount Desert, ME: Beech Hill.

Foner, A., & Schwab, K. (1981). Aging and retirement. Monterey: Brooks/Cole.

Gardner, E. F., & Monge, R. H. (1977). Adult age differences in cognitive abilities and educational background. Experimental Aging Research, 3, 337-383.

George, L. K., (1980). Role transitions in later life. Monterey: Brooks/Cole.

George, L. K., & Bearon, L. B. (1980). Quality of life in older persons: Meaning and measurement. New York: Human Sciences Press.

Gershon, S., & Raskin, A. (Eds.). (1975). Genesis and treatment of psychologic disorders in the elderly. New York: Raven Press.

Granick, S., Kleban, M. H., & Weiss, A. D. (1976). Relationships between hearing loss and cognition in normally hearing aged persons. Journal of Gerontology, 31, 434-440.

Gribbin, K., Schaie, K. W., & Parham, I. A. (1980). Complexity of life style and maintenance of intellectual abilities. Journal of Social Issues, 36(2), 47-61.

Gurland, B. J., & Wilder, D. E. (1984). The CARE Interview revisited: Development of an efficient, systematic clinical assessment. Journal of Gerontology, 39, 129-137.

Gurland, B., Golde, R. R., Terest, J. A., & Challop, J. (1984). The SHORT-CARE: An efficient instrument for the assessment of depression, dementia, and disability. Journal of Gerontology, 39, 166-169.

Herrmann, D. J. (1982). Know thy memory: The use of questionnaires to assess and study memory. Psychological Bulletin, 92, 434-452.

Hultsch, D. F., & Plemons, J. K. (1979). Life events and life-span development. In P. B. Baltes & O. G. Brim, Jr. (Eds.), Life-span development and behavior. Vol. 2 (pp. 1-36). New York: Academic Press.

Kahn, R. L., & Miller, N. E. (1978) Adaptational factors in memory function in the aged. Experimental Aging Research, 4, 273-289.

Kihlstrom, J. F. (1981). On personality and memory. In N. Cantor & J. F. Kihlstrom (Eds.), Personality, cognition, and social interaction (pp. 123-149). Hillsdale, NJ: Lawrence Erlbaum.

Labouvie-Vief, G. (1980). Adaptive dimensions of adult cognition. In N. Datan & N. Lohmann (Eds.), Transitions of aging (pp. 3-26). New York: Academic Press.

Lazarus, R. S., & Launier, R. (1978). Stress-related transactions between person and environment. In L. A. Pervin & M. Lewis (Eds.), Perspectives in interactional psychology (pp. 287-327). New York: Plenum Press.

Maehr, M. L., & Kleiber, D. A. (1981). The graying of achievement motivation American Psycologist, 36, 787-799.

Malatesta, C. Z., Izard, C. E. (Eds.). (1984). Emotion in adult development. Beverly Hills: Sage.

Monge, R. H. (1975). Structure of the self-concept from adolescence through old age. Experimental Aging Research, 1, 281-291.

Mussen, P., Honzik, M. P., & Eichorn, D. H. (1982). Early adult antecedents of life satisfaction at age 70. Journal of Gerontology, 37, 316-322.

Neisser, U. (1978). Memory: What are the important questions? In M. M. Gruneberg, P. E. Morris, & R. N. Sykes (Eds.), Practical aspects of memory (pp. 3-24). New York: Academic Press.

Nesselroade, J. R., & Reese, H. W. (1973). Life-span developmental psychology: Methodological issues. New York: Academic Press.

Pearlin, L. I., & Schooler, C. (1978). The structure of coping. The Journal of Health and Social Behavior, 19, 2-21.

Perlmutter, L. C., & Monty, R. A. (1979). Choice and perceived control. Hillsdale, NJ: Lawrence Erlbaum.

Pervin, L. A., & Lewis, M. Perspectives in interactional psychology. New York: Plenum Press.

Popkin, S. J., Gallagher, D., Thompson, L. W., & Moore, M. (1982), Memory complaint and performance in normal and depressed older adults. Experimental Aging Research, 8, 141-145.

Reisberg, B. (1981). Brain failure: An introduction to current concepts of senility. New York: Free Press.

Ryff, C. D., & Heincke, S. G. (1983). Subjective organization of personality in adulthood and aging. Journal of Personality and Social Psychology, 44, 807-816.

Salthouse, R. A. (1982). Adult cognition: An experimental psychology of human aging. New York: Springer-Verlag.

Salthouse, T. A., & Somberg, B. L. (1982a). Isolating the age deficit in speeded performance. Journal of Gerontology, 37, 59-63.

Salthouse, T. A., & Somberg, B. L. (1982b). Skilled performance: Effects of adult age and experience on elementary processes. Journal of Experimental Psychology: General, 111, 176-207.

Saltzman, C. (1982). A primer on geriatric psychopharmacology. American Journal of Psychiatry, 139, 67-74.

Schaie, K. W. (Ed.) (1983). Longitudinal studies of adult psychological development. New York: Guilford Press.

Schmitt, J. F., & McCroskey, R. L. (1981). Sentence comprehension in elderly listeners: The factor of rate. Journal of Gerontology, 36, 441-445.

Schultz, R. (1976). Effects of control and predictability on the physical and psychological well being of the institutionalized aged. Journal of Personality and Social Psychology, 33, 563-573.

Schultz, R., & Hanusa, B. H. (1980). Experimental social gerontology: A social psychological perspective. Journal of Social Issues, 36(2), 30-46.

Sinnott, J. H., Harris, C. S., Block, M. R., Collesano, S., & Jacobson, S. (1983). Applied research in aging: A guide to methods and resources. Boston: Little, Brown.

Spirduso, W. W. (1980). Physical fitness, aging, and psychomotor speed: A review. Journal of Gerontology, 35, 850-865.

Storandt, M. (1983). Counseling and therapy with older adults. Boston: Little, Brown.

Tausig, M. (1982). Measuring life events. Journal of Health and Social Behavior, 23, 52-64.

Thomae, H. (Ed.). (1975). Patterns of aging: Findings from the Bonn longitudinal study of aging. Basel: Karger.

Thomas, P. D., Hunt, W. C., Garry, P. J., Hood, R. B., Goodwin, J. M., & Goodwin, J. S. (1983). Hearing acuity in a healthy elderly population: Effects on emotional, cognitive, and social status. Journal of Gerontology, 38, 321-325.

Vaillant, G. E. (1977). Adaptation to life. Boston: Little, Brown.

Yordi, C. L., Chu, A. S. Ross, K. M., & Wong, S. J. (1982). Research and the frail elderly: Ethical and methodological issues in controlled social experiments. Gerontologist, 22, 72-77.

Additional Sources

Aker, J. B., Walsh, A. C., & Beam, J. R. (1977). Mental capacity: Medical and legal aspects of the aging. Colorado Springs: Shepard's Inc.

Barton, E. M., Baltes, M. M., & Orzech, M. J. (1980). Etiology of dependence in older nursing home residents during morning care: The role of staff behavior. Journal of Personality and Social Psychology, 38, 423-431.

Bennett, E. S., & Eklund, S. J. (1983). Vision changes, intelligence, and aging: Part I. Educational Gerontology, 9, 255-278.

Botwinick, J. (1981). We are aging. New York: Springer.

Brinkman, S. D., Smith, R. C., Meyer, J. S., Vroulis, G., Shaw, T., Gordon, J. R., & Allen, R. H. (1982). Lecithin and memory training in suspected Alzheimer's disease. Journal of Gerontology, 37, 4-9.

Burnside, I. M. (Ed.). (1978). Working with the elderly: Group processes and techniques. North Scituate, MA: Duxbury Press.

Busse, E. W., & Pfeiffer, E. (Eds.). (1969). Behavior and adaptation in late life. Boston: Little, Brown.

Caplan, R. D. (1983). Person-environment fit: Past, present, and future. In C. L. Cooper (Ed.), Stress research (pp. 35-78). New York: Wiley.

Coelho, G. V., Hamburg, D. A., & Adams, J. E. (Eds.) (1974). Coping and adaptation. New York: Basic Books.

Costa, P. T., Jr., & McCrae, R. R. (1976). Age differences in personality structure: A cluster analytic approach. Journal of Gerontology, 31, 564-570.

Cox, H. (1984). Later life: The realities of aging. Englewood Cliffs: Prentice-Hall.

Freeman, J. F. (1979). Aging: Its history and literature. New York: Human Sciences Press

Fry, C. L., & Keith, J. (1980). New methods for old age research: Anthropological alternatives. Chicago: Loyola University, Center for Urban Policy.

Garfunkel, F., & Landau, G. (1981). A memory retention course for the aged. Washington, DC: National Council on the Aging.

Gilhome-Herbst, K. R. (1980). The social consequences of acquired hearing loss. Hearing, 35(2), 54-57.

Gilhome-Herbst, K. (1983). Psycho-social consequences of disorders of hearing in the elderly. In R. Hinchcliffe (Ed.), Hearing and balance in the elderly (pp. 174-200). London: Churchill Livingstone.

Gilhome-Herbst, K. R., & Humphrey, C. M. (1980). Hearing impairment and mental state in the elderly living at home. British Medical Journal, 281, 903-905.

Golden, R. R., Teresi, J. A., & Garland, B. J. (1984). Development of indicator scales for the Comprehensive Assessment and Referral Evaluation (CARE) Interview Schedule. Journal of Gerontology, 39, 138-146.

Hultsch, D. F., & Deutsch, F. (1981). Adult development and aging: A life-span perspective. New York: McGraw-Hill.

Iler, K. L., Danhauer, J. L., & Mulac, A. (1982). Peer perceptions of geriatrics wearing hearing aids. Journal of Speech and Hearing Disorders, 47, 433-438.

Kastenbaum, R. (Ed.). (1981). Old age on the new scene. New York: Springer.

Kohut, S., Jr., Kohut, J. J., & Fleishman, J. J. (Eds.). (1983). Reality orientation for the elderly (2nd ed.). Oradell, NJ: Medical Economics Books.

Lopata, H. Z. (1973). Widowhood in an American city. Cambridge, MA: Schenkman.

McReynolds, L. V., & Kearns, K. P. (1983). Single-subject experimental designs in communicative disorders. Baltimore: University Park Press.

Neugarten, B. L. (Ed.). (1964). Personality in middle and late life. New York: Atherton Press.

Kohut, S., Jr., Kohut, J. J., & Fleishman, J. J. (Eds.). (1983). Reality orientation for the elderly (2nd ed.). Oradell, NJ: Medical Economics Books.

Lopata, H. Z. (1973). Widowhood in an American city. Cambridge, MA: Schenkman.

McReynolds, L. V., & Kearns, K. P. (1983). Single-subject experimental designs in communicative disorders. Baltimore: University Park Press.

Neugarten, B. L. (Ed.). (1964). Personality in middle and late life. New York: Atherton Press.

O'Neil, P. M., & Calhoun, K. S. (1975). Sensory deficits and behavioral deterioration in senescence. Journal of Abnormal Psychology, 84, 579-582.

Osgood, N. J. (1982). Life after work: Retirement, leisure, recreation, and the elderly. New York: Praeger.

Perlmutter, L. C., & Langer, E. J., (1982). The effects of behavioral monitoring on the perception of control. Clinical Gerontologist, 1, 37-43.

Puff, C. R. (Ed.). (1982). Handbook of research methods in human memory and cognition. New York: Academic Press.

Savage, R. D., Britton, P. G., Bolton, N., & Hall, E. H. (1973). Intellectual functioning in the aged. London: Methuen.

Schaie, K. W., & Marquette, B., (1972). Personality in maturity and old age. In R. M. Dreger (Ed.), Multivariate personality research: Contributions to the understanding of personality in honor of Raymond B. Cattell (pp. 612-632). Baton Rouge: Claitor's.

129

Siegler, I. (1975). Terminal drop hypothesis: Fact or artifact. Experimental Aging Research, 1, 169-185.

Sprott, R. C. (1980). Age, learning ability, and intelligence. New York: Van Nostrand Reinhold.

Suls, J., & Mullen, B. (1982). From the cradle to the grave: Comparison and self-evaluation across the life-span. In J. Suls (Ed.), Psychological perspectives on the self (pp. 97-125). Hillsdale, NJ: Erlbaum.

Sunderland, A., Harris, J. E., & Baddeley, A. D. (1983). Do laboratory tests predict everyday memory? A neuropsychological study. Journal of Verbal Learning and Verbal Behavior, 22, 341-357.

Tamir, L. M. (1979). Communication and the aging process: Interaction throughout the life cycle. New York: Pergamon.

Thomas, A. J., & Gilhome-Herbst, K. R. (1980). Social and psychological implications of acquired hearing loss for adults of employment age. British Journal of Audiology, 14, 76-85.

Thompson, S. C. (1981). Will it hurt less if I can control it? A complex answer to a simple question. Psychological Bulletin, 90, 89-101.

Vitaliano, P. P., Breen, A. R., Albert, M. S., Russo, J., & Prinz, P. N. (1984). Memory, attention, and functional status in community residing Alzheimer type dementia patients and optimally healthy aged individuals. Journal of Gerontology, 39, 58-64.

Weinstein, B. E., & Ventry, I. M. (1982). Hearing impairment and social isolation in the elderly. Journal of Speech and Hearing Research, 25, 593-599.

Wolanin, M. O., & Phillips, L. R. F. (1981). Confusion: Prevention and care. St. Louis: C. V. Mosby.

Woodruff, D. S. (1983). The role of memory in personality continuity: A 25 year follow-up. Experimental Aging Research, 9, 31-34.

Social Aspects of Aging and Health in Late Life

Tom Hickey
University of Michigan

and

Patrice Cruise
Andrews University, Missouri

A growing interest in aging and in the social context of old age and older persons has emerged in American society over the past several years. The processes of aging are being studied more intensely now than ever before. Researchers are employing a variety of theoretical frameworks and methodologies in attempting to explain these often elusive phenomena. The number of articles on aging in professional journals has risen dramatically in the recent past. In fact, most of what we know about aging and older persons has been reported or written in the last 20 years. The media has also picked up the aging theme, as evidenced by numerous articles in newspapers and magazines. An increasing number of television commercials and programs, and even box-office movies, are featuring older people, highlighting various aspects of aging and exploring problems and concerns faced in retirement and in late life.

Several factors appear to be related to this increasing interest in aging. Perhaps most obviously, people are living longer. Life expectancy at birth has increased from 49 years in 1900 to almost 74 years in 1981; the older person who reaches age 65 or 70 today more likely than not will live well into his or her 80s. The number of elderly 65 years of age and older has risen from 3 million in 1900 to 27 million in 1982 (U.S. Bureau of the Census, 1983). Surging advances in science, technology, and medicine have given seemingly unlimited possibilities, not only to prolong life but to improve its quality as well. In an era of huge national deficits and a shrinking economy, this steady increase in numbers of elderly is forcing our society to scrutinize age entitlement programs, such as Social Security and Medicare, in an effort to develop creative ways of allocating scarce resources.

In our traditionally "youth-oriented" society, with its emphasis on productivity and the "body-beautiful," we have generally tended to view the elderly as frail and in need of help in carrying out their activities of daily living. Retirement has often been characterized as a period of inactivity and rolelessness, despite the fact that most people remain relatively vigorous and healthy throughout the 7th decade of their lives. Moreover, for many of these people retirement at age 65 provides an opportunity to pursue fulltime activities which require much physical energy and intellectual skill (Hendricks & Hendricks, 1981; Hickey, 1980).

Recently, in an attempt to counter negative views of old age and justify cost-containment of social programs, the pendulum has begun to swing the other way. Consequently, the elderly are now often characterized as generally healthy and well-off. In actuality, the elderly are a diverse and heterogeneous group. Although many are fairly healthy, they remain at increasing risk of chronic diseases and the need for long-term care (Hickey, 1980).

In order to understand the services needed by the elderly in today's society, and the role of professionals in working with the elderly, it is important to consider the demographics of the elderly population.

Aging of the Population

The proportion of older to younger members in the U.S. has more than doubled since the turn of the century. In 1900, there were about 7 persons 65 years of age and older for every 100 person aged 18-64. By 1982, there were about 19 per 100; it is projected that by 2050 this ratio will double again (Allan & Brotman, 1981; U.S. Bureau of the Census, 1983).

The "very old," those 75 years of age and older, warrant special attention. Though less than 5% of the total population in 1982, by 2030, when the present college-age cohort reach 65, they may well constitute 10% of the population. The percentage of those 85 years of age and older is projected to jump from 1% in 1982 to more than 5% in 2050 (U.S. Bureau of the Census, 1983).

The implications of an aging population for care and services, as well as overall impact on resource utilization, is most evident when looking at population numbers. There are approximately 2.2 million people over age 85 in the United States today, a number likely to rise to 15 million people within 50 years (U.S. Bureau of the Census, 1983). The over 85 group are most at-risk, and likely to be frail and dependent upon others for care, assistance, and services. One out of every three in this age group reside in an institution (Hickey, 1980).

Therefore, young people beginning their adult lives and careers today can expect to have a lot of company in their old age, if not a great deal of competition for scarce resources. If anything, such demographic projections are conservative. The sharp rate of decline in mortality since 1970 suggests that most demographic projections have underestimated the "geriatric population boom" of the future. For example, for some time now demographers have been saying that half of the elderly population will be over 75 by the year 2000. However, the median age of the over 65 population has now reached age 72, and is climbing rapidly. Thus, with nearly 15 million people over age 75 in the United States today, there is legitimate concern for their personal needs and health dependencies.

The proportion of the population which is elderly varies by race and sex. In 1982, 8.5% of the population age 65 years and older was Black. Females 55 years of age and older comprised approximately 12% of the total U.S. population, while males 55 years of age and older accounted for almost 9% (see Figure 1). An example of the effects of migration on population age can be seen when examining the age distributions of different ethnic groups in the U.S. population. The median age of the Hispanic population is about 22 years, compared to 24 for Blacks and nearly 30 years for the White population. Yet,

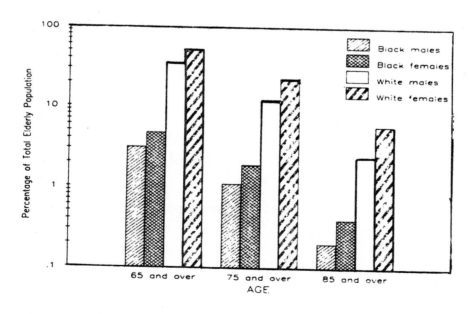

Figure 1. Population 65 years and over, by race and sex: 1982*

133

as a result of migration patterns, Cubans living in the U.S. are generally much older than other Hispanics.

Life expectancy at birth has increased, but differs according to race and gender, with much of the difference being attributed to socioeconomic status (see Figure 2). The average life expectancy at birth for Blacks was 16 years less than that for the White population in 1900; by 1978, the difference had narrowed to 5 years. Life expectancy is lower for males than for females, resulting in an increased incidence of health, social, and economic problems in the elderly female population.

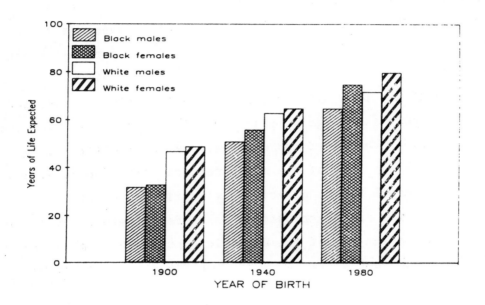

Figure 2. Expectation of life at birth, by race and sex: 1900 to 1980*

The average American woman experiences 11 years of widowhood and is more than twice as likely to be in a nursing home than a man (Brotman, 1980). Moreover, for the single, elderly woman, institutional care is extended over a longer period of time, if not for the remainder of her life. Men, on the other hand, are more likely to return from the nursing home to the care of a spouse. Only 12% of the present nursing home population are married, whereas 69% are widows (Hickey, 1980).

Economics of Aging in American Society

Income levels and financial status of the elderly population vary widely. Indeed, some elderly persons are among the richest in the country. However, a disproportionate number are among the poorest. For many elderly, retirement is accompanied by a reduced, fixed income, which results in less purchasing power as inflation increases. This, in turn, impacts on almost every area of life, including health status. Although a higher income does not necessarily cause an older person to experience good health, higher income and better health are definitely correlated. Forty percent of those with annual incomes over $25,000 report excellent health as compared with others of their own age. However, less than 25% of those with incomes below poverty level report excellent health (Schulz, 1980; U.S. Bureau of the Census, 1983).

There is a strong relationship between advancing age and declining income. The income of 1 out of every 7 elderly persons falls below poverty level, while the ratio is 1 to 10 for the younger population (U.S. Bureau of the Census, 1983). It should be noted, however, that income is not a precise measure of economic well-being. Simple comparisons between the older and younger population are incomplete and do not account for the fact that some elderly have considerable assets. Also, older people in the future are likely to be better-off financially than their parents were. Similarly, noncash benefits, such as in-kind public transfers of food, housing, and medical care are not included when ascertaining income levels. Statistical documentation of this phenomenon, however, seems to be generally inadequate or lacking (Schulz, 1980).

Generally, income tends to increase until about age 55; as people begin to retire, there is a steady decline in income (Beattie, 1983; Weeks, 1984). In 1980, 9.7% of those in the 65-69 age group were still employed fulltime, while only 2.5% of those 70 years and older were. This difference in employment status accounts significantly of the declining income associated with advancing age. However, older persons who do continue to work fulltime tend to have incomes similar to those of younger persons of the same sex and race. Such individuals represent only a small percentage of the elderly, and tend to be self-employed, such as physicians, lawyers, and other professionals (Weeks, 1984). What becomes apparent is that income differences which existed between a cohort of people when they were younger continue to persist into old age (Schulz, 1980).

Sex and Race

Women tend to be more economically disadvantaged throughout most of life than men, and this is particularly true in old age. Women typically have shorter work histories than men, and they tend to earn less. In a system which bases Social Security and other pension benefits on the length of time worked and on earned wages, women have been at a clear disadvantage, resulting in far less income in old age than men (Beattie, 1983; Schulz, 1980).

Until recently, many private pension systems had no form of survivor benefit; that is, the unemployed housewife of a wage-earner would not be eligible to receive his pension after his death. The Social Security system, however, does provide some benefits for nonworking spouses. In the event of death, the survivor is entitled to the working spouse's full benefits (Beattie, 1983; Schulz, 1980).

Even so, in 1981, women aged 65 and older had a median income of $4,800 compared to an income of $8,200 for their male age-peers, which means that the median income of older women was only 58% of the income of older men (U.S. Bureau of the Census, 1983). The gap almost parallels the difference that persists between men and women in younger age groups, again emphasizing that the financial inequities in their younger years are not diminished in old age (Schulz, 1980).

Just as sex differences in income persist throughout the life span, so do race differences. Based on ethnic origin, Native Americans and Blacks are the most economically disadvantaged groups with respect to retirement income. Minority women, in turn, are the poorest elderly. Thus, although the proportion of elderly poor has been decreasing over time, the proportion of elderly female-headed families below poverty level, particularly among the Black population, has been increasing (Gelfand, 1982; Jackson, 1980).

In the White population, poverty distribution across age groups is not evenly distributed (Figure 3). The elderly account for the largest proportion below poverty level. However poverty is more evenly dispersed across age groups in the Black population, suggesting that many elderly Blacks living below poverty level may have lived in poverty most of their lives (Gelfand, 1932; Jackson, 1980).

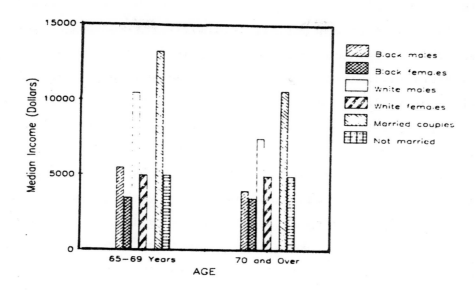

Figure 3. Median annual incomes of persons 65 years and over, by age, race, marital status and sex*

Other Factors

Some other factors which affect income of the elderly include household size, geographic location, background characteristics, and health status (Weeks, 1984). Although older families are usually smaller, they tend to have less income per person than do middle-aged families, but only slightly less than younger families. However, many elderly are widowed and live alone; thus, their incomes are typically less than those of married couples in any age group (U.S. Bureau of the Census, 1983).

There are wide ranges in the cost-of-living expenses in different geographic locales (e.g., it costs almost $2,000 more annually to live in Boston than in Baton Rouge). Generally, the sunbelt region is less expensive than the northern areas. Despite the age migration to places like Florida and Arizona, a majority of the elderly do not migrate, choosing to remain close to family and friends, regardless of economic advantages elsewhere (U.S. Bureau of the Census, 1983). Regional variation in the distribution and cost of services can impact on the "purchasing power" which older people have with their incomes. Although there are only inadequate data to describe service distribution inequities, service access is generally reduced in rural areas, where there is likely to be a proportionately higher older population. However, the presence of a stronger informal support system in such areas may offset gaps in services.

Background characteristics, such as socioeconomic status and educational level, can play a significant part in determining an adequate income after retirement. Higher socioeconomic status and educational level tend to result in higher retirement income. In addition, those with higher educational levels tend to work longer; thus their income is usually higher than for their nonworking counterparts. Furthermore, many elderly who have been marginally poor before retirement (i.e., with cash incomes 125% below the poverty level) tend to fall below poverty level after retirement because of fewer employment opportunities and fixed incomes. In addition to working longer, those with higher educational levels tend to be able to "work the system" better; that is, they may be able to put their knowledge to practical use and negotiate the system through tax breaks, investments, and similar opportunities (Beattie, 1983; Schulz, 1980).

Health status also plays a significant role in determining income level in late life. Long-term care for chronic illness and impairment can be very costly. The phenomenon of "spend-down" (or using up the majority of one's personal resources in order to qualify for governmental subsidy and reimbursement) places an additional burden on the chronically-ill populations and their families. This needs-test criterion tends to promote an institutional bias for long-term care of the elderly, rather than allowing for choices or real alternatives in their care (Butler, 1978; Mueller & Gibson, 1976).

Income Sources

Sources of income among the elderly are more diverse than for any other age group. Pension benefits, including Social Security, are the single largest source of income for the elderly, with savings and investments as their second resource. Salary and wages continue to be a source of income for some elderly persons, particularly for those in the 65-69 age range, and for those with higher educational levels. Only 10% of the elderly receive income from public assistance (Brotman, 1980; Hendricks, & Hendricks, 1981; Schulz, 1980; Weeks, 1984).

Pension Income

Social Security payments are the single most important income resource of the elderly and are nontaxable. However, Social Security was never intended to be the sole source of support for retirement; yet, between 20% and 30% of the elderly rely on Social Security for 90% or more of their income (Brotman, 1980). Social Security is subject to the earnings limitation test, which means that a person can earn only a certain amount and still receive full Social Security benefits. After age 70, however, the earnings limitation test is dropped and a person can earn any amount and still receive full benefits. Yet, by this age, many people are unable to work or find employment (Schulz, 1980; Weeks, 1984).

Social Security benefits depend on the length of time worked and wages earned. Benefits are computed using a formula which is designed to produce a "delicate balance between two competing principles: adequacy and equity" (U.S. House Select Committee on Aging, 1980, p. 55). Adequacy refers to replacing a lower percentage of the higher wage earner's income, whereas equity refers to provision of higher benefits for higher wage earners. Thus, although Social Security benefits do not replace as high a percentage of high wage earner's income as of low wage earner's income, low wage earner's tend to be much more dependent upon Social Security. In 1979, almost 25% of all elderly with incomes below poverty level had Social Security benefits as their only source of income (Weeks, 1984). It should be noted here that even though Social Security benefits are indexed to inflation, a significant proportion of elderly remain below the poverty level (Schulz, 1980).

There are also other public and private pension systems to which wage earners may contribute during their working years in order to receive benefits in retirement, with eligibility criteria and benefits varying from employer to employer. Federal, military, and railroad pensions are public pensions which are separate from the Social Security system. State and local government pension plans can either be separate from, or in combination with the Social Security system. Benefits from public pensions are typically higher than those of most other pension systems, whereas benefits of private pensions are typically lower. Because many people change employment during their working years, some may be "double-dipping," or drawing benefits from a combination of Social Security, public, and private pension depending on where they worked. Similarly, most public and private pension systems have no earnings limitation test, resulting in another form of "double-dipping," that of receiving pension benefits while still being employed (Schulz, 1980; Weeks, 1984).

Employment Earnings

Earnings make a great difference in the economic position of the elderly. As noted earlier, those elderly who remain employed fulltime tend to earn as much as younger persons of the same race and sex. In 1981, about 41% of those aged 55-64 worked fulltime, 10% aged 65-69 worked fulltime, and 2% aged 70 years and older worked fulltime (Weeks, 1984). The primary reasons for either continued employment or retirement are related to whether one can make more from work than from Social Security or other pension benefits. The earnings limitation test for Social Security has acted as a rather strong disincentive to work, despite the fact that it has been liberalized considerably. Thus, the majority of elderly who are employed, are only employed part-time (Schulz, 1980; Weeks, 1984).

Public Assistance

The proportion of elderly who are below the poverty level has decreased in the past few decades, from over 33% 25 years ago to approximately 16% today. This is somewhat deceiving, however; if the "near-poor" are included, the poverty rate for the elderly population jumps to 30%. Likewise, the relative numbers have increased because of the greater numbers of elderly in the population. Despite large increases in the number of impoverished elderly people, only 10% of the elderly receive any kind of public assistance (U.S. Bureau of the Census, 1983).

In 1981, more than $437 billion was spent for both cash and noncash benefits under both governmental and private programs; yet, the issue of poverty persists among the aged (Beattie, 1983).

Cash Benefits

The Supplemental Security Income Program (SSI) is a means-tested program. It is the primary source of public assistance to poor elderly. Administered through the Social Security Administration, the SSI program replaced three state-administered public assistance programs (Old Age Assistance, Aid to the Blind, and Aid to the Permanently and Totally Disabled) and provided much broader eligibility criteria. States are permitted to supplement SSI payments, which is done in about one-half of the states.

The goal of the SSI program is to provide eligible persons with a guaranteed income level. Eligibility requirements include being 65 years of age or disabled and a U.S. citizen or legal permanent resident with a total income of less than that estimated as the SSI benefit level. Typically, however, the total income for many SSI recipients reaches that of poverty level, partially because eligibility does not preclude home ownership and a small savings account. The SSI program has nearly doubled the number of low income elderly who are now eligible for supplemental income benefits (Schulz, 1980).

Noncash/In-Kind Benefits

Noncash benefits, in the form of in-kind public transfers for food (food stamps), housing (publicly owned or subsidized rental housing), and medical care (Medicaid), have expanded much in the past decade. The value of these in-kind transfers are not included, however, when figuring income levels. Therefore, many poor elderly who are below poverty level are in actuality receiving noncash benefits with a value that might increase their income to above poverty level (Beattie, 1983; Schulz, 1980).

Implications

Because income level impacts on almost every area of life, it is important to identify those groups who are most likely to become poor in late life. As stated earlier, poverty rates are highest among the "old-old," women, and minorities. Those who live alone, are not married, do not work, depend exclusively on Social Security benefits, and live in small towns and rural areas also have high poverty rates. Because this latter group is typically comprised of the "old-old," women, and minorities, the cycle continues.

The Federal government spent almost $200 billion in 1982 for programs benefitting the elderly, with the majority of money (59%) going to Social Security. Although this may sound like a lot of money, many elderly continue to remain below the poverty level because a large percentage who are eligible for means-tested programs do not apply or participate in them. As the distribution indicates, most of the federal expenditures for the elderly are through entitlement programs (Social Security and Medicare) which are not means-tested. Although they may aid the low-income elderly, these programs are not specifically targeted towards them. The principal means-tested program, SSI, pays maximum benefits which are below the poverty level.

The implications of their economic status for the poor elderly's health care are obvious. The poorest among them depend upon Medicaid. The marginally, or near poor, which comprise a much larger segment of the elderly population, have fewer choices in seeking care and services in the high-costing private sector. Neither of these groups is likely to afford important preventive care and services from specialists or ancillary health provides (e.g., vision screening and eye care, hearing aids, mental health assistance, foot care, and rehabilitation services). Finally, a large proportion of the lower-income elderly have restricted access to health care due to unavailability or cost of necessary support services such as transportation (Hickey, 1980).

Education

Educational levels of the elderly population are below that of the younger population. However, this gap has narrowed considerably in the past 30 years and is expected to almost close by 1990. This is because the proportion of those 55-64 years of age with a high school education is almost the same as that of the younger population, due primarily to the educational opportunities which were available after World War II. Another factor appears to be immigration patterns. The elderly population today has a much higher proportion of immigrants with correspondingly lower educational levels than does the younger population (U.S. Bureau of the Census, 1983).

Educational levels between Blacks and Whites are significantly different. Thirty-three percent of the White population age 65 and over, and almost twice that percentage of elderly Blacks have never gone beyond elementary school; when looking at the elderly over 75 years of age, almost 50% of elderly Whites and 75% of elderly blacks never completed high school. As noted earlier, education and income are significantly related, and those with higher educational levels tend to earn more; therefore, they tend to be better-off after retirement than those with lower educational levels (Schulz, 1980).

Marital Status and Living Arrangements

There are significant differences between elderly men and women in terms of marital status and living arrangements. Over 80% of men aged 65 and over live in family settings, whereas under 60% of elderly women live in families. Similiarly, only 40% of elderly females are married and living with their husbands; however, more than 75% of elderly men are married and living with their wives. Almost 50% of elderly females are widowed, compared with 12% of elderly males. After 75 years of age, the figures increase to nearly 70% of the women who are widowed, with an increase to 20% of elderly widowers (U.S. Bureau of the Census, 1983).

These differences between men and women are due not only to the higher age-specific death rates of men, but also to the fact that men tend to marry younger women. Another point worth noting is that elderly widowed males have remarriage rates which are seven times higher than those of females. Approximately 6% of elderly women have never married, compared with 4% of elderly men. When looking at differences between Blacks and Whites, Blacks are more likely to be single, separated, or divorced than are Whites, although the differences between males and females are similar to those found in the White population.

Almost 30% of the elderly population live alone and most of these are women. Approximately 40% of elderly women live alone, compared with 14% of elderly men. Over 75 years of age, however, the percentage dramatically increases, especially for women—50% of the women in this age category live alone, whereas 20% of the men live alone. Although the striking differences between males and females are apparent, just as in the discussion of marital status, there are few differences in the percentage of Blacks and Whites who live alone (U.S. Bureau of the Census, 1983).

Regardless of race or sex, the proportion of aged living alone is increasingly apparent. This phenomenon may be due to better income, greater availability of age-segregated housing, and/or a general decline in intergenerational living arrangements among kin. Similarly most research suggests that the elderly prefer living alone or only with their spouse as long as they can (Jackson, 1980).

On the other hand, elderly who live in isolation and are without family ties often experience more serious problems, both in terms of health and finances. One study discovered that those who are widowed are five times more likely to be institutionalized than are married people (Butler & Newacheck, 1981). Elderly persons who have never been married, or are divorced or separated, are 10 times more likely to be institutionalized. In addition, these striking differences in risk of institutionalization do not appear to be related to functional disability. Vicente, Wiley, and Carrington (1979) report similar findings, that being unmarried and living alone were positively correlated with institutionalization. They also found that those who were White with low incomes, chronic illnesses and disabilities, in addition to being unmarried and living alone, were at higher risk for institutionalization of a longer duration.

Housing

Among the elderly population, only 5% are institutionalized, 4-5% live in specialized planned housing, and the remaining 90% live in the community at large (Lawton, 1980). It is important to note that the percentage of elderly persons likely to be institutionalized during the course of a given year is far higher than the much publicized 5% rate. Close to 10% of the population over age 65 spend some portion of time in an institution during the course of a year. This percentage is two to three times higher for the 75 years and over age group.

Although 71% of the elderly own their own homes, with 84% of these homes being mortgage-free, these figures can be misleading (Allan & Brotman, 1981; Brotman, 1980). Home ownership may provide financial and emotional security to some elderly, but for many others it can become a burden they are not prepared to deal with. Fixed incomes may not provide much flexibility in dealing with home ownership. Large old homes are usually not well-insulated and utility costs can be prohibitive; likewise, taxes may be high. Upkeep and maintenance may not only be costly, but difficult for the elderly to manage; there may be stairs that are not easily negotiable by those with increasing frailty. Although the neighborhood may have once been relatively pleasant and secure, it may now be in a high crime area. Selling is not a simple solution to this problem, because the home may be difficult to sell and may not provide enough money for subsequent rental costs (Allan & Brotman, 1981; Brotman, 1980.

In recent years, urban renewal, conversion to condominiums, and race-integration policies have threatened the housing status of many elderly. There appears to be a noticeable lack of affordable rental housing in some areas, which has affected not only the low-income elderly, but the middle-income elderly as well. It has been estimated that elderly renters now spend 5%-15% more of their income on housing than the general population (Sherman, in press; Weeks, 1984).

Sherman (in press) has categorized types of planned housing which may be available for the elderly person according to the amount of independence required by the typical occupant. The categories include retirement villages (communities), mobile homes, retirement hotels which are often called Single Room Occupancies, (SROs), independent apartments, congregate housing, shared housing, licensed boarding homes and domiciliary care. Retirement villages reflect the highest degree of independence and the domiciliary care the least. The following descriptions, based largely on Sherman's (in press) framework, do not represent clearcut categories or distinctions between housing types. There continues to be some overlap in the definition and labeling of planned housing for the elderly.

Retirement Community

Age-segregated retirement communities tend to set the elderly apart from much of society to the perceived advantage of the elderly (Weeks, 1984). These communities provide housing (houses/condominiums, apartments, mobile homes) within a short distance of a "haven" of services (i.e., grocery store, drugstore, medical facilities, recreational facilities, social services, and restaurants).

Retirement Hotels/SROs

Retirement hotels are varied and can range from very expensive to cheap; some may offer meal service. Although SRO housing can be found in retirement hotels, it is also found in large commercial hotels and rooming houses. SROs are typically furnished rooms, usually without kitchens or baths. Many facilities which offer SRO housing are old and dilapidated, and are usually found in inner city areas. Although SRO and retirement hotels are similar, retirement hotels tend to be more luxurious and are more likely to offer meals as a service.

Independent Apartments

Independent apartments are frequently referred to as senior highrises. This is age-segregated apartment housing for those elderly who are usually capable of living independently. Although these highrises may sometimes serve as a nutrition site for a daily hot meal, many residents do not take advantage of this more than a few times each week.

Congregate Housing

Congregate housing may resemble independent apartments for the elderly, but the one essential difference is a central kitchen with common dining options. Residents may also have individual kitchens in their own apartments. Many congregate housing sites are involved in other supportive services, such as activity programs, outpatient clinics, and transportation. As more and more supportive services become a part of congregate housing, they will be less distinguishable from homes for the aged. Presently however, congregate housing is for the more independent, whereas homes for the aged (or domiciliary homes) provide more help with functional activities of living on a 24-hour basis (Sherman, 1984).

Illnesses of an Aging Population

One of the more significant aspects of aging is the changing health status of the population and the implications for dependency upon society. Although there is a lower incidence of acute illness among the elderly population, they average more days of restricted activity and almost as many days of bed disability due to acute conditions than do people aged 17-64 (National Center for Health Statistics, 1982).

One reason for the greater impact of acute conditions on the elderly is that they are much more likely to have one or more chronic, or long-term, conditions that may aggravate their acute problems, thus prolonging recovery. Foremost among these chronic conditions are the various forms of arthritis, cerebrovascular disease, and hypertension (see Table 1). In addition, many other chronic diseases cause varying degrees of distress, such as arteriosclerosis, diabetes, and cancer. The leading causes of death for the elderly differ somewhat from the mortality figures of the population as a whole (see Tables 2 and 3). However, chronic conditions clearly prevail as the leading cause of death among the elderly (National Center for Health Statistics, 1982).

Table 1. Rate per 1,000 persons of 10 leading chronic diseases, by age: 1979.*

		Age		Ratio of
Rank	Chronic disease	17-64	65+	65 to 17-64
1.	Arthritis	150	443	9:2
2.	Cerebrovascular disease	137	385	6:5
3.	Hypertensive disease	83	274	7:2
4.	Chronic sinusitis	169	156	1:0
5.	Arteriosclerosis	11	124	124:0
6.	Varicose veins	35	89	4:7
7.	Diabetes mellitus	34	80	8:9
8.	Hemorrhoids	57	66	1:3
9.	Frequent constipation	19	64	5:8
10.	Hernia of abdominal cavity	24	63	7:9

*Adapted from National Center from Health Statistics, (1979). Current estimates from the National Health Interview Survey. In S. Jack & P. Ries (Eds.), Vital & health statistics. Series 10, No. 136, Public Health Service, Washington, DC: U.S. Government Printing Office.

Table 2. Deaths (per 100,000) for the 10 leading causes of death in the total population.*

Rank	Cause of death	Rate	Ratio of Male to Female	Black to White
	All causes	878	1:8	1:5
1.	Diseases of heart	336	1:1	1:3
2.	Malignant neoplasmas	184	1:5	1:3
3.	Cerebrovascular diseases	75	1:2	1:8
4.	Accidents and adverse effects	47	2:9	1:2
5.	Chronic obstructive pulmonary diseases	25	2:9	0:8
6.	Pneumonia & influenza	24	1:8	1:6
7.	Diabetes mellitus	15	1:0	2:0
8.	Chronic liver disease & cirrhosis	14	2:2	1:1
9.	Atherosclerosis	13	1:3	1:1
10.	Suicide	12	3:3	0:5

*Adapted from National Center for Health Statistics: (1) Advance Report, Final Mortality Statistics, 1979. Monthly Vital Statistics Report, Vol. 31, No. 6, Supp. DHHS Pub. No. (PHS) 821120. Hyattsville, MD: Public Health Service, September, 1982, Table 5, pp. 25 and 26; (2) Advance Report, Final Mortality Statistics, 1980. Monthly Vital Statistics Report, Vol. 32, No. 4, Supp. DHHS Pub. No. (PHS) 831130. Hyattsville, MD: Public Health Service, August, 1983, Tables B and C, pp. 4 and 6.

Table 3. Deaths (per 100,000) for the 10 leading causes of death in the population age 65 years and over.*

Rank	Cause of death	Rate
	All causes	5,157
1.	Diseases of the heart	2,299
2.	Malignant neoplasms	1,005
3.	Cerebrovascular diseases	588
4.	Chronic obstructive pulmonary diseases	155
5.	Pneumonia & influenza	148
6.	Atherosclerosis	112
7.	Accidents & adverse effects	98
8.	Diabetes mellitus	97
9.	Nephritis, nephrotic syndrome, & nephrosis	48
10.	Chronic liver disease & cirrhosis	36

*Adapted from National Center from Health Statistics: (1) Advance Report, Final Mortality Statistics, 1979. Monthly Vital Statistics Report, Vol. 31, No. 6, Supp. DHHS Pub. No. (PHS) 821120, Hyattsville, MD: Public Health Service, September, 1982, Table 5, pp. 25 and 26; (2) Advance Report, Final Mortality Statistics,1980. Monthly Vital Statistics Report, Vol. 32, No. 4, Supp. DHHS Pub. No. (PHS) 831130. Hyattsville, MD: Public Health Service, August, 1983, Tables B and C, pp. 4 and 6.

Physical/Functional Disabilities

Health concerns in late life are the result of the longer disability which tends to occur with acute diseases, and the increased incidence of chronic conditions. At age 70, for example, an individual can expect to experience at least two or three chronic conditions. Moreover, gender, race, and socioeconomic status are significant predictors of disability and play an important role in determining how dysfunctional chronic illness will be (Hickey, 1980).

Most types of impairments are more prevalent in those aged 65 and older than in the younger population. Hearing losses are the most common impairment of the elderly, followed by vision problems, ambulatory problems, paralysis, speech impairments, and the loss of limbs. It is evident that normal, age-related sensory losses create a significant functional impairment for many older persons as they pursue their daily activities. Visual and hearing impairments restrict mobility, ranging from the gradual inability to drive a car to difficulties involved in using buses and other forms of public transportation to, eventually, isolation in their homes caused by auditory and visual uncertainties and fears about walking in public places. Serious loss of vision and hearing can further isolate them from such meaningful activities and contacts with the larger world as visiting with other people, watching television, and reading newspapers and magazines. The social isolation experienced by older persons with hearing and vision impairments has gone relatively unnoticed in the research literature and in clinical geriatric writings.

Definitions of health vary according to whether physical, mental, or social criteria are used. However, "health status" among the elderly usually means either (a) the presence/absence of disease, or (b) the degree of functional disability (Hickey, 1981; Weeks, 1984). Functional disability implies a social definition of health that examines departures from normal role functioning instead of focusing primarily on medical or biological functioning (Chappell, 1981). Weeks (1984) notes that a person's ability to function independently is one of the most important aspects of disease and disability because "dependence upon other brings with it a trail of social and economic consequences" (p. 230).

The extent to which the elderly are in need of functional assistance increases with age. Five percent of those aged 65-74 years need help in one or more basic physical activities, compared with 23% of those 75 and over who need this type of assistance. In addition, 30% of those 75 years and over need the help of another person in performing activities of daily living, compared with only 7% of those aged 65-74 (National Center for Health Statistics, 1983).

Functional abilities vary widely in the elderly, even between individuals with basically the same physical disorders. Such factors as future perspective or motivation, past health behaviors, the encouragement and support of others, and related psychological and personal characteristics are important determinants of functional health status. Thus, functional assessment is as important as physical diagnosis in establishing the health status and prognosis of most elderly persons. In this regard, the compounding effects of multiple health problems should not be minimized. The dysfunction caused by a single disorder is likely to be much greater in the person who has one or two other significant health problems than in someone healthier (Hickey, 1980).

Informal Support Networks

Although only 5% of the elderly are institutionalized, some assert that this is too low a proportion when compared to those who actually need the type of services that only an institution can provide. Many elderly living in the community are more functionally impaired than those who are institutionalized. They are maintained in the community setting primarily through informal support networks, such as family members, relatives, and friends. However, the actual extent of informal help provided by these support networks has been difficult to document (Archbold, 1982; Shanas, 1979).

For years it was thought that many elderly were abandoned by their families. Shanas (1979) demonstrated that most families do not abandon their older members, and, if anything, they err too long in keeping their dependent members from institutionalization.

On the other hand, minority elderly historically have had to rely more on family support because they are excluded from, or are poorly served by, many social programs; thus, minority families were primarily responsible for their aged, including their economic and health needs, this is a somewhat different situation than that of their White cohorts. Presently, however,

151

even though the extended family may exist, not all Black, Asian-American, or Hispanic-American elderly can count on them for support (Gelfand, 1982).

With this in mind, it is still family members rather than friends who provide help first, with spouses likely to be the primary helpers. After spouses, adult children, especially daughters and daughters-in-law, are the most likely helpers. Elderly men tend to receive help from their wives, whereas more elderly women receive help from their children (Archbold, 1982; Brody, 1981; Shanas, 1979).

The fact that the majority of informal caregivers are women has been well-documented (Archbold, 1982; Brody, 1981). However, it is unclear just what will happen to the informal support network system due to the growing proportion of females in the workforce.

Many kinds of support services are available to the elderly. The most frequent of these appear to be social and emotional support and assistance to help the elderly maintain their independence, such as transportation, shopping, household chores, and home maintenance (Eustis, Greenberg, & Patten, 1984). The widespread development of social support services for the elderly in the community reflect a growing recognition of the importance of such services in maximizing independence and delaying institutionalization.

One area of concern which receives little acknowledgement in the literature is the elderly's diminished capacity to replenish their psychological and social resources. The loss of friends through death and serious illness, and reduced contact with family members who live at a distance represent a serious blow to their personal support. While younger persons have many opportunities to make new friends and to maintain active social roles, the elderly experience a shrinking social world and a reduction in psychological support which accompanies this age-related phenomenon.

Health and Social Services Utilization

Financing Issues

Medical and health care costs have risen dramatically in the past several years; this is especially true in relation to the elderly population. Although the elderly constitute only 10-12% of the total

U.S. population, they now account for more than 30% of the total costs of health care in this country. Medicare and Medicaid cover many of the costs incurred by the elderly; however for those elderly without Medicaid, Medicare pays less than half of their medical bills. Coverage problems due to certain restrictions such as eligibility requirements, limited duration of illness periods, and the increasing need for coinsurance from private carriers emphasizes the fact that health care costs can be a potential threat to the elderly who rely on relatively fixed incomes. The increasing prevalence of chronic illness in the elderly, with the subsequent need for expensive long-term care, only increases the reality of this economic threat (Butler & Newacheck, 1981; Hickey, 1980).

Health care resources are provided through a combination of public and private funds. The enactment of Medicare and Medicaid legislation in 1965 is primarily responsible for the increase in public expenditures for health care; before 1965, public funds accounted for only one-third of the health-care dollar (Mueller & Gibson, 1976). Medicare and Medicaid expenditures, $53.2 billion in 1981, accounted for more than 80% of all health outlays; private funds (including out-of-pocket payment and private insurance) accounted for the balance (Kutza, 1981). From the consumer's perspective, however, the distribution of public and private resources varies widely. Medicare and Medicaid are primary resources for the institutionalized and the poor; private resources, on the other hand, account for a much larger proportion of the health care expenditures of the noninstitutionalized elderly and those above poverty levels.

Medicare

Medicare (Title XVIII of the Social Security Act, 1965) is a health insurance program for those aged 65 and over as well as for some disabled persons under 65 years. Both parts are a form of insurance; however, Part A (hospital insurance) is compulsory for all participants in the Social Security system and Part B (medical insurance) is voluntary. Part A is financed through standard employee payroll deductions and mandatory contributions by employers, Part B requires payment of a monthly premium, similar to that of private insurance (U.S. DHEW, 1965).

The goal of Part A coverage is to provide the best care in the most appropriate (or approved) setting, whether that care be in a hospital,

153

skilled nursing facility (SNF), or at home. This coverage is defined in terms of a benefit period, which begins when a person enters the hospital and ends 60 days after that person has been out of a hospital or SNF. Although there are limits to the volume of certain services a person is entitled to within a benefit period, there is no limit on the number of benefit periods. There are presently 90 days of hospital care and 100 days of SNF care per benefit period; however, the SNF care must follow a hospital stay of at least three days. If someone uses more than 90 days during a given benefit period, they can draw from their 60-day lifetime reserve. There is no stipulation of hospital admission or maximum number of visits for home health care under Part A. However, individuals must be "home-bound" and require intermittent (or part-time) skilled care, which includes nursing, physical therapy, occupational therapy, or speech-language pathology. Home health aide services and medical supplies and appliances are also included as part of the covered services in home health care.

Part B coverage applies to various outpatient services and treatments and is subject to deductibles and time limitations. Part B pays for 80% of the "reasonable" charge for a number of services--physicians' services, medically necessary equipment and supplies, medical therapies, diagnostic tests, necessary ambulance services, and some prosthetic devices related to the loss of an internal organ. Inpatient hospital services not covered under Part A may be covered by Part B. Treatment by a dentist, podiatrist, or chiropractor is covered only if there is a specific health problem which requires necessary medical care that only one of these professionals can provide.

Reimbursement of outpatient mental health services is presently limited to $250 per year. Part B does not pay for out-of-hospital drug costs, eyeglasses, hearing aids, dental services, routine foot care, routine physical examinations, or immunizations. This is ironic because many of these services are those which are a high priority need for the elderly, and which contribute to their continued independent living in the community. Butler (1977-1978) discusses this paradox, noting that Medicare seems to have been designed in terms of the health care needs of the younger population, rather than the elderly. Covered services do not include dentures, which could significantly reduce the problem of malnutrition, or hearing aids, which could reduce the prevalence of depression and paranoia associated with isolation from hearing loss.

Because Medicare rulings change, questions regarding coverage in particular cases can best be answered by a Medicare representative. Although Medicare has entitled the elderly to good hospitalization and major medical insurance benefits, Medicare pays for only 40-45% of the medical care expenditures of the elderly.

Medicaid

Medicaid (Title XIX of the Social Security Act) was enacted along with Medicare in 1965 as a program of medical assistance for the poor and medically indigent individuals of any age. Medicaid eligibility is based on income level and absence of resources and is financed through federal, state, and local funds. For the indigent, it is most often the only resort for health care. For the larger population of lower socioeconomic and marginally poor elderly, Medicaid care is the eventual option as other resources become exhausted (Hickey, 1980; Schulz, 1980).

Each state administers its own Medicaid program within federal guidelines and regulations. Certain basic services must be provided, including inpatient and outpatient hospital service, diagnostic services, nursing home care, home health services, screening, diagnostic, and treatment services for young people, family-planning services, and physicians' services. However, states may limit the extent of mandatory covered services, such as the number of hospital days and visits which will be covered. Many states restrict reimbursement rates for physician visits. In some states, for example, they are so low (e.g. 30% of prevailing rates) that many physicians will not accept Medicaid patients. Some states supplement the mandatory covered services to include prescription drugs, dental care, chiropractic care, eyeglasses, podiatric services, and private duty nursing, although the services offered by each state can change annually as state plans are modified in line with budget constraints.

Reimbursement Systems

Hospitals are the primary institutions for medical care and, as such, are the major recipients of reimbursement for that care. Hospital care accounted for more than 46% of all health care expenditures in 1981, which was provided by federal funds 75% of (Gibson & Waldo, 1982; McCarthy, 1981). A prospective reimbursement system, called Diagnostic Related Groups (DRGs), was recently initiated as a regulatory mechanism to curb spiraling hospital costs. DRGs provide the basis for a classification system by which data on the cost of patient care can be formulated and standardized. The system uses the patient's medical diagnosis, prescribed treatments, and age to categorize and define the services a hospital provides. This restructuring of hospital reimbursement formulas is a prospective reimbursement system for Medicare and a drastic departure from the traditional retrospective reimbursement system of per diem costs.

The prospective reimbursement system was initially established in the 1982 Tax Equity and Fiscal Responsibility Act (TEFRA), subsequently refined in the 1983 amendments to the Social Security Act (PL 98-21), and will be phased in over a 4-year period which began October 1, 1983. Although the system presently applies only to Medicare, many people believe that Medicaid and private insurance coverages will eventually be included. In addition, it is likely that covered services under these programs other than hospital care (home health care, etc.) will move toward a prospective reimbursement system. One can expect more thoughtful and detailed analyses of this major change in fiscal policy to begin to appear in the literature in the near future.

Under the prospective reimbursement system, cost control is paramount, and fiscal constraints are pervasive. The recent implementation of this program makes it too early to predict the full impact of this type of reimbursement scheme on the health care delivery system, especially for the elderly. Earlier discharges are likely, possibly resulting in "sicker" elderly persons being transferred to skilled nursing facilities (SNFs) earlier than in the past. This, in turn, should lead to an increase in the level of care needed which the SNF may or may not be prepared to provide. On the other hand, some "sicker" people will be sent home earlier to recuperate, which will lead to an increase in the need for home health and related community support services. It remains to be seen whether the SNFs and community settings will be able to respond to this need for "short-term, long-term" care that is likely to result from the introduction of DRGs.

A Continuum of Services: Noninstitutional to Institutional

Noninstitutional services are frequently referred to as "alternatives" to institutional care or "community-based" services. Eustis, Greenberg, and Patten (1984) point out that these terms are misleading. The term "alternative" implies that these are services for preventing or delaying institutionalization. However, many elderly not necessarily "at risk" of institutionalization can nonetheless benefit from noninstitutional services. Likewise, for some elderly, the services provided in an institution may be more appropriate because of the level of care they require. Thus, noninstitutional and institutional services should be seen as a continuum of flexible options, which provide for the elderly and their families several choices depending on the degree of chronic disability and health dependency experienced (Butler, 1978; Eustis, Greenberg, & Patten, 1984).

Community Supports/Aging Service Networks

Area Agencies on Aging

Established through Title III of the Older Americans Act, Area Agencies on Aging were intended to function as a service planning and coordination unit at the local level. In practice, their functions, auspices, and responsibilities differ widely, subject to local interests, service needs, and politics. Generally, however, Area Agencies enjoy a broad mandate "to develop area service plans, to expand services by pooling resources, to coordinate existing services, and, where necessary, to fund gap-filling services for the aged" (Estes, 1979, p. 39).

Multipurpose Senior Centers

Several different kinds of services are offered in the community to serve the elderly. One of the most visible is the multipurpose senior center. Although senior centers differ greatly, their basic purpose remains centered around the social functioning of independent elderly--those able to participate in self-directing programs. Centers initially offered more recreation and socialization opportunities which are so important for the elderly to remain connected and involved in and with the community. Many have become more oriented toward health and social services however, increasingly more are offering services such as counseling, health screening, legal aid, and information and referral services. Many senior centers serve as nutrition sites for congregate meals; most offer transportation services. In addition, monitoring services, such as calling and checking-up on the elderly who live alone, are now being offered through many senior centers. Anecdotal reports suggest that use of senior centers by elderly members of minority groups is proportionately lower than among the White population.

Adult Day Care

Adult day care services are provided in a centralized location for chronically-impaired elderly. Although clients are generally in need of specific health interventions to assist in rehabilitation or restorative activities (Koff, 1982), different day care programs vary a great deal, ranging from those with a social or activity orientation to those which are aimed more toward health and medical care, rehabilitation, and the provision of psychological services. Adult day care may be provided through a hospital, nursing home, or extended care facility, where the provision of services merge with those of the sponsoring facility. Services usually include physical therapy, speech-language pathology, occupational therapy, group therapy, specific nursing procedures, dentistry, podiatry, and personal care. "The aim of day care services is to dissociate the 'hotel' element of hospital care from therapeutic content, leaving only the latter" (U.S. DHEW, 1972). Since its inception, adult day care has constantly struggled for financial stability. As a so-called "add on" social or health care service, public support for day care is minimal. Programs which have been a fiscal success have relied on such mechanisms as private subsidies and foundation grants, eligibility and fee restrictions targeted at the less-impaired and more affluent (i.e., " for profit" programs), or located within a health care institution to reduce staffing costs (Eustis, Greenberg, & Patten, 1984; Hickey, 1980; Koff, 1982).

Outpatient Health Care

Medical personnel and facilities tend to be used more by the elderly than by the younger population, due in large part to the greater prevalence of chronic disease among the elderly population. The elderly average over six physician visits per year for every five made by the rest of the population (U.S. Bureau of the Census, 1983). Although physician visits are not a very good indicator of health status, physician care is usually linked to sick care, and not well care. Thus, it is assumed that the more physician visits one has, the sicker one is.

A concept which has been gaining more attention in recent years is that of Health Maintenance Organizations (HMOs). The development of HMOs was seen as a major mechanism for assuring access to health care in the absence of a policy on national health insurance, while at the same time decreasing costs of social health programs. The concept of HMOs developed from holistic philosophies of health care with emphasis on prevention. In reality, HMOs have often demonstrated their similarity to the traditional medical model, with emphasis on cure rather than prevention. Although it is likely that the concept of Health Maintenance Organizations will spread, the fiscal status of HMOs remain questionable given the aging of the U.S. population (Eustis, Greenberg, & Patten, 1984).

Home Care

A vital link in the continuum of long-term care services in the community is that of home care. Home care is an attempt to aid the elderly in physical, mental, and social functioning, and to maximize their independence as long as possible. This is done through a variety of services, which are classified as home health care, personal care, and homemaker and chore services. Home health care and personal care are directed at the individuals themselves and are known as health or medically oriented services; homemaker and chore services are aimed at helping the elderly maintain their homes and are more socially oriented services (Eustis, Greenberg, & Patten, 1984).

In the history of public funding for long-term care, institutional care has traditionally been favored over home care. Consequently, home care and other aspects of a coordinated continuum of long-term care have not thrived (Koff, 1982). A study which compared home services to institutionalization found that until the elderly become extremely impaired, cost for home services (including the large portion provided by family/friends) is less than the cost of institutionalization (Comptroller General of the U.S., 1977). However, the portion of costs borne by family/friends is

significantly higher at all impairment levels. Figure 4 shows a comparison
of costs for home care borne by family/friends and agencies at each
impairment level and well illustrates this point.

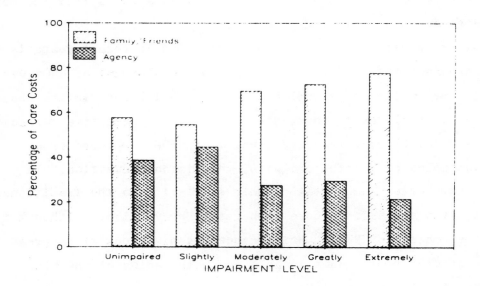

Figure 4. Distribution of care costs for impaired elderly between
family/friends and agency* by impairment level: 1977.

Home Health Care Services

Home health care services which are reimbursable under Medicare include
skilled nursing care, physical therapy, speech-language pathology,
occupational therapy, and home health aide services. Services must be
provided by a Medicare-certified agency that offers skilled nursing care and
at least one other service. Strict eligibility requirements limit home
health care services under Medicare. These services, therefore, are usually
provided only on a short-term basis, with the average number of visits in
1977 being 23 (Eustis, Greenberg, & Patten, 1984).

Skilled nursing care and home health aide services are the only
mandatory services which states must offer under Medicaid to persons who
are eligible for skilled nursing care at home by the order of a physician
(U.S. DHHS, 1981). Like Medicare, Medicaid usually covers physical therapy,
speech-language pathology, occupational therapy, and medical social services
for those who are eligible. Although Medicaid regulations are

160

somewhat more liberal than Medicare, states have the freedom to determine their own eligibility criteria and services provided, and many states tend to support Medicaid less than Medicare. As the cost of Medicaid has risen, especially in poor economic times, service availability and eligibility have declined across the board.

Personal Care Services

Personal care services are related to home health care services, and are intended to help the elderly perform activities of daily living, such as bathing and dressing. Activities related to their medical problems, such as dressing changes, are also included. These services are usually funded through Medicaid, Title III of the Older Americans Act, and the Social Services Block Grant (Title XX) (Eustis, Greenberg, & Patten, 1984).

Homemaker and Chore Services

Homemaker and chore services include laundry, housecleaning, shopping, minor repairs around the house, errands, yard work, and basic financial management (U.S. DHHS, 1981). These services are generally not funded through Medicare or Medicaid, but instead through Title III of the Older Americans Act and the Social Services Block Grant (Title XX). Therefore, fewer restrictions regarding eligibility apply, although there are variations from state to state (Eustis, Greenberg, & Patten, 1984).

Hospital Care

When comparing hospital utilization by the elderly with that of the younger population, it is evident that the elderly are hospitalized almost twice as often, stay twice as long, and use twice as many prescription drugs. Since the 1965 enactment of Medicare, the elderly have increased their utilization of hospitals by more than 50% compared with an 11% increase in the general population. The average hospital stay of the elderly is about 12 days, compared with 6 days for the rest of the population. Again, this is due to the greater prevalence of chronic disease conditions among the elderly and the fact that chronic conditions tend to cause more frequent hospitalizations and for longer periods of time (Eustis, Greenberg, & Patten, 1984; Hickey, 1980).

Nursing Home Care

The rate of nursing home use by the elderly has risen dramatically as a result of the enactment of Medicare and Medicaid, doubling from 2.5% to 5% in the population over 65 in the past 20 years. Almost 75% of those who are institutionalized are not married, compared with 40% of the noninstitutionalized who are unmarried. The risk of institutionalization increases with age: 1.5% of those 65-74 are institutionalized; 6% of those 75-84; and 23% of those who are 85 years and older (U.S. Bureau of the Census, 1983).

The terminology surrounding nursing homes is often confusing. Extended care refers to the type of care found in Medicare-approved skilled nursing facilities (SNFs), which provide aftercare, including intense medical assistance, following a stay in an acute care hospital. However, many patients do not require skilled nursing care after a period of time, but do need some form of maintenance care. Intermediate care facility (ICF) designates a less intense type of care provided on a long-term basis and is more representative of the traditional nursing home.

When patients are discharged from the hospital, but continue to need constant medical supervision, they are transferred to the SNF for extended care. This is reimbursable under Medicare only after a minimum 3-day stay in a hospital and includes 24-hour nursing services as an extension of hospital care, establishment of a nursing care plan, and dietary and medical care for a maximum period of 100 days. At times, patients can be discharged home during this period; however many are often transferred to an ICF bed where Medicaid funding takes over if the person is medically indigent. Consequently, ICFs became the domain of Medicaid, and many nursing homes designate parts of their facilities as either ICF or SNF.

The "spend-down" phenomenon, described earlier in this chapter, helps explain why there are so few discharges from nursing homes back into the community. It is not uncommon for the elderly to deplete their resources to qualify for Medicaid coverage of their institutional care; thus, they have no resources for returning to the community. This is also part of the "institutional bias" of public funding practices for long-term care.

Summary

In order to better understand the services needed by the elderly in today's society, and the professional's role in planning and delivering needed services to the elderly, the social and environmental context of aging was presented. Demographic trends were explored, and it was noted that the increasing numbers of elderly are creating more pressure for increased services. Financing of health care for the elderly, primarily through Medicare and Medicaid, was discussed in the context of how financing influences the continuum of services which are available to the elderly. We also noted that the elderly at greatest risk for various health and social problems were the low-income, single, "very old," isolated (few support networks), women, and minorities. The following case histories are typical, and represent situations which place the elderly at high risk.

Mr. E. retired several years ago from his job as a salesman; he and his wife then left their apartment in the city and moved to their cottage in the country. Recently, Mr. E. had a stroke, which left him partially paralyzed on his left side, partly aphasic, and confused. He is incontinent of urine most of the time. He is receiving speech-language pathology, and physical therapy, but will not practice on his own. The E's have no children and they have made few friends since moving to this rural community. Mrs. E. has become increasingly frustrated with the situation--this man whom she is taking care of is certainly not her energetic, articulate husband of several months earlier. She begins experiencing chest pain and is hospitalized. Because there is now no one to care for Mr. E., he must be institutionalized in a nursing home. When Mrs. E. is discharged, she realizes that she cannot care for him, at least for the time being. However, she does not drive and the nursing home which he is in is more than 1 hour away. There is no public transportation and she has few friends to help her. She is experiencing guilt and increasing anxiety over this, knowing her husband is unhappy and wants to come home, yet not knowing what she can or should do.

The fact that Mr. and Mrs. E. have few informal or formal support systems places them both at high risk--him for institutionalization (which has happened) and she for increased stress which, in turn, increases the chances for health problems. They have few options available at this point. If Mrs. E. brings her husband back home, she realizes that the burden of caring for him is likely to be too much for her to handle. However, the guilt that she is experiencing is not easy for her to live with.

Home health care is an option in this situation if Mrs. E. can handle the responsibility of caring for him the majority of the time. A home health aide could possibly come in 3 times per week to help Mr. E. with his personal care. Physical therapy and speech-language pathology, could possibly be provided, along with regular nursing care. The situation is fragile, however, and requires consistent monitoring to help Mr. and Mrs. E. adapt to their situation and choose the most viable option.

Miss T, an 88-year-old single woman, has lived alone in the "family home" since her parents died almost 30 years ago. The neighborhood used to be in a "nice" section of town, but in the past several years the old houses have been subdivided into apartments, and the crime rate has been steadily rising. Though her niece has urged her to move to one of those "nice and safe senior highrises," Miss T. has refused because she thinks "it would just be too much trouble." Her hearing has diminished considerably in the past several years. Although her niece has urged her to have it checked, Miss T. has refused because she says, "I don't have enough money for that." After her house has broken into several months ago, Miss T. has become increasingly isolated and suspicious, and will not open the door for anyone who has not called first; and even if she does hear the phone ring, she won't always answer it because she knows she probably cannot hear what the person is saying. Her niece signed her up for Home-Delivered Meals (which delivers hot lunches to her home 5 days a week), but because she would not answer her door, they stopped coming.

The fact that Miss T. does have a fairly strong support system in her niece has probably enabled her to remain independent in her home for as long as she has. Her niece, however, is approaching retirement and planning to move south with her husband. This will probably force Miss T. to be institutionalized, although she has vowed she "would die first, rather than be institutionalized."

This situation does not provide many alternatives. If finances were not a problem, perhaps a sitter could be hired to stay with Miss T., or to at least look in on her when her niece moves away. Taking Miss T. to visit one of the senior highrises and introducing her to some of the residents might be another option. If at all possible, institutionalization should be avoided until no other options exist.

Growing numbers of elderly in the population are forcing professionals who work with the elderly to study the phenomenon of aging in order to increase both their knowledge of aging issues and their skills in working with the elderly and the aging services network. Assessment of need in the elderly population, in addition to the responsibility of professionals in responding to this need, remain critical issues. Speech-language pathologists and Audiologists are crucial resources for the elderly. As can be seen from the above case histories, sensory losses in the elderly, especially hearing losses, impact significantly on lifestyle and social interaction pattern. Because hearing losses are usually so progressive, the elderly are often unaware of the problem and may gradually withdraw, becoming confused, angry, hostile, depressed, or paranoid. They may be considered senile by their family and friends. Speech difficulties often cause isolation of the affected person, not only from family and friends who no longer feel that they can communicate with the person, but also from the larger society. The role of the professional who deal with communication problems goes beyond dealing with the specific problem. It includes helping the elderly person with these deficits to adapt to their environment and facilitating interaction between the affected person and the aging service networks to promote the optimal level of functioning.

Finally, it is somewhat unfortunate that the social problems and caretaking issues raised here must become more complex when viewed from the context of social policy. From a humanistic and ethical perspective, we are committed as a society to remediating the social and physical ills of the last stage in life. Some would even claim that there is an ethical as well as a demographic imperative. Yet, there are other needs and problems in society, as well as many more people under age 70 than past it. Thus, our resources will continue to place a realistic limit on the ethical commitments of society and generate continuing political debate.

Although this chapter has not addressed social policy issues directly, such a context is necessary for understanding the implications of demographic factors and patterns of service design and use. Outcomes from current debate over the following questions will directly affect the roles of various professions in providing services to the elderly.

- o Should the long-term care population be defined in terms of age or need?
- o Should older persons be "mainstreamed" or given special consideration in the design and delivery of health care and social services.
- o How should society's responsibility be divided between the private and the public sectors, and between federal and local levels?

o What kind of reimbursement mechanisms are best for which segments of the population?

o How much regulation is desirable?

o Who is entitled to services in the home or in the institution?

These and related policy questions will continue to shape this society's formal response to the social and health needs of its elderly population.

Self-Study Questions

1. How would you characterize the age of the U.S. population?

2. What are the economic implications of living longer today for the individual? For society? How might these questions be answered differently 25-30 years from now?

3. In what ways do the concepts of illness and health status change or remain the same over the adult lifetime?

4. In what ways do socioeconomic characteristics change or remain the same over the adult lifetime?

5. Describe the several ways in which their greater longevity works to the disadvantage of women.

6. List and define various residential living options available to the elderly.

7. How do Medicaid and SSI payments differ from Medicare and Social Security benefits?

8. Differentiate Medicare from Medicaid. How do the coverages under Parts A and B Medicare apply to the elderly?

9. What is meant by Diagnostic Related Groups? How do the DRGs differ from the payment mechanisms previously in place?

10. Describe the various supportive programs available to the noninstitutionalized elderly. How would one determine what services and programs are available in a given community and their eligibility and qualification requirements?

11. What is the institutional bias in public funding programs for long-term care?

12. What are the implications of multiple impairments both to the elderly and to service providers in the community?

REFERENCES

Allan, C., & Brotman, H. B. (Compilers, 1981). Chart book on aging in America. White House Conference on Aging.

Archbold, P. G. (1982). An analysis of parentcaring by women. Home Health Care Services Quarterly, 3(3), 5-25.

Beattie, W. M. (1983). Economic security for the elderly: National and international perspectives. The Gerontologist, 23(4), 406-410.

Brody, E. M. (1981). "Women in the middle" and family help to older people. The Gerontologist, 21(5), 471-480.

Brotman, H. B. (1980). Every ninth American. Draft prepared for "Developments in Aging, 1980" for the Special Committee on Aging, U.S. Senate.

Butler, L. H., & Newacheck, P. W. (1981). Health and social factors relevant to long-term care policy. In J. Meltzer, F. Farrow, & H. Richman (Eds.), Policy options in long-term care. Chicago: University of Chicago Press.

Butler, P. A. (1978). Financing non-institutional long-term care services for the elderly and chronically ill: Alternatives to nursing homes. Washington, DC: Legal Services Corp.

Butler, R. N. (1977-1978). Nursing home care: An impossible situation unless... International Journal of Aging and Human Development, 8(3), 291-294.

Chappell, N. (1981). Measuring functional ability and chronic health conditions among the elderly: A research note on the adequacy of three instruments. Journal of Health and Social Behavior, 22(2), 90-102.

Comptroller General of the U.S. (1977, December). Report to the Congress: Home health--The need for a national policy to better provide for the elderly. Washington, DC: U.S. General Accounting Office.

Estes, C. L. (1979). The aging enterprise. San Francisco: Jossey-Bass.

Eustis, N., Greenberg, J., & Patten, S. (1984). Long-term care for older persons: A policy perspective. Monterey, CA: Brooks/Cole.

Gelfand, D. E. (1982). Aging: The ethnic factor. Boston: Little, Brown.

Gibson, R. M., & Waldo, D. R. (1982). National health expenditures, 1981. Health Care Financing Review, 4(1) 1-35.

Hendricks, J., & Hendricks, C. D. (1981). Aging in mass society: Myths and realities (2nd ed.). Cambridge, MA: Winthrop.

Hickey, T. (1980). Health & aging. Monterey, CA: Brooks/Cole.

Jackson, J. J. (1980). Minorities and aging. Belmont, CA: Wadsworth.

Koff, T. H. (1982). Long-term care: An approach to serving the frail elderly. Boston: Little, Brown.

Kutza, E. A. (1981). The benefits of old age: Social-welfare policy for the elderly. Chicago: University of Chicago Press.

Lawton, M. P. (1980). Environments and aging. Monterey, CA: Brooks/Cole.

McCarthy, C. (1981). Financing for health care. In S. Jonas (Ed.), Health care delivery in the United States (2nd ed.). New York: Springer.

Mueller, M. S., & Gibson, R. M. (1976). Age differences in health are spending, fiscal year 1975. Social Security Bulletin (U.S. DHEW) publication. Washington, DC: U.S. Government Printing Office.

National Center for Health Statistics. (1982, October). Current estimates from the national health interview survey, United States, 1981. In B. Bloom (Ed.), Vital and health statistics. Series 10-No. 141. DHHS Pub. No. (PHS) 83-1569. Public Health Service. Washington, DC: U.S. Government Printing Office.

National Center for Health Statistics. (1983, September). Americans needing help to function at home. In B. Feller (Ed.), Advance data from vital and health statistics, No. 92. (DHHS Publication No. PHS 83-1250). Hyattsville, MD: Public Health Service.

Schulz, J. H. (1980). The economics of aging (2nd ed.). Belmont, CA: Wadsworth.

Shanas, E. (1979). The family as a social support system in old age. The Gerontologist, 19, 169-174.

Sherman, S. R. (in press). Housing. In A. Monk (Ed.), Handbook of gerontological services. New York: Van Nostrand Reinhold.

U.S. Bureau of the Census. America in transition: An aging society. Current population reports. Series P-23, No. 128. Washington, DC: U.S. Government Printing Office.

U.S. DHEW. (1972). Home care for persons fifty-five years and over: United States, July 1965-June 1968. In Vital and health statistics (Series 10, No. 73). Washington, DC: National Center for Health Statistics.

U.S. DHEW. (1965). Economic security act and social security bulletin. Washington, DC: U.S. Government Printing Office.

U.S. DHHS. (1981). Health Care Financing Administration. Long-term care: Background and future directions. Washington, DC.

U.S. House Select Committee on Aging. (1980, December). Retirement: The broken promise: A report by the committee. Washington DC: U.S. Congress.

Vicente, L., Wiley, J. A., & Carrington, R. A. (1979). The risk of institutionalization before death. The Gerontologist, 19, 361-367.

Weeks, J. R. (1984). Aging: Concepts and social issues. Belmont, CA: Wadsworth.

Suggested Readings

Binstock, R. H. (1983). The aged as scapegoat. The Gerontologist, 23(2), 136-143.

Carp, F. M. (1976). Housing and living environments of older people. In R. H. Binstock & E. Shanas (Eds.), Handbook of aging and the social sciences. New York: Van Nostrand.

Gikow, F. F. (1981). A decision model: How to determine appropriate community services for the elderly. Nursing and Health Care, 322-326.

Kuypers, J. A., & Bengtson, V. L. (1973). Social breakdown and competence: A model of normal aging. Human Development, 16, 191-201.

Neugarten, B. L. (Ed.). (1982). Age or need? Public policies for older people. Beverly Hills, CA: Sage.

Willis, D. P. (Ed.). (1983). Special issue: "Aging: Demographic, health, and social prospects." Milbank Memorial Fund Quarterly: Health and Society, 61(3).

Implications of Physiological, Psychological,
& Sociocultural Changes in Aging
for Communication

Linda Jacobs-Condit

American Speech-Language-Hearing Association, Rockville, Maryland

The previous chapters have addressed the aging process as reflected in physiological, psychological, and sociocultural change. Taken alone or even collectively, these changes may have a significant impact upon the elderly person's lifestyle and patterns of interaction with specific implications for communication.

For example, any or all of the physical changes which reduce mobility or limit activities (i.e., arthritis, fatigue, health problems, motor slowness) may result in limited accessibility to interpersonal and social interactions ultimately leading to reduced opportunity for communication. Similarly, hearing and vision changes may effect limitations of communication. Negative responses in others may be elicited by changes in speech or vocal characteristics or by alterations in physical appearance which are common to the aging process. Further, preoccupation with self as well as fear and anxiety about current or possible future health problems may not contribute to good communicative patterns.

It has been stated that, in essence, the elderly have a reduced ability to adapt especially in communicative situations. However, the elderly may develop alternate strategies to better adjust to linguistic or cognitive shifts as well as to sensory losses. On the other hand, negative psychological adjustment to life changes or to a reduction in the number of communication partners may effect reduced interpersonal communication. In the same vein, anxieties about actual or perceived cognitive decline may lead to a withdrawal from communication situations.

This unconscious yet self-imposed isolation as well as the isolation occasioned by altered lifestyle patterns significantly reduce opportunities for communicative interactions. Other barriers to communication may include artificial physical environs as may be found in nursing homes or elderly housing facilities, as well as the attitude of many elderly towards communication disorders (i.e., denial, rejection of treatment, false expectations, or even fear).

At a time when there is a growing demand for greater life-satisfaction and at a time when other groups of handicapped older persons have benefitted from significant advances, large numbers of elderly may face a profound diminution of quality of life due to reduced opportunity for communication for any number of reasons. As a result, the elderly may be unable to share perceptions or memories, unable to inform others of how to best meet physical needs, or unable to enjoy communication-based activities such as meetings, movies, religious services, newspapers or even card games. If these effects of aging and implications for communication are to be significantly reduced, educational programs and therapeutic approaches must exist that are specifically designed for appropriate intervention with older persons within the context of the aging process itself.

General Considerations in the Management
of Older Persons With Communication Disorders

Jess Dancer
University of Arkansas, Little Rock

Assessment of the elderly requires comprehensive assessment
of the physical, emotional, and social status of the
individual. Common medical diagnostic knowledge is
often inadequate for assessing the elderly since multiple
physical problems can be present accompanied by some normal
age-related physical changes which affect function. The
patient's social and emotional problems must be acknowledged
if the treatment plan is to be effective (Beck, 1981).

The purpose of this chapter is to outline and discuss the general
management considerations that professionals in communicative disorders
should know and use in the evaluation of older persons with speech,
language, and hearing problems. General management considerations include
those aspects within the client, the clinician, the test environment, and
the client's environment that can affect the assessment and management of
an older person's communication handicap.

The task of presenting general management guidelines for use with older
persons is not a simple one. As Oyer and Oyer (1976, p. 3) pointed out, age is
virtually the "only common denominator of this heterogeneous group."
Similarly, Butler and Lewis (1982) stated that old people become more diverse
rather than similar as they age. Thus, each attempt to provide a general
management guideline can be countered with the objection that such guidelines
are often inappropriate for any given older person. In dealing with older
persons on a regular basis, one is struck by the extreme differences in the
performance of two older individuals in the context of a clinical evaluation.
Person #1 might enter the assessment situation and perform all tasks given in a
standard manner with no apparent difficulties whatsoever. Person #2 might
enter the same assessment situation and perform so poorly on the tasks that the

professional is hard-pressed to specify what modifications in assessment procedures are appropriate.

For the clinician, the key words in the assessment of the communication needs of older persons are Knowledge and Flexibility. Clinicians need to know (a) the major age-related normal structural and functional changes that affect communication skills, (b) typical client-clinician communication barriers that retard the assessment process, and (c) the data base appropriate for facilitating the assessment process. In addition, the clinician needs to anticipate potential problems in the assessment of the individual and to be flexible in adapting examination procedures to the abilities of the person. Lastly, the clinician needs to educate the family and significant others in their role of helping the older person with a communication disorder.

Normal Age-Related Changes That Affect Communication Skills

Clinicians who work with older persons quickly become aware that the communication skills of older persons are often markedly different from the skills of younger or middle-aged adults. Problems such as hearing loss (presbycusis), visual acuity loss (presbyopia), poor memory or cognitive functioning, slow response time, fatigue, complaints of physical distress, and poor manual dexterity may be present to complicate the communication assessment. In this regard, the clinician must try to keep the normal aspects of aging within each older individual separate from the abnormal aspects that represent communication pathology. At present, this is not an easy task for the clinician, because . . ."we simply do not know much about old age, especially about healthy old age" (Ford & Sbordone, 1980, p. 575).

Although a great deal of research has and is being done on the effects of normal aging on communication (Beasley & Davis, 1981), normative data on many facets of speech, language, and hearing performance in older persons are presently unavailable. For example, Bergman (1980, p. 2) reviews the area of auditory performance in older persons and comments that before we can meet the problems of declining communicative functioning in aging persons, . . ."we must learn specifically what changes in auditory skills and performance tend to occur with aging." The same general sentiment that much more needs to be learned is also expressed in regard to the peripheral speech mechanism (Kahane, 1981), aging speech (Kent & Burkard, 1981), neuromuscular control of speech

(Kent & Burkard, 1981), histologic correlates of aging (Nadol, 1981), and language skills in healthy older people (Obler & Albert, 1981).

Although the normal effects of aging on communication obviously require a great deal more study, one point is clear. Clinicians responsible for the assessment and management of older persons with speech, language, and hearing problems must account and compensate for the common problems in assessment that result from the normal aging processes within each individual, regardless of their primary communicative disorder. As examples, a person with aphasia may also have an age-related hearing loss (presbycusis), and the clinician should identify such a loss and modify the assessment of aphasia to compensate for such a loss. A person with presbycusis may also have an age-related visual problem (presbyopia), and the clinician should be able to modify a speechreading task to account for the loss in visual function. A person with a laryngectomy might also have a hearing loss that interferes with the ability to perceive a stoma-blast, which must be identified and remediated.

Communication Barriers in the Assessment of Older Persons

General management considerations actually go far beyond the tasks that we require of older persons within the context of the formal test situation. If the ultimate aim of the assessment process is a . . . "definitive statement of the factors involved in the presenting problem (communication handicap) and the degree to which each is involved (Brooks, 1978, p. 133)," then clinicians must be willing to correct any barriers in the transfer of information between the older person and themselves. Here, general management considerations are a part of the clinician's interpersonal skills and attitudes.

Even as clinicians we are likely to harbor many of the negative attitudes toward older persons that society in general holds. When we encounter older persons in the context of our professional roles, Mean (1977, p. 73) indicates that we may respond in a variety of negative ways:

1. We may react emotionally to our own feelings of aging and death;
2. We may feel threatened or discouraged by the older person's lack of motivation;
3. We may want to return to work with younger or middle-aged persons who have a "future;"

4. We may feel threatened by the emotional demands of the older person;

5. We may see the person as senile, inflexible, intolerant, talkative, mentally ill, hypochondriacal, and so forth.

We are not alone among health professionals in our tendency to apply labels and stereotypes to older persons that ultimately interfere with our realistic assessment of their communication skills. In a study of psychiatrists, Ford and Sbordone (1980) found that these professionals (a) considered older patients less ideal to work with than younger patients, (b) gave poorer prognoses to older patients than to younger patients with the same degree of impairment, and (c) used psychotherapy less often and prescribed drugs more often to older patients than to younger ones. We must realize and accept that part of the effective management of older persons is the management of our own attitudes and behaviors toward older persons.

A particularly valuable clinical skill is the appropriate use of interpersonal communication, defined as the "process of sending and receiving messages between two persons, or among a small group of persons, with some effect and some immediate feedback" (DeVito, 1983, p. 5-6). In the process of interpersonal communication, a source (clinician, older person) formulates a message and sends the message via a number of message channels (auditory, visual, tactile, kinesthetic) to a receiver (clinician, older person) who interprets the message. The receiver may then respond to the message with another message (feedback). Such feedback is necessary between clinician and older person for effective communication, because it allows each person to modify communication behaviors in appropriate ways.

Surrounding the source-message-receiver (feedback) process is the field of experience which indicates that effective communication takes place only to the extent that the participants share common experiences. Although we cannot always share the direct experiences of others (those of us who are not old or have communicative disorders), can learn to empathize with people different from ourselves (Dancer & Keiser, 1980; Dancer & Keiser, 1981) and thus extend our field of experience. Communication with older persons may be particularly difficult because of cultural as well as personal differences between the client and the clinician (Monfils, 1979). A knowledge of effective interpersonal and intercultural communication should help the clinician to facilitate the information-gathering stage of the assessment process.

Older persons themselves are also likely to harbor ageist attitudes toward themselves and their abilities. One can hardly escape the negative messages about aging that pervade our culture. Butler and Lewis (1982) indicated that in our Western civilization, <u>decline</u> has been the key concept in relation to aging and <u>neglect</u> has been the major treatment. Whereas Butler and Lewis point out that in many older persons old age can be an emotionally healthy and satisfying time of life with a minimum of physical and mental impairment, . . ."the healthy aged tend to be invisible in the psychology of human development, and this is in accord with the general public avoidance of the issues of human aging" (p. 23). Thus, older persons are likely to be unduly pessimistic about their communication abilities and reluctant to seek or respond positively to our intervention. Such pessimism is fostered in those older persons who realize that their own aging is accompanied by sensory decrements, declining social support, financial difficulties, and multiple chronic illnesses. Small wonder that many older persons are difficult-to-test and lack sufficient motivation for change.

Data Base Appropriate for Facilitating the Assessment Process

According to Hull (1980), the data base necessary for the adequate management of the communication needs of an older person will vary depending upon the overall characteristics of the population served and the setting within which that service takes place. For example, an audiologist who serves the hearing needs of healthy and secure older persons in the higher socioeconomic levels might need little information beyond that which is discipline-specific. Thus, an audiologic case history form, a protocol for the audiologic assessment of impairment (Maurer & Rupp, 1979) and of handicap (Ventry & Weinstein, 1982), and a communication skills assessment/hearing aid evaluation and fitting (Alpiner, 1982) may be the primary components in the overall management plan which in turn lead to specific recommendations for aural rehabilitation. Even in this situation, the audiologist must consider the many nonauditory factors that enter into successful management. The success or failure of rehabilitation often depends upon the audiologist's ability to deal with factors such as motivation, visual and manual dexterity problems, attitudes toward amplification, and so forth (Rupp, Higgins, & Maurer, 1977).

More and more, we are serving older persons in settings that require an exhaustive interdisciplinary data base from many disciplines other than our own--social workers, psychologists, physicians, nurses, pharmacists, nutritionists, gerontologists, dentists, occupational therapists, and physical therapists as examples. Such a data base may appear as part of a comprehensive Problem-Oriented Health Record (Ferguson, 1980). In such an interdisciplinary setting, the professional in communicative disorders functions as a member of a health care team. The team members cooperatively explore the problems of an older person from many perspectives.

o Audiologists see a confused older person who does not understand or follow instructions and explore the possibility that a hearing loss may be the primary cause.

o Speech-language pathologists see the same person and look for a loss in linguistic processing.

o Pharmacists see the same person and look for drugs or drug interactions.

o Physicians look for signs of organic brain syndrome.

o Psychologists look for signs of depression.

o Nutritionists look for poor eating habits.

Only within the context of team discussion and debate can a diagnosis emerge that takes into account all of the relevant information from all disciplines. The professional in communicative disorders has a pivotal role on any interdisciplinary health care team, and it becomes imperative that we understand and apply the concepts of team dynamics. Not only do we serve in team meetings as an advocate for the communication needs of the older persons we have assessed, but we also serve as the only member of the team with specific training in both the normal processes of communication and their pathologies. The education of other team members as to the importance of communication in the life of the older person and in the appropriate methods/strategies for better communication with older persons will significantly enhance the collection of information which underlies the data base. We should not underestimate the importance of our role in the ultimate team management of older persons, and we should work to acquire the characteristics and skills of successful team members (Dancer & Thomas, 1983).

Adapting Examining Procedures to the Individual

The general protocol of the speech-language or audiologic assessment of an older person does not differ greatly, in principle, from that used in younger age groups (Krueger & Cicciarelli, 1981; Maurer & Rupp, 1979). Indeed, Giolas (1982) recommends that we begin by assuming that the standard assessment procedure is appropriate and by allowing the situation and the performance of the individual to dictate the necessary modifications. Such modifications may be based on specific problems which occur during the testing process. Schow, Christensen, Hutchinson, and Nerbonne (1978) offer a specific listing of problems which might occur such as confusion, anxiety, memory loss, fatigue, bizarre responses, and so forth. For each problem, they offer some possible solutions. For example, they suggest that when confusion over the task occurs, the clinician may (a) repeat instructions, giving examples or demonstrations where possible, (b) present information more slowly, and (c) allow for adequate response time. As another example, if anxiety over the test situation is present, suggestions include (a) familiarization with the examiner and testing situation, (b) a brief period of conversation before examination, and (c) positive reinforcement and encouragement during testing.

For audiological testing, Kopra (1982, p. 319) suggests that the underlying principle in the modification of traditional audiologic techniques is. . . "if a listener is not able to respond reliably to a given auditory task, progressively simplify the task until the listener is able to respond reliably." Thus, if the older person cannot reliably respond to the traditional single-tone presentation because of tinnitus, the clinician may use a pulsed or warbled tone to simplify the task. If the older person cannot reliably respond to spondee words, more redundant units such as paired digits might be used. Of course, once a modification has been made, the validity of that modification must be known. That is, does the modification produce the same test results as the more traditional technique? In the case of pulsed-tone thresholds, a number of studies (Dancer & Conn, in press; Dancer, Ventry, & Hill, 1976; Waltzman & Hochberg, 1972) show that such thresholds do not differ significantly from those obtained with single-tone presentations.

Thus, clinicians must keep in mind that the ultimate purpose of the assessment is to determine a reliable and valid picture of the older person's communication skills. Any modification that enhances or clarifies a person's functional abilities adds to the success of the overall management plan.

Education of Family and Significant Others

A necessary component in the overall management of older persons with communicative disorders is the education of family members and significant others of their role in facilitating the assessment/management process. Dancer and Keiser (1980) give three purposes of programs that focus on the family or significant others. Such programs should (a) lead to a better understanding of the impact of speech, language, or hearing disorders on the everyday communicative abilities of the affected individual, (b) increase the person's willingness to help the older person with a communicative disorder, and (c) provide specific suggestions that persons can use to increase the likelihood of successful communication.

Dancer and Keiser view empathy training as an important first step in motivating support persons to learn and apply effective communication behaviors. The concept of empathy is one of placing ourselves in another person's position, sharing their experiences, and thinking and feeling as that person thinks and feels. Thus, empathy training allows us to become more sensitive to and aware of the needs and values of others, even though those needs and values may be different from our own. Such training is often necessary to counter the generally negative attitudes that persons hold toward communication impairments and toward the elderly. Fortunately, empathy appears to be a skill or trait that can be enhanced through appropriate educational experiences (Dampier, Dancer, & Keiser, in press; Dancer & Keiser, 1981).

If we assume that empathy toward older persons with communicative disorders can be enhanced by developing perceived similarities in ourselves and in older persons, then we can structure learning activities that promote empathic responses. One particularly effective demonstration is a simulation experience in which family members/significant others assume the role of a person with a communication handicap. For example, the person plays a game of Bingo recorded on an audiotape in which filtering has been used to make the numbers and letters all but unintelligible (Dancer & Keiser, 1980). After failing to Bingo on the task, the point that hearing-impaired persons often "hear, but can't understand" is not difficult to make.

Health professionals in general need to be made aware of the strong correlation between decreased auditory acuity and lower scores on the Mental Status Questionnaire (Ohta, Carlin, & Harmon, 1982). The Mental Status Questionnaire is a commonly-used measure to assess the degree of organic brain syndrome. Ohta et al. (1982, p. 1) interpret their findings as indicating . . ."a causal relationship between sensory acuity and test performance and indicating that the cognitive capabilities of elderly individuals may be underestimated as a result of reduced sensory acuity." Family members are also likely to interpret confusions or misinterpretations on the part of an older family member as evidence of cognitive changes ("Grandpa must be getting senile") rather than as evidence of hearing or vision changes.

A recent text by Shadden, Raiford, and Shadden (1983) offers the professional in communicative disorders a complete in-service program on speech, language, and hearing disorders. The program offers numerous exercises and an audiotape that allows persons to experience through simulation the communication difficulties and frustrations of persons with aphasia, hearing loss, and Parkinson's disease. Similarly, the Dancer-Keiser audiotape on hearing loss (1980) offers simulation exercises that place the individual in listening situations that have been filtered to provide the experience of reduced speech understanding.

Successful management requires that families/significant others not only be sensitized to the problems but also be offered specific suggestions for enhancing successful communication. The suggestions are easy, simple to use, and oftentimes mean the difference between success and failure in any given communication situation. It is wise to remember that what seems obvious to professionals in communicative disorders might not have occurred to family members/significant others.

   o Get the person's attention before beginning to talk
   o Talk in a face-to-face manner with the person
   o Make sure the lighting is appropriate

o Speak a little louder and a little more slowly

o Make questions or statements simple and straightforward and rephrase, rather than repeat, if necessary

o Allow the person more time for a response

o Avoid distracting or noisy backgrounds

o If you are not sure that the person understood, ask a verification question (e.g., "What time should you take your pill?")

o Find a listening area that reduces reverberations to a minimum

o Use assistive communication devices, if necessary

o Above all, <u>ask</u> the person what helps most in communication.

Rather than just providing these suggestions, you will need to insure through role-playing activities that family members/significant others can actually perform the suggestions you have offered.

Summary

In summary, speech-language pathologists and audiologists interested in working with communicatively handicapped older persons need extensive academic preparation and practical experience in a number of areas:

1. Clinicians must account and compensate for the common problems in assessment that result from the normal aging processes within each individual, regardless of their primary communicative disorder;

2. Clinicians must have a knowledge of effective interpersonal and intercultural communication strategies that are facilitative to the information-gathering stage of the assessment process;

3. Clinicians must be able to function within an interdisciplinary team effort and must be able to effectively advocate the communication needs of older persons to other team members;

4. Clinicians must be able to modify the standard tests to take into account the special problems encountered when assessing older persons;

5. Clinicians must function as educators of family/significant others in their role as facilitators of the communication process.

Self-Study Questions

1. Outline the academic coursework and practicum experiences necessary for speech-language pathologists or audiologists to manage the communication problems of older persons.

2. Outline an assessment/management protocol appropriate for use with older persons in your particular work setting (or assumed work setting).

REFERENCES

Alpiner, J. (1982). Handbook of rehabilitative audiology. (2nd ed.). Baltimore: Williams & Wilkins.

Beasley, D., & Davis, G. (1981). Aging, communication processes and disorders. New York: Grune & Stratton.

Beck, C. (1980). Assessment of the elderly. In W. Thomas (Ed.), Student oriented learning outlines in interdisciplinary geriatrics. Little Rock, AR: University of Arkansas for Medical Sciences.

Bergman, M. (1980). Aging and the perception of speech. Baltimore: University Park Press.

Brooks, D. (1978). Evaluation of hard-to-test children and adults. In Diagnostic procedures in hearing, language, and speech. Baltimore: University Park Press.

Butler, R., & Lewis, M. (1982). Aging and mental health. (3rd ed.). C. V. Mosby.

Dampier, K., Dancer, J., & Keiser, H. (in press). Changing attitudes toward older persons with hearing loss: Comparison of two audiotapes. American Annals of the Deaf.

Dancer, J., & Conn, M. (in press). Effects of two procedural modifications on the frequency of false alarm responses during pure-tone threshold determination. Journal of Auditory Research.

Dancer, J., & Keiser, H. (1980). The hearing-impaired elderly: Training others to help. Hearing Aid Journal, 33, 10, 36-37.

Dancer, J., & Keiser, H. (1981). The effect of empathy training on geriatric-care nurses. Journal of Self Help for Hard-of-Hearing People, 2, 3-4, 9.

Dancer, J., & Thomas, W. (1983). Beyond the boundaries: Interdisciplinary health care of the elderly. Asha, 25, 25-30.

Dancer, J., & Ventry, I., & Hill, W. (1976). Effects of stimulus presentation and instructions on pure-tone thresholds and false-alarm responses. Journal of Speech and Hearing Disorders, 41, 315-324.

Devito, J. (1983). The interpersonal communication book. (3rd ed.). New York: Harper & Row.

Ferguson, D. (1980). Problem oriented records. In W. Thomas (Ed.), Student oriented outlines in interdisciplinary geriatrics. Little Rock, AR: University of Arkansas for Medical Sciences.

Ford, C., & Sbordone, R. (1980). Attitudes of psychiatrists toward elderly patients, American Journal of Psychiatry, 137, 571-575.

Giolas, T. (1982). Hearing handicapped adults. Englewood Cliffs, NJ: Prentice-Hall.

Hull, R. (1980). Aural rehabilitation for the elderly. In R. Schow & M. Nerbonne (Eds.), Introduction to aural rehabilitation. Baltimore: University Park Press.

Kahane, J. (1981). Anatomic changes in the aging peripheral speech mechanism. In D. Beasley & G. Davis (Eds.), Aging, communication processes and disorders. New York: Grune & Stratton.

Kopra, L. (1982). Modifications of traditional techniques for assessment of the elderly client. In R. Hull (Ed.), Rehabilitative audiology. New York: Grune & Stratton.

Kent, R., & Burkard, R. (1981). Changes in the acoustic correlates of speech production. In D. Beasley & G. Davis (Eds.), Aging, communication processes and disorders. New York: Grune & Stratton.

Krueger, K., & Ciccareilli, T. (1981). Protocol for the assessment of older persons with speech-language problems. Unpublished assessment protocol, Little Rock Veterans Administration Medical Center, Little Rock, AR.

Maurer, J., & Rupp, R. (1979). Hearing and aging. New York: Grune & Stratton.

Mean, B. (1977). How to relate to the elderly patient. Geriatrics, 11, 73-77.

Monfils, B. (1979). Verbal communication patterns of the elderly. Paper presented at the meeting of the Speech Communication Association convention, San Francisco, CA.

Nadol, Jr., J. (1981). The aging peripheral hearing mechanism. In D. Beasley & G. Davis (Eds.), Aging, communication processes and disorders. New York: Grune & Stratton.

Obler, L., & Albert, M. (1981). Language and aging: A neurobehavioral analysis. In D. Beasley & G. Davis (Eds.), Aging, communication processes and disorders. New York: Grune & Stratton.

Ohta, R., Carlin, M., & Harmon, B. (1982). Auditory acuity and performance on the mental status questionnaire in the elderly. Unpublished manuscript, West Virginia University.

Oyer, H., & Oyer, J. (1976). Aging and communication. Baltimore: University Park Press.

Rupp, R., Higgins, J., & Maurer, J. (1977). A feasibility scale for predicting hearing aid use with older individuals. Journal of the Academy of Rehabilitative Audiology, 10, 81-104.

Schow, R., Christensen, J., Hutchinson, J., & Nerbonne, M. (1978). Communication disorders of the aged. Baltimore: University Park Press.

Shadden, B., Raiford, C., & Shadden, H. (1983). Communication disorders of the aged: A workshop. Tigaard, OR: C. C. Publications.

Ventry, I., & Weinstein, B. (1982). The hearing handicap inventory for the elderly: A new tool. Ear and Hearing, 4, 128-134.

Waltzman, S., & Hochberg, I. (1972). Comparison of pulsed and continuous tone thresholds in patients with tinnitus. Audiology, 2, 337-342.

Rehabilitation of Speech and Language Disorders

G. Albyn Davis
University of Massachusetts, Amherst

and

Terry W. Baggs
Memphis State University, Tennessee

With the expanding number of elderly persons in the United States, there is an accompanying increase in the number of people with communication disorders that are in general, unique to adulthood, and old age in particular. Speech disorders of adulthood include apraxia of speech, dysarthria, and alaryngeal speech due to laryngectomy. Language impairments of adulthood include (a) the primary language disorders of aphasia, and (b) secondary deficits that reflect primary impairments of intellect and more specific cognitive functions. The main reason that these communication disorders occur in adulthood can be traced to their causes, which include medical conditions that either are occasional unfortunate consequences of adult living (e.g., automobile accidents, excessive smoking) or are exaggerations of subtle disease processes that are characteristic of older persons (e.g., stroke).

In this chapter, we shall be concerned with many of the unique issues that age and aging bring to bear on the identification, assessment, and treatment of communication disorders. We shall use the term "aging" to refer primarily to characteristics of old age rather than to its more literal meaning as a lifelong process of development, culmination, and decline. In order to provide an initial frame of reference, we have listed most of the disorders and their mean ages of onset in Table 1. These ages indicate that some disorders are more likely to be seen after age 65 than other disorders. At least, communicatively impaired subjects in basic and applied research are most likely to be elderly only with certain disorders. In addressing the clinical literature for writing this chapter, our experience has been that most case presentations involve clients younger than age 60; but, when clients are older than 65, authors do not express anything particularly unique about assessing or treating the elderly age group. This inattention points to the need for

writing such a chapter in which much is based on our individual clinical
experience and intuition.

Table 1. Mean ages for the different language and speech disorders.

	Mean age
Language disorders	
Aphasia: General	50-60
Wernicke's aphasia	62-67
Dementia of Alzheimer's disease	58-74
Speech disorders	
Apraxia of speech (in Broca's aphasia)	50-56
Ataxic dysarthria	48
Hypokinetic dysarthria (Parkinson's)	> 67
Mixed dysarthrias: Multiple Sclerosis	30 *
Amyotrophic Lateral Sclerosis	57
Alaryngeal speech (laryngectomy)	58-62

Note. Mean ages were determined from examination of a variety of large-N
studies (N = number of subjects) and articles reporting demographic data. The
ranges are ranges of means. These figures represent a mixture of age at onset
and age at hospital admission. *Represents peak age.

Primary and Secondary Deficits

An understanding of certain relationships between aging and communicative
disorders depends upon understanding the distinction between primary deficits
and secondary deficits. This distinction is based on the recognition that
motor systems and cognitive systems interact with each other; and within each
of these major systems, there are motor and cognitive subsystems that interact
as well. It is relevant at all levels of differential diagnosis, namely, in
distinguishing among different disorders and among different patterns of
deficit within a disorder category. In other words, the primary deficit of
dysarthria (i.e., neuromuscular impairment) can be distinguished from the
primary deficit of aphasia (i.e., cognitive impairment of language function).
Moreover, within the dysarthrias, flaccid dysarthria is based on a primary
deficit (i.e., lower motor neuron impairment) that differs from the primary
deficit of spastic dysarthria (i.e., upper motor neuron impairment). These
primary impairments of the nervous system produce varied secondary deficits of
speech production.

At the heart of this matter is the definition of what is a speech or language disorder requiring services of the speech-language pathologist. Decisions pertain to identifying problems for which the clinician has a rehabilitative role and, then, to defining what that role should be depending on the communicative phenomenon under consideration. Relative to aging, if Alzheimer's dementia is considered to be a communication disorder, we should understand that linguistic and other communicative problems are often secondary to the primary intellectual deficits of dementia. Efficient medical and/or behavioral treatment of any disorder is directed at the primary deficit(s). Regarding Alzheimer's dementia, the primary deficits may not in many cases be a speech or language disorder per se.

Language Disorders

Language disorders may occur in the absence of a speech disorder and in the absence of any other modality-specific disorder such as hearing loss or vision loss. Because of the dependence of language function on basic cognitive structures and processes, impairment of language is a "central" disorder manifested through all peripheral modalities (auditory, visual, oral, and graphic). However, an older language-impaired adult is more likely than a younger adult patient to possess additional disorders affecting communicative ability, such as sensory impairments or memory problems.

Aphasia

The primary language disorder of adulthood is aphasia. Aphasia, an impairment of central processes contributing specifically to language function, is caused by damage to areas of the brain that are primarily responsible for the language function. These areas are located in the left cerebral hemisphere for most people. (For convenience, and to be consistent with prevailing common practice, the "left hemisphere" will be identified as the verbal hemisphere; and the "right hemisphere" will be designated as the nonverbal hemisphere).

The average age of current clinical populations of persons with aphasia appears to be between 55 and 57 years, as indicated by large-N studies dominated by victims of stroke (Davis & Holland, 1981). When large-N studies are dominated by head injury, as in the studies of war-injured populations, most subjects are below age 50 with some averaging in their 20s (e.g., Wepman,

1951). There can still be some variation in the central tendencies of large groups dominated by stroke. Of the 357 standardization sample for the current Porch Index of Communicative Abilities (PICA) test norms (Porch, 1981), only the original group of 150 were thoroughly described (Porch, 1967). The mean age of this group was 61 years. The mean age of the 281 patients studied by Basso, Capitani, and Vignolo (1979) was 50 years. Detailed characteristics of large samples often are not presented (Goodglass & Kaplan, 1983; their revised standardization sample), and so age characteristics of samples in important clinical research are sometimes difficult to determine.

The Syndromes and Age

The language function consists of multiple subsystems that have been identified primarily with respect to the linguistic descriptors of syntax, semantics, and phonology. It appears that these components can be selectively impaired depending on location of damage within the left hemisphere, as determined by modern methods of linguistic analysis and lesion location. When brain damage occurs in a particular location (which certainly is not the case in all instances of aphasia), recognizable patterns of secondary symptoms occur. These patterns are referred to as syndromes reflecting the multifarious nature of aphasia. Several classification schemes have arisen throughout the historical development of aphasiology. The most common classification system currently in use by researchers is the neoclassical scheme associated with the Boston group of investigators (see Goodglass & Kaplan, 1983). Because the syndromes do not always occur in "pure form" and aphasias occur in varied mixes, the syndromes should be considered as prototypes of the ways in which aphasic patterns can differ from each other, thereby contributing to the uniqueness of each patient.

Several demographic investigations of aphasia have indicated that there is a relationship between the syndromes and age (Harasymiw, Halper, & Sutherland, 1981; Holland, 1980; Kertesz & Sheppard, 1981; Obler, Albert, Goodglass, & Benson, 1978). The most consistent finding is that the average of persons with Wernicke's aphasia is 10-12 years older than persons with Broca's aphasia. Persons with Broca's aphasia are usually younger than the overall mean age of aphasic persons (e.g., 56 years in Obler's study and around 59 years in Harasymiw's study), while persons with Wernicke's aphasia are generally older than the mean age for aphasia. For example, in a review of 398 cases in

188

Boston, Obler et al. (1978) found the median age of Broca's aphasia to be 51 years and the median age of Wernicke's aphasia to be 63 years. In Harasymiw's perusal of 358 case records in Chicago, male and female cases of Broca's aphasia averaged nearly 56 years of age, while male Wernicke's aphasias averaged 67 years and females averaged about 62 years.

Different explanations for this age difference have been proposed, such as Brown and Jaffe's (1975) theory that organization of function in the cerebral cortex continues to evolve into the later adult years. Eslinger and Damasio (1981), having found similar age differences in a smaller sample, suggested that stroke in the middle cerebral artery may shift posteriorly with advancing age. However, they added that there was no verification of this possibility with the localization of lesions in their sample. Another possibility is that the biological and cognitive/sensory changes of aging interact with a focal lesion in the left temporal lobe to produce the unique characteristics of Wernicke's aphasia. Even if such a theoretical notion cannot be proved, the clinician should at least expect that a person with Wernicke's aphasia is likely to possess additional problems characteristic of old age. The severe difficulties with comprehension in this type of aphasia may be compounded by the sensory losses of aging.

Etiology, Aging, and Recovery

The most frequent cause of aphasia in the elderly is stroke, the prevalence of which triples between the ages of 45 to 54 and 65 to 74 from 2% to 6%. Among people over age 75, the prevalence of CVA approaches 10% (Sahs, Hartman, & Aronson, 1976). The increasing prevalence of stroke with advancing age has been attributed to the idea that stroke is often a sudden and dramatic aberration of changes occurring in the aging central nervous system. These changes include an increase in blood pressure due in part to changes in arteries resulting from arteriosclerotic disease processes. Therefore, stroke may arise from unrecognized incipient disease processes that accompany aging but are not components of normal aging. It has been suggested that cerebral blood flow diminishes with advancing age; however, the presence of age-related differences is often influenced by the presence of older persons with dementia and arteriosclerosis in the sample studied (Valenstein, 1981). When these confounding factors are eliminated, age differences in blood flow are not observed.

Stroke, especially ischemic CVAs, produces a characteristic recovery pattern that influences the clinician's prognosis for improvement of language functions (Davis, 1983). Immediately after onset, a temporary period of generalized reduction of blood flow causes impairments of functions remote from the site of lesion (called "diaschisis"). After 2-3 weeks, the pattern of spared and impaired functions becomes discernible; and recovery of impaired functions can begin to be more clearly measured. However, the period of diaschisis has been shown to be longer for persons older than age 60 than for persons younger than age 60 (Meyer, Kanda, Fukuuchi, Shimazu, Dennis, & Ericsson, 1971). Some degree of recovery after stroke is inevitable, tempered by initial severity of the overall deficit. This inevitable recovery is called "spontaneous recovery." Most recovery occurs during the initial 2 months after onset. Rate of recovery of overall language function begins to slow down after these 2 months, and some leveling of recovery has been observed from 6 to 12 months post-onset.

A picture of recovery in terms of overall language function is incomplete. Although auditory comprehension may show large and rapid early gains during the first 2 months, verbal function appears to improve at a slower rate and for longer period of time. Amount of auditory gain has been measured to be greater than verbal gain within 4 months after onset. However, at 12 months post-onset, the amount of verbal gain is likely to be greater than the amount of measured auditory gain, except for severely impaired aphasic persons. Treatment may produce improvements in verbal, graphic, and gestural functions beyond the first year after onset.

Amount and rate of improvement is subject to wide variation, depending in part on factors that accompany the aging process. Chronological age has been considered to be a powerful factor in the clinician's decisions about prognosis (Davis, 1983; Wertz, 1983). However, relatively large-N research (with a reasonably broad age range) has not been of much support in proving that recovery and age are correlated in patients with stroke (Basso, Capitani, & Vignolo, 1979; Kertesz & McCabe, 1977). An exception is a study of 80 CVA patients ranging from 35 to 73 years of age, in which age was one of six variables that predicted good or poor "terminal speech performance" (Marshall & Phillips, 1983). One reason for negative findings regarding age and recovery is that age generally is not controlled in the initial design of a recovery study. For example, assurances that all age levels are comparable with respect to education, living status, medical status, and other confounding variables are not provided. Marshall and Phillips found that one of the other six significant variables was general health, which varies with age. Another reason for apparently contradictory findings is that chronological age is often a poor predictor of status with respect to these other variables. Aging occurs, of course; but it is difficult to characterize the typical 70-year-old, because aging occurs at different times and rates among individuals.

A reviewer of the literature should consider these issues, but look beyond the investigator(s) conclusions to examine the basis for these conclusions. For example, Pickersgill and Lincoln (1983) concluded that recovery is independent of age; but no subject was older than 69, thereby removing much of the elderly population from consideration. Such conclusions, therefore, are not wrong; they simply apply to characteristics of materials, processes, or subjects that were studied.

When thinking about age in predicting recovery with aphasia, the clinician should consider using chronological age only as an index of the client's status relative to other factors that accompany aging. Therefore, consideration is given to medical status, psychological status, availability of a support system, motivation, living environment and so on, in order to decide upon the possible influence of "age." The clinician should not conclude that the age of 75 is necessarily a negative indicator regarding recovery. It might be negative if the particular 75-year-old is a person who has arteriosclerosis, diabetes and arthritis, is depressed, living in a nursing home without family visitation, and not interested in talking to anyone. It may be taken lightly if the 75-year-old were living at home in a thriving 50-year marriage, playing golf regularly, and writing his memoirs. As Davis (1983) concluded, "aging probably does provide a magnet which draws recovery backward to some extent...However, it is aging and not age that makes a difference" (p. 107). One reason for well-controlled studies of normal aging are needed is to determine whether the second type of 75-year-old harbors subtle changes that have impacted in relatively minor ways on his or her lifestyle and, yet, still may serve as a low-power magnet that might affect recovery.

Focal Nonverbal Impairments

During the past 5 years or so, speech-language pathologists have become interested in people with right (nonverbal or minor) hemisphere damage. This concern has paralleled interest in pragmatics as a means of characterizing a complete view of language as it is used for natural communicative purposes. As we are learning about how language function interacts with context, we are learning about how left hemisphere functions interact with right hemisphere functions. Pragmatics is becoming the framework by which we are learning that people with right hemisphere damage may have communication problems.

Because right hemisphere problems arise from the same etiologies that produce aphasia, age-related factors pertaining to stroke apply to the "other" hemisphere as well. A consideration unique to this clinical population is the speculation that the right hemisphere may be more susceptible to aging than the left hemisphere. This speculation is based primarily on behavioral measures that are indicative of hemisphere use, such as the observation that verbal skills "hold" and nonverbal skills "don't hold" with advancing age (Johnson, Cole, Bowers, Foiles, Nikaido, Patrick, & Woliver, 1979; Kocel, 1980). Rather than there being greater structural or physiological change in the right hemisphere, these observations may be a function of shifts in cognitive strategy with age or a function of the manner in which nonverbal skills are often tested (e.g., speed tasks).

Persons with damage to the right hemisphere may have disturbances of orientation in time and space, visuospatial integration, music perception, and emotional recognition and expression (Myers, 1984). A common characteristic of these disturbances is that they reflect difficulties in the use of the integrative or holistic cognitive style attributed to the right hemisphere. These primary deficits, which occur in various combinations in different patients, may affect utilization of the contexts of language function and, therefore, the interaction of language with these contexts (Foldi, Cicone, & Gardner, 1983; Gardner, Brownell, Wapner, & Michelow, 1983; Millar & Whitaker, 1983). For example, amusia and/or muted emotions may be responsible for impairments of paralinguistic context (i.e., prosody) in the comprehension and expression of emotion. When comprehending the intent of an utterance involves relating language to extralinguistic or linguistic context, persons with right hemisphere-damage have some trouble. They tend to be literal in their interpretations of metaphor. They miss the point of stories, and sometimes do not stay on the point when telling a story. They may miss the point of a joke. These communication disorders are only beginning to be defined, and there has been minimal organized attempt as yet to examine treatments of these problems.

Dementia of Alzheimer's Disease

In her review of language in dementia (or "generalized intellectual impairment"), Bayles (1984) cited research showing that 10% of persons over age 65 suffer from mild dementia, with 1% suffering from severe dementia. With about 25 million Americans presently older than 65, this is a substantial number of people. (It also may be necessary to note that, therefore, 90% of persons over age 65 may not be suffering from dementia.) The symptoms of dementia, involving a generalized reduction of a wide range of cognitive functions, do not necessarily originate from progressive diseases with gradual onset. A person may accumulate several small ischemic CVAs producing what is commonly called "multi-infarct" dementia. Some dementias are treatable (e.g., the alcohol abuse and vitamin B deficiency of Korsakoff's syndrome), and others might be thought of as "pseudodementias" due to depression or excessive medication. Both treatable and untreatable dementias occur frequently in old age, because depression and excessive medication are problems frequently encountered by the elderly. Etiologies may not necessarily be cortical in location, as Albert (1978) has referred to subcortical dementias (e.g., (Parkinson's disease). In studies of persons with dementia, it may become important to specify the etiology as precisely as possible, or, as in Bayles and Tomoeda's (1983) study of naming, differentiate among groups of persons with dementia.

Alzheimer's disease is the principal cause of dementia in late adulthood. Usually diagnosed by a process of eliminating other more obvious causes, subject groups may be labeled as having "suspected Alzheimer's disease" (Martin & Fedio, 1983). The label has been used to refer to a progressive dementia beginning prior to age 65 (pre-senile dementia), with "senile dementia" occurring after age 65. Because the underlying pathology of both is the same, the arbitrariness of the age 65 division has been recognized. Alzheimer's disease is now considered to represent a progressive dementia due to several changes in the central nervous system that can occur at any age of middle through late adulthood. Furthermore, since the central nervous system changes

193

in this disease are seen to a lesser degree in normally aging brains, Alzheimer's disease sometimes has been used as a means of examining normal aging "under a microscope." Although possible qualitative differences between normal aging and Alzheimer's disease have yet to be determined, one possibility lies in the chemical composition of normal and pathological brains (Valenstein, 1981). The pathology causes progressive deterioration of cognitive functions involved in orientation, memory, intelligence, and judgement. Pyramidal tract dysfunction (i.e., hemiparesis, hyperreflexia) and loss of primary sensory functions are "exceedingly rare" in this disorder (Fernandez & Samuels, 1982).

It may be difficult to expect a single characterization of the deficits in Alzheimer's dementia. In a single patient, the disease progresses from a very mild to a very severe form over several months or years. This progression has been described with respect to three stages: early, intermediate, and later stages (Obler & Albert, 1981). The linguistic behavior of the early stage has been compared to anomic aphasia, whereas the late stage in some individuals may give the appearance of Wernick's aphasia. Therefore, comparisons of these patients with the normal elderly or with aphasic adults should be made with an identification of stage of progression in the subjects with dementia. Bayles and Tomoeda (1983), for example, distinguished between mild and moderate cases of Alzheimer's disease in their study of naming behavior.

The speech and language deficits of Alzheimer's dementia are becoming better understood through clinical scrutiny and formal research. The mechanics of speech production are not impaired; however, other causes of dementia, such as Huntington's disease and Parkinson's disease, produce speech disorders. As noted by Bayles (1984), the linguistic components of phonology, syntax, and semantics are not uniformly impaired. With dementia, the linguistic problems appear to be centered on the semantic component which is closely related to more general conceptual aspects of cognition. Although naming difficulty is a central characteristic of even the mildest forms of aphasia, persons with mild Alzheimer's disease, as well as other mild dementias, have not shown a deficit in confrontation naming (Bayles & Tomoeda, 1983). Naming errors of moderate dementias are common and increase in severity. These errors were once characterized as reflecting perceptual deficits, but more comprehensive research has shown that most errors are semantically related to targets and become less related with increasing severity of deficit (Bayles & Tomoeda, 1983; Martin & Fedio, 1983). Pragmatic dimensions of language function (i.e., use of language in context) become severely disrupted in the late stage of dementia, with failure to establish eye contact and socially inappropriate utterances. Some of the most severely impaired persons may be essentially mute and may show no interest in communicating.

Speech Disorders

Speech disorders include impairments of the mechanics of speech production, with language comprehension and the capacity to produce language remaining intact. When limb impairment is absent or minimal, persons with speech disorders are able to use language normally through the writing modality. Speech disorders may occur at a number of levels of the production system, including respiration, phonation, resonance, and articulation.

Apraxia of Speech

Apraxia of speech is a disruption of the volitional coordination of oral movements for the purpose of speech production, usually without damage to the neuromuscular system for speech (Werz, LaPointe, & Rosenbek, 1984). It is primarily an impairment of articulation. Without damage to the neuromuscular system, vegetative uses of the oral mechanisms remain intact except for infrequent occurrence of cortical dysphagia; and, intact subpropositional speech is usually much more fluent than propositional speech production. Because a lesion in the frontal cortex causes apraxia of speech, this disorder often accompanies Broca's aphasia. Some neurologists consider apraxia of speech to be a definitive component of this nonfluent aphasia. However, apraxia of speech may occur without clear evidence of language disorder; conversely, Broca's aphasia may occur without demonstrative evidence of verbal apraxia. Apraxia of speech is caused by the same etiologies that produce aphasia, and so our discussion of stroke applies to this speech disorder as well.

Dysarthria

Dysarthria, an impairment of the neuromuscular system that is used for the production of speech (Darley, Aronson, & Brown, 1975), it may affect all levels of the production system in a single patient. Paralysis of these muscles impairs vegetative functions as well; for example, impairing the swallowing function, a disorder called "dysphagia." Age characteristics of this population in general are difficult to find; in one large-N study, with 212 subjects, ages of subjects were not reported (Darley, Aronson, & Brown, 1969). As in aphasia, age characteristics will follow from etiology with many cases stemming from head injury in teenagers as well as from the strokes typical of older age.

Dysarthria may be caused by damage to the central and/or peripheral nervous systems; thus, depending on site of damage, dysarthrias of different types may occur. For example, damage to the peripheral nervous system results in muscle weakness as the primary disorder, and is observed as a "hypo-reflexia." A person will talk slowly and with slurred articulation if he or she has this flaccid dysarthria. Damage to the central nervous system can produce some weakness, but can also cause rigidity of the muscles and a "hyper-reflexia." A mild slurring of speech may be disrupted by bursts of loud and forceful production in these cases of spastic dysarthria. Ataxic dysarthria occurs when the coordination center (cerebellum) is damaged and causes difficulty in controlling the speed, range, and direction of speech muscle movement. Prognosis for recovery depends to a great extent on the etiology, with many causes of dysarthria concentrated in the middle-aged and older adult population (Brown, Darby, & Aronson, 1970).

Parkinson's disease usually begins between the ages of 50 to 70. Appel (1981) suggested that the mean age of onset is 67 years. It produces a speech dysfunction called hypokinetic dysarthria. The most frequently cited cause is damage to the midbrain (substantia nigra) which reduces dopamine levels. Dopamine acts to inhibit electrical action potentials in the corpus striatum, a subcortical structure in the cerebrum that is part of the extrapyramidal motor system. Another cause may be drug-induced, which would be of concern to elderly persons receiving multiple medications. In particular, long-term large doses of phenothiazine, typically prescribed for sedation or nausea, can result in central nervous system damage (Hildick-Smith, 1983). Hypokinetic dysarthria is characterized by tremor of muscles while at rest as well as reduced range and variable speed of articulatory movement. It is one of the most frequently studied forms of dysarthria (Hunker & Abbs, 1984; Ludlow & Bassich, 1984).

Mixed dysarthrias are produced by multiple sclerosis (MS) and amyotrophic lateral sclerosis (ALS), both of which are progressive disease processes. MS usually is first diagnosed in early adulthood, between the ages of 20 and 40, and has a prognosis for survival of several years, even decades. In Darley, Brown, and Goldstein's (1972) study of 168 persons with MS, ages ranged from 17 to 73 years with 40 being about the median age. This cannot be considered to be the median age of onset, however, about one-third of the subjects had been with the disease for 10 years or more. The median duration of MS in a group of 656 subjects was 10 years with the longest being 31 years (Freal, Kraft, & Coryell, 1984). Therefore, a client with MS is likely to be seen at any age of adulthood, but the 20s or 30s is near estimated time of onset.

ALS, on the other hand, usually begins between 40 to 60 years of age, with an average age of onset at 57 years (Janiszewski, Caroscio, & Wisham, 1983). It consists of atrophy, weakness, and spasticity from upper and lower motor neuron disease and is characterized by the absence of sensory signs. The cause is unknown but Appel (1981) has theorized that Alzheimer's disease, Parkinson's disease, and ALS may all have a common etiology. He suggested that all three are characterized by a deterioration of pre-synaptic neuronal input that is seen in normal aging, and so proposed that all three are due to "lack of a disorder-specific neurotrophic hormone." Differences among the syndromes were attributed to location of the hormone reduction. In ALS the site of this reduction would be in the muscles themselves, resulting in the impaired function of anterior horn cells in the spinal column that is characteristic of ALS. Prognosis for survival is generally only 3-5 years.

Alaryngeal Speech

Adults may be confronted with surgical removal of larynx (total laryngectomy), resulting in loss of the source of sound for speech. A life-saving necessity usually employed as a treatment for laryngeal cancer, the surgery may also be required after traumatic injury to the laryngeal region. The goals of rehabilitation for the laryngectomized individual are to provide a substitute sound source and to facilitate psychological adjustment to this dramatic physical change.

Laryngeal cancer comprises less than 2% of all cancers (American Cancer Society, 1984), the incidence of which increases with age. For males, the incidence is 9.2 per 100,000 persons in the mid-30's and 41.9 per 100,000 in the 60s. For females, incidence is considerably less but the relationship to age is similar (Young, Percy, & Asire, 1981). Depending on its size and location within the larynx, the neoplasm poses a treat to airway and may cause changes in vocal function (Boone, 1983). Because elderly persons are often high surgical risks, radiation therapy may be the preferred choice of treatment (Clifford & Gregg, 1981). Radiation therapy, laser surgery, and partial laryngectomy may be preferred in order to save as much of the laryngeal mechanism as possible. These treatments may leave an impaired laryngeal mechanism, and the patient may then be referred to the speech-language pathologist for standard voice therapy. Total laryngectomy, on the other hand, requires some rather unique treatment strategies.

There are a few indications of the age characteristics of the laryngectomee population typically seen by a speech-language pathologist. In one large-N study of laryngectomees who had received voice training, 118 patients averaged 58 years of age with a range of 26 to 80 years (Shames, Font, & Matthews, 1963). Most of these subjects were males. In a study of 237 female patients, 31% were in their 40s and 35% were in their 50s (Gardner, 1966).

Diagnosis and Assessment

When identifying the communication problems of an elderly client, the clinician is faced with deciding, in one case, the degrees to which a primary communication disorder and normal aging are contributing to the problems observed and, in another case, the degrees to which the communication disorder and pathological aging (i.e., dementia) are contributing to the observed problems. In some cases, whether the aging phenomena are normal or are pathological is unclear; and the diagnostic team does its best to make this determination.

Aphasia Versus Normal Aging

Normal changes in the central nervous system may contribute to a proportion of the language deficit that is measured in aphasia. This proportion may be relatively small in some cases, especially in more severely impaired aphasic individuals. Nevertheless, if aging does indeed contribute to the language behavior of an elderly person with aphasia, simplistically our treatment maybe directed primarily to the proportion of deficit that is due to a focal lesion, and not to the component that is subject to the processes of aging. At least, our prognoses may be tempered by our ability to recognize the proportion of behavior due to primary communication disorder and the proportion due to normal aging. Unfortunately, we have been outlining a decision-making process that has little support from carefully investigated fact. Our concern stems as much from mythological expectations about normal aging as it does from experimental observations of changing language function across the lifespan.

The difficulties of investigating normal aging have been reviewed extensively elsewhere (Schaie, 1980). These difficulties include controlling for the possible influence of education (because age-defined groups differ in amount of formal education) and controlling for health status when comparing different age-defined groups. Only a few random and sundry studies of the psycholinguistics of aging have been conducted (see Davis, 1984). Most normative data accompanying aphasia assessment tools, for example, are from average performances of an adult population ranging in age from around 20 to 80 years. Such data do not indicate which subtest performances are susceptible to changes simply as a function of normal again. Standardization of some aphasia tests has included correlation of the age of aphasic subjects to test scores (Porch, 1967). When normal subjects were compared with each other according to age-decade, a slight drop in scores after age 60 was observed (Borod, Goodglass, & Kaplan, 1980a, 1980b). The normative research that should precede wise clinical application should be encouraged.

The study of aging language functions was reviewed by Davis (1984). From studies of intelligence testing, aging has been seen as a process in which verbal functions "hold" and nonverbal functions "don't hold" throughout the lifespan. However, a few investigations have indicated that language processing may be affected in subtle ways with respect to speed of processing, familiarity of semantic content, and complexity of the language task. When the language task involves recall of new learning, as in answering questions about a paragraph, an element of normal decline may be involved in a small portion of an aphasic client's performance. The clinician may suspect that aging could be a component of performance in the following tasks found in common comprehensive tests for aphasia:

Minnesota Test for Differential Diagnosis of Aphasia (Schuell, 1972)
1. Reading rate
2. Paragraph reading

3. Oral and written spelling

4. Writing sentences

Porch Index of Communicative Ability (Porch, 1981)

1. Describing object function

2. Writing sentences

Boston Diagnostic Aphasia Examination (Goodglass & Kaplan, 1983)

1. Repetition of low-probability sentences

2. Word fluency

3. Writing sentences

4. Parietal lobe tests (nonverbal)

Communicative Abilities in Daily Living (Holland, 1980)

1. Overall score

It is important to realize that the above possible aging effects pertain to changes in the central language function, and are not intended to signal possible influences of sensory and motor reductions that can occur with normal aging. Also, reduced performance on the above tasks may be a function of educational background. These particular subtests were singled out as the result of inferences made from the examination of studies of normal elderly persons, and from standardization studies of the tests themselves. Goodglass and Kaplan (1983) have determined that special cut-off scores should be considered for patients over age 60 for certain subtests of the BDAE (i.e., nonverbal oral agility and animal naming).

Size of the age-effect is unknown; however, with respect to most basic tests of language ability, we suspect that it would be small without influence from low motivation, depression, sensory reductions, or motor problems such as arthritis. Usually, experiments that compare aphasic subjects to age-matched normal controls involve substantial differences. Often these studies use aphasic and normal groups with mean ages in the middle to late 50s with a weak representation of elderly patients or normal elderly controls. For example, Gewirth, Shindler, and Hier (1984) compared aphasic groups with dementia groups and normal controls. While the dementia groups averaged around 70 years of age, the aphasic subjects were in their 50s (Wernicke's about 58; Broca's 45), and the normals averaged 58 years.

We are aware of only one study of aphasic subjects who were compared with both a geriatric group and a young adult group so that a possible aging effect could be observed. Yorkston and Beukelman (1980) found that the speaking rate of aphasic subjects (mean age of 45) was reduced relative to geriatric subjects (mean age 73), but there was no age effect on this parameter. An age effect occurred in communicative efficiency (i.e., content units per minute), in which elderly subjects were much less efficient than younger adults (mean age 31). Even the mildly impaired aphasics were still much worse than the elderly group on this measure. Nevertheless, with such an experimental design, we can see that aging might be a factor in such a measure if it were taken on elderly aphasic persons. Proportion of the age factor relative to aphasia might have been estimated if the study had also included an elderly aphasic group.

Aphasia Versus Dementia

There has been a common failure to distinguish between primary and secondary deficits with dementia. The literature is filled with references to aphasia in patients with dementia. A speech-language pathologist might be referred a patient with "expressive aphasia" or similar dated designation who might also have a history of alcoholism, seizures, and frequent psychiatric admissions. Another possibility is that a daughter, having discovered the existence of a speech clinic in the community, may bring her 75-year-old mother who is mute (with severe dementia) to the clinic because her mother cannot talk. However, for some reason, a few physicians have gotten the idea that any deviation of language behavior or any poor performance on a "test for aphasia" necessarily means that the person has aphasia. Although an Alzheimer patient may score like a person with Wernicke's aphasia on a test for aphasia, this patient may not have Wernicke's aphasia. Speech-language pathologists receive enough referrals of persons with "expressive aphasia," merely because of unusual speech, for this to be an important issue. Clinicians need to be prepared to inform physicians (or families) that the individual referred does not have aphasia and, therefore, does not warrant the kind of treatment that these physicians (or families) might be expecting.

Whereas the brief history in the previous paragraph might be suggestive of a misdiagnosis regarding aphasia, such a patient might have also suffered a stroke in the left middle cerebral artery, thereby making the existence of aphasia along with dementia a very likely possibility. Determining the primary basis for deviant language behavior is vital, at least, for prognosis. If the basis is focal cortical infarction, there indeed may be some chance for improvement; although improvement may be held back by confounding problems. If the basis is progressively deteriorating dementia, the prognosis would be less encouraging. Although it may be valuable for the clinician to assess the client no matter what the problem is, it is very important for the assessment of such clients to be done after information is obtained regarding a neurological evaluation and a neuropsychological evaluation. Because language-focused behavioral observations of clients with apparent dementia do not often present clear-cut distinctions, as much medical background as possible can be extremely informative.

Distinguishing between one patient with only aphasia and another patient with only dementia is often fairly easy. Medical history should be fairly suggestive as to whether the patient is likely to have one problem or the other. The clinician will in all likelihood see a focal lesion with sudden onset as the basis for aphasia and insidious onset of a generalized disease process (or of unknown origin) as the basis for dementia. When basing a decision upon language behaviors, diagnostic aphasia test manuals are of little assistance. The interpretation manual for the Porch Index of Communicative Ability (Porch, 1981) does provide sample patterns of patients with bilateral brain damage. These patterns contain deficits across all subtests, nonverbal as well as verbal, and do not show the characteristic pattern of aphasia which generally follows in order of difficulty on the language tasks. Clinicians should apply what is generally known about dementia to the interpretation of behaviors on language tests. Persons with Alzheimer's dementia will be without problems of phonology and syntax, and mild dementias will show no impairment of confrontation naming. More severely deficient persons with dementia are likely to be difficult to test, and identifying them is based on observation of their general behavior.

Without adequate medical history, which unfortunately is sometimes unavoidable, the clinician can observe distinctions during an initial interview with the client. In fact, it is our belief that formal language testing, especially tests for aphasia, is not necessary or very helpful for the purpose of differential diagnosis at this level. Except for Wernicke's aphasia, the aphasic person will recognize communicative difficulty, be frustrated by it out

202

of a desire to communicate, and be eager to be evaluated and treated. The person with aphasia will be oriented as to time and place, and will recall events of the past while having difficulty expressing these memories through language. This patient is likely to show concern about personal appearance and, except for visible evidence of hemiplegia in many cases, is likely to look like the average person on the street. The person with mild dementia, on the other hand, will have essentially normal phonology and syntax in their expressive language. The individual may appear interpersonally distant or somewhat hyperactive and euphoric. The individual may be restless, distractable, irritable, disinterested, and a little confused as to orientation. More severe cases may produce streams of jargon and engage in bizarre behaviors. They may wander aimlessly about the room or may want to leave the room without apparent reason. They may appear to have paid little attention to grooming and dress.

Another dimension of distinction is time. Aphasic persons tend to improve spontaneously and with treatment, and many improve a substantial amount in the first month or two after a clearly identifiable date of onset. Elderly aphasic persons, who are aging normally, will show these characteristics. Persons with Alzheimer dementia will gradually worsen and various treatments have been shown to be unable to reverse this trend. Therefore, distinction between these two disorders comes from comparison of multiple testing done over time. A value of language testing of persons with dementia may lie in the documentation of rate of decline with a sensitive and reliable measure.

Difficult differential diagnosis comes when a single patient has both dementia and aphasia. The situation is a likely occurrence in the evaluation of elderly clients with a history of focal CVA. The clinician will suspect the possibility of dementia in persons with a medical history of gradual onset of deficits that are general in nature. Moreover, there is always the possibility that an elderly aphasic individual will also possess what deVries (1983) called <u>unrecognized incipient disease processes</u> in which the early stages of progressive dementia have begun but have not yet been recognized from observing behavior. From behavioral observation, however, a person with overt dementia and aphasia is likely to exhibit the symptoms of dementia described in the previous paragraph. Aphasia and dementia will be mixed together in this client's language behavior.

Our ability to make linguistic distinctions in these patients is currently limited. More research on the characteristics of language in dementia is needed. More current research has dealt primarily with naming behavior, and a more comprehensive approach to language should be taken using methodologies that are not biased by virtue of having been created to measure aphasia. Comparisons between subjects with aphasia and subjects with dementia are a bit "unfair," when the test is one that was devised for and normed on subjects with aphasia. Linguistic and psycholinguistic methods should be brought to bear on the study of all linguistic levels of behavior in dementia.

Right Hemisphere Damage Versus Dementia

In terms of behavior, the muted affect, indifference, disorientation, normal phonology and syntax, and wandering from the point in telling a story found in persons with right hemisphere damage may present a picture that is similar to persons in the early stage of dementia. Again, medical history may be helpful in that the person with right hemisphere damage is likely to have been diagnosed as having suffered a focal lesion (e.g., stroke) of sudden onset. As would be the case with aphasia as well, specific sensory and motor signs of unilateral cortical damage (e.g., hemiparesis) might be present with right hemisphere damage. Also, the person with dementia may display language comprehension deficits and word retrieval difficulties that would not be seen after right hemisphere damage, in addition to a medical history of gradual onset and lack of unilateral damage.

Speech Disorders Versus Normal Aging

In examining an elderly client with a motor speech disorder, the speech-language pathologist should be aware that a component of observed function is likely to include effects of aging as well as the primary speech disorder. Unfortunately, these two origins of reduced function will not be manifested through discretely distinguishable observations. That is, age-related effects on speech will be "masked" by the primary speech disorder. In this section, we shall point out where age-related changes of speech production might be a component of the behaviors observed in speech-disordered persons.

We know that speech production changes with age partly because listeners can make reasonably accurate judgements as to whether a speaker is a young adult or an elderly adult. The distinction is based on perceptual features indicative of inefficient laryngeal valving (breathiness, harshness, and vocal tremor), changes in pitch, imprecise consonants, and slow rate of articulation (Hartman & Danhauer, 1976; Ryan & Burk, 1974). However, significant effects on common clinical measures of production (i.e., syllable production rates) are hard to find (Kreul, 1972; Shanks, 1970). Normal aging does not critically impair intelligibility.

Just as dysarthria reflects impairment at all levels of the production system, aging impacts on most of these levels, especially on articulation, phonation, and respiration (see Curtis & Fucci, 1983; Kahane, 1981). When assessing an elderly client's speech mechanism and speech function, the clinician should keep in mind that age-related changes might be involved in several levels of speech production. We shall begin our discussion with the level of articulation. As a subtle perceptual feature of articulation, voice onset time (VOT) is reduced more in males than females (Benjamin, 1982; Weismer & Fromm, 1983), reflecting similar sex differences in structural changes of the larynx (Kahane, 1983). Reduced VOT may contribute to the perception of imprecise articulation, making voiceless plosives, for example, sound like voiced plosives. Phoneme and phrase durations are longer (Benjamin, 1982; Weismer, 1984), possibly contributing to measured reduction of speaking rate (Ramig, 1983). In one study where persons with Parkinsonian dysarthria were compared with young and old control groups, the rate of this dysarthric speech was comparable to the rate of the younger group but was faster than the geriatric control group (Weismer, 1984). This throws some confusion into how the speech rate in Parkinson's disease might be interpreted with respect to the reduction of rate in normal persons of the same age. The Parkinsonian rate might be thought of as being "normal" when compared to young adults and as being "abnormal" with respect to the opposite pull on rate that is characteristic of aging.

Next, let us consider phonation and respiration. Pitch changes differ between males and females, with rising fundamental frequency in elderly males, especially those in poor health (Ramig & Ringel, 1983), and decreasing fundamental frequency in females beginning with menopause (Stoicheff, 1981). Phrase length and, therefore, duration are related to the respiratory cycle for speech; and the elderly show a reduction of vital lung capacity from younger adulthood. The actual effects of reduced capacity on speaking are unclear but one effect might be the increases in intra- and intersentence pause duration measured by Ramig (1983). All of these changes are likely to be components of the speech behavior observed in an elderly patient with a speech or language disorder.

We are discussing the speech changes in this section, because they present differential diagnostic problems within patients with speech disorders. With very mild dysarthrias, it may be difficult to tell the difference between dysarthria and aging. The diagnoses of dysarthria often depends upon identification of a neurological condition or disease that causes dysarthria. This may be a problem primarily in the initial stages of a dysarthria with insidious onset, as in Parkinson's disease. In his comparison among Parkinsonian patients and old and young control groups, Weismer (1984) concluded that the shortened voiceless interval, which includes VOT, is the only speech characteristic of these patients that is also an effect of aging.

With respect to other etiologies and levels of dysarthria, the problem becomes one of identifying the aging component. This component is likely to be small, as we had discussed with aphasia, in a patient without other confounding health problems. However, the medical problems and/or medication administered for these problems, both of which are so prevalent in the elderly population, may substantially compound the speech deficits produced by a dysarthria. The elderly patient's general health status should contribute to the clinician's prognosis for speech improvement. The clinician should ask the patient's physician whether, for example, medication might be having a certain effect on speech and, if so, whether a change of medication might be possible.

Test Administration

Testing the elderly aphasic patient is likely to involve some considerations not applicable to the testing of middle-aged and younger adults. Even if age-effects on language function are small, the elderly patient may carry enough extra "baggage" accumulated from aging in general to require the clinician to make adjustments. These adjustments might pertain to the selection of tests, the number of tests administered, and the manner in which they are administered.

When assessing aphasia, the clinician wants as unimpeded a look at language function as possible. However, the elderly aphasic patient may possess auditory and visual sensory reductions demanding that the clinician be sure that a client's hearing aid is present and functioning and that glasses are also present. Auditory stimuli may need to be louder and clearer than is needed for younger adults, and visual stimuli may need to be large and uncluttered. Whenever the client has arthritis, tasks requiring fine motor coordination should be minimized and writing performance should be interpreted with respect to this motor overlay. There is a much greater need to use a room that is free from distractions. In order to minimize the influence of fatigue, relatively short tests are chosen such as the Sklar Aphasia Scale (Sklar, 1973) or the Aphasia Language Performance Scales (Keenan & Brassell, 1975). For neuropsychological testing of elderly persons, Lezak (1983) recommended elimination of the need for visual search, use of tests with high face validity, and use of norms that are appropriate for older persons.

The clinician should also be sensitive to the psychological orientation that elderly persons may bring to a test situation. Lezak (1983) noted that the most important factor may be enlisting their cooperation, as follows:

> With no school requirements to be met, no jobs to prepare for, and usually little previous experience with psychological tests, a retired person may very reasonably not want to go through a lot of fatiguing mental gymnastics that may well make him look stupid to the youngster in the white coat sitting across the table. Particularly if they are not feeling well or are concerned about diminishing mental acuity, elderly persons may view a test as a nuisance or an unwarranted intrusion into their privacy. (p. 118)

It is important to anticipate these feelings and let the patient know that such misgivings are perfectly natural and understandable. The clinician should spend extra time explaining the purpose of testing and familiarizing the patient with the test situation. Lezak suggested testing elderly people with meaningful and nonthreatening materials such as playing cards. Elderly persons sometimes have little patience for activities that have no apparent relevance to their daily lives, and many formal aphasia tests are filled with such unfamiliar activities.

Treatment of Elderly Patients: A General Comment

A few attributes of old age are influential for treatment of any of the language and speech disorders reviewed in this chapter. One is the reduction of physical working capacity (PWC), perceived by the elderly as a loss of vigor (deVries, 1983). The reduction of PWC has been measured with respect to vital air capacity in the lungs, elasticity during expiration, muscle strength, muscle fatigue, and aerobic capacity (i.e., maximal oxygen consumption). Aerobic capacity is considered to be the best single measure of PWC; and, for men, a gradual decline begins in early adulthood and reaches less than half of peak values at a mean age of 75. This substantial decline may be attributed not only to normal aging but also to unrecognized incipient disease processes or to "hypokinetic disease." Hypokinetic disease is a reduction of vigor and associated mental difficulties stemming simply from disuse. According to deVries (1983), the reductions of PWC seen in aging"...can also be brought about in young, well-conditioned men in as little as three weeks by the simple expedient of enforced bed rest" (p. 291). Therefore, reduced vigor in older persons can be compounded when elderly individuals are generally inactive and engage in little or no physical exercise.

Language and speech treatment is hard work. Usually it entails repetitive drills, and may be most effective when performed several times per week for a period of a few months. Certain speech therapies are physically taxing, such as "pushing" exercises to improve voice or the practice of esophageal voice or increasing phrase lengths. Most speech therapies involve repetitive exercise of articulatory, phonatory, and respiratory muscles that are susceptible to the declining strength and increasing fatigue that accompany aging. This means that treatment sessions may tend to be shorter and, if possible, more frequent for elderly clients. Tasks should be carefully paced with rest periods between tasks. Furthermore, light physical exercise on a regular basis should be encouraged, especially in nursing homes where residents may spend a lot of time in bed or just sitting around. Group treatment is a fine time to have clients engage in a brief period of arm and leg raising and other mild exercises "to stimulate the circulation." Research has shown that elderly persons (mean age = 69.5) can be trained to increase their PWC (deVries, 1983).

Treatment of Aphasia

Most direct treatment of the language impairments in aphasia has been based on the assumption that aphasia represents a reduction in processing capability rather than a loss (or disappearance) of linguistic competence from long-term memory. The distinction between impairment of performance versus loss of competence becomes less clear in severely impaired cases. Therefore, procedures that might be logically derived from either assumption may be employed. Basic treatment is structured around a variety of tasks designed to allow the patient to exercise receptive and/or expressive language modalities.

Basic Approaches

Most traditional treatments of aphasia may be characterized generally as cognitive or behavioral approaches. Clinicians often use a combination of blending of these orientations, because interaction with the client is basically the same in both.

Cognitive approaches have been identified as "stimulation-facilitation" approaches by other reviewers (LaPointe, 1983; Sarno, 1981). These approaches generally have been based on a theoretical formulation of the nature of the aphasic deficit. In terms of procedures, the cognitive tradition originated with Schuell's "stimulation" methodology, in which improvements in expression are considered to be the result of intensive and extensive stimulation of the auditory language modality (Darley, 1982; Schuell, Jenkins, & Jimenez-Pabon, 1964). Variations of this theme have developed from a recognition that different types of aphasia may entail different goals and/or methods of stimulation (Davis, 1983).

Procedures are directed toward the facilitation of impaired language processes by means of careful selection of stimuli in a stimulus-response-feedback form of interaction with the client. A stimulus is planned to be powerful enough to naturally elicit a particular response, whether it be pointing to a picture in a comprehension task or verbalizing in an expressive task. Tasks are planned to be easy enough for the client to be accurate in most responses, with feedback upon occasional errors intended simply to improve the response. Specific lexicon may vary from day-to-day, because the intent is to exercise a process at a level of success rather than to teach a specific lexicon. A task may be designed around a particular sentence structure, not to "teach" that structure, but because the targeted structure is relatively easy for the patient to process. Specific examples of stimulation include "deblocking" (Weigl & Bierwisch, 1970), "intersystemic reorganization" (Luria, 1970), and "thought-centered therapy" (Wepman, 1976). Relatively recent expansion of stimulation has been encouraged by Chapey (1981) who recommended stimulation of "divergent" language involving numerous creative responses to single stimuli.

Although behavioral approaches have refined cognitive methodology, there are some differences in orientation which result in slight differences of procedure. Whereas behavioral methods are derived from theories about learning, their proponents do not base procedures on theoretical assumptions about language function, aphasia, or recovery. Treatment begins with identification of relevant linguistic behaviors, and proceeds according to principles of behavior change. More emphasis is placed on the consequent event as influencing behavior change (operant conditioning) than on the antecedent event (i.e., stimulus) in cognitive approaches. Because of this focus on response consequences, the production of errors is somewhat more permissible. Improvements come from the shaping of responses based on the reinforcement of those that come closest to targeting behavior. Also, in contrast to cognitive approaches, a task often involves a small set of words or phrases that are presented or expected repeatedly over several trials or sessions (Thompson, McReynolds, & Vance, 1982). The goal is to achieve generalization or "acquisition" to linguistic units that were not used in treatment (Prescott, Selinger, & Loverso, 1982; Salvatore, 1982; Thompson & Kearns, 1981).

Marriage of cognitive and behavioral orientations has been labeled as the "programmed-stimulation" approach (LaPointe, 1983). Principles of programming have been borrowed from strict operant procedures for the planning of "task hierarchies" by more cognitively oriented clinicians. A long-term treatment program may entail a planned progression of tasks moving from easier to more difficult levels of language performance. Adjacent tasks may differ from each other by only one stimulus variable. Common examples of programs include Visual Action Therapy (VAT) for severely impaired clients (Helm-Estabrooks, Fitzpatrick, & Barresi, 1982) and Melodic Intonation Therapy (MIT), a procedure for Broca's aphasia in which fluent verbal expression is achieved by melodically intoning an utterance (Sparks, 1981). MIT contains elements of intersystemic reorganization, whereas VAT targets gestural behavior for training. In the usual program, success at one task is an essential prerequisite for achieving success at the next step or level.

Innovations and the Elderly

In a previous section, we presented the speculation that aging may impact more on the right hemisphere that on the left or, at least, more on nonverbal cognitive processes than on verbal processes. This speculation relates to additional speculations about the role of the right hemisphere in recovery, and in the use of musical intoning and visual imagery in treatment (Fitch-West, 1983; Helm-Estabrooks, 1983). Bringing the right hemisphere into the language process is one of the more innovative assumptions in the cognitive orientation. This is not the substitution theory, namely, that the right hemisphere "takes over" language function. Instead, treatments have been suggested that may invoke nonverbal processes (e.g., music, visual imagery) as a means of facilitating the left hemisphere's language function and perhaps, eventually leading to an "intersystemic reorganization" of an impaired language function. This possibility has been raised relative to Melodic Intonation Therapy (see Helm-Estabrooks, 1983). In addition, Fitch-West (1983) has postulated that "arousal of visual imagery" may facilitate verbal expression in aphasia treatment. However, actual treatment procedures, beyond simply the suggestion to use concrete words, have not been fully developed to capitalize on this hypothesis. Moreover, old age may reduce the effectiveness of such procedures.

Innovations with basic approaches have included technological advances in the manner by which these procedures are administered or delivered to patients. The "language laboratory," providing supplemental stimulation or training, has been around since the 1960s with automated teaching machines and the Language Master by Bell and Howell. Microcomputer technology has extended this concept to more flexible and creative levels. Computers provide not only supplemental independent practice, but they also enable treatment to be delivered over telephone lines to patients for whom a clinician is not readily available (Fitch & Cross, 1983). So far, programs (software) have focused on presentation of reading stimuli and multiple choice responding (Katz, 1984; Weiner, 1984). Hardware may be added so that digitalized speech can be presented (Mills & Thomas, 1983). Other developments from microprocessing include a small recording device with which the client may practice repeating stimuli (Boone & Campbell, 1983). Elderly patients may have some difficulty with synthesized auditory presentations (however, digitalized speech is superior) and with the motoric dexterity needed for keyboards or joysticks. Also, great pains should be taken to avoid using machines to replace supportive interaction with a clinician, especially for elderly clients who already have suffered reductions of human contact.

Pragmatics and Treatment

Pragmatics is the study of how language processes interact with context. Treatment based on pragmatic principles is a treatment of language impairment. In a sense, a pragmatic orientation is a modification of cognitive and behavioral approaches so that these two traditional methods may be carried out "pragmatically" (Wilcox & Davis, in press). Therefore, pragmatics does not necessarily represent a mutually exclusive methodology, even though it may entail the addition of some relatively new procedures. Pragmatics adds a new variable to traditional approaches. This new variable simply is context, added to more familiar variables such as sentence length, familiarity of vocabulary, and syntactic complexity.

Applied pragmatics is intended to address a basic clinical problem, namely, the generalization of facilitation achieved in the clinic to the natural communicative environments and demands of individual aphasic patients. This clinical problem is addressed by shaping clinical methods so that stimulus presentations and response expectations reflect the varied uses of language within natural contexts (see Spradlin & Siegel, 1982). Stimuli and responses are defined with respect to extralinguistic contexts (settings and people), linguistic contexts (discourse structure and coherence devices), and paralinguistic contexts (prosody) that modulate language function for the individual. Although clinicians traditionally have been practical (called "being pragmatic") by stimulating clients in homebased settings, the systematic application of normal adult research on contextual variables has not yet been fully explored or implemented.

Pragmatic Content and Aging

One of the principal implications of considering context to its fullest lies in the selection of semantic content for stimulation tasks and of topics for conversational interactions in individual or group sessions. Elderly persons present options that often differ from options available with middle-aged and young adults. The individualization of content and topics usually comes from the client's "horizontal" and "vertical" contexts, both of which include people and settings (Wilcox & Davis, in press). Horizontal contexts include current people and settings involved in the client's communicative environment, and are common sources of content that would be most relevant to the individual. Vertical contexts include people and settings primarily from the client's past, and are less common sources of content when such matters are discussed in the treatment literature. Of the adult age groups, the elderly have the longest vertical contextual dimension and sometimes a narrowed horizontal dimension.

An elderly person's horizontal context may differ from the social sphere of younger adults. Social contexts include the family, occupation, and community; and usually by age 65, occupation can be subtracted from this equation. The elderly differ among themselves as to community involvement. Some prefer "disengagement" from social stimulation while others desire to maintain activity levels with involvement not achieved before retirement. Census statistics show that most elderly persons live in a family arrangement, with more women living alone than men. In fact, in the United States 69% of females and 23% of males over age 75 are widowed; 50% of females and 77% of males live with families. Nearly 48% of females over age 75 live alone, while only 21% of males live alone. These figures represent substantial increases over the population aged 65-74 (Deming & Cutler, 1983). As people grow older, family constellations change with children leaving home, introduction of grandchildren, changing distances between parents and children, and so on. Therefore, if the clinician is to draw upon family names for naming exercises, in many cases these names will be from the client's vertical context or past. Topics might entail what the children did, rather than what they are doing.

The elderly person's personal history provides a wealth of meaningful ideas for content to be used in direct stimulation. Older persons have difficulty encoding and retaining new information, and so attempting to relate to them from a younger clinician's current perspective may be difficult also. Informational cues to the client's earlier years, when the client was encoding at his or her best, can be derived from a familiarity with history of the periods coincident with the client's young adult years. The clinician should find out about famous people and events that were prominent when the client was going to school, starting a job, and raising a family (Davis & Holland, 1981). Older people like to recall the past and are able to do it well. Reminiscence therapy or Life Review therapy have been valuable mechanisms in the counseling of elderly persons (Ronch, 1981).

PACE

Pragmatic procedures that have been implemented include attempts to bring conversational structure and communicative dynamics to the stimulation of language function in the clinic. One such procedure is PACE therapy, or Promoting Aphasics' Communicative Effectiveness (Davis & Wilcox, 1981; Wilcox & Davis, in press). This procedure changes the interaction between clinician and client in subtle ways in order to achieve conversational dynamics such as turn-taking and the communication of new information. PACE is intended to provide the experience of successful communication within a framework that is more like natural conversation than the traditional direct stimulation framework. It permits the practice of conversational acts such as hint-and-guess sequences and the repair of communicative breakdowns. The patient can practice verbal skills under a variety of circumstances created by varying extralinquistic contexts such as participants and knowledge of the topic. The interaction between participants and shared knowledge is a powerful determinant of communicative success. This interaction can be imagined when one considers a patient conversing with the clinician or spouse about topics such as news events or the patient's family history. The patient can easily engage in PACE with persons other than the clinician and with message stimuli selected according to topics of high or low shared knowledge.

When considering the use of PACE as a communication exercise with a variety of other persons, the clinician soon realizes that the elderly patient may not have a spouse or other readily available family member with whom to engage in such practice. In a nursing home setting, the clinician may enlist the cooperation of staff members who communicate frequently or infrequently with the aphasic client. Also, when developing topics, the clinician should explore subjects from the client's past that are easily and, sometimes, gladly remembered.

One advantage of PACE with the elderly is that the client communicates as an independent individual without direct interference from the clinician.

According to the principles of this procedure, the clinician does not direct the client to perform in any way and encourages the use of certain behaviors through modeling when taking a turn as the sender of a message. This takes pressure off of the client. Older people are less flexible than younger people and often have a difficult time dealing with stress. PACE does not have some of the stress that can occur with direct stimulation and training.

Group Treatment

Group treatment of aphasia varies widely depending the clinician's goals in instituting this form of treatment. In some clinical programs, group interaction may be a by-product of informal social periods that are intended to provide relaxation in the middle of an extensive clinical schedule. Sometimes groups are arranged for the purpose of psychological adjustment, and which are usually managed by a psychologist or psychiatrist. Another goal of group treatment may involve the same goals of individual treatment, namely, to improve communicative ability. In meeting each of these three goals, group treatment may be a valuable supplement to individual treatment by virtue of the special support system created among persons with similar problems, including the problems created by aphasia and the problems created by aging. Aphasic persons possess an empathy for each other that cannot be achieved by a clinician who is not only unaffected by brain injury but also who is often much younger. An aphasic client may be more likely to accept encouragement and criticism from someone who is faced with the same situation.

Treatment of Secondary Language Deficits

The speech-language pathologist may not be as directly involved in the treatment of secondary language disorders. The section indicates some reasons for this and presents some issues pertaining to the treatment of language impairments due to other primary deficits.

Right Hemisphere Damage

As discussed earlier in this chapter, primary deficits after right hemisphere damage are defined with respect to the nonverbal functions commonly associated with this half of the brain. Impairments of perception, cognition, and personality have traditionally been assessed by the neuropsychologist.

Treatment for these disorders has also been developed within neuropsychology, and has been referred to most frequently as "cognitive retraining" (Adamovich, Henderson, & Auerbach, 1984; Ben-Yishay & Diller, 1983; Diller, 1976). If we are to ascribe to the notion that appropriate treatment is directed to primary deficits, then there may be some question as to who is ultimately responsible for providing cognitive retraining. Speech-language pathologists are trained in general principles of remediation, such as behavioral modification techniques, and are often more available then neuropsychologists in many settings for elderly patients. Also, a comprehensive on primary deficits usually entails addressing secondary deficits. In these cases, pragmatic communicative interactions between language and context may be treated by the speech-language pathologist. However, treatment protocols for pragmatic communicative impairments, if they exist, have not received wide circulation. People with right-hemisphere damage are generally not referred to speech-language pathologists.

If referrals were to increase and treatment protocols were developed for pragmatic language impairments, then the speech-language pathologist may still have to deal with potential aging factors in the elderly patient. The suggestion that right hemisphere functions age more than left hemisphere functions may be a factor in the success of treatment of right hemisphere damaged patients. Performance (nonverbal) functions have been observed to recover more slowly than verbal functions in younger adult head-injured patients (Mandleberg & Brooks, 1975).

Dementia

One key to assisting persons with dementia is to identify the cause. Physicians are not so quick to label someone as having "organic brain syndrome" or "senile dementia" as they once were especially when the etiology is uncertain. Follow-up testing is often done until various possibilities have been ruled out. If the individual appears to have a treatable dementia or a "pseudodementia," then improvement of cognitive function may be noticed after a change of diet, adjustment of medication, or psychological adjustment to loss of family and/or home. However, if the cause is the relentless progression of Alzheimer's disease, then outlook for the improvement of cognitive function is not favorable.

Behavioral methods for dementia and milder problems of old age have not
been known to be successful in reversing the trend of deterioration with
Alzheimer's disease and other progressive etiologies. Various milieu and other
therapies, such as "reality orientation," have been attempted (Barns, Sac, &
Schore, 1973). Bayles (1984) suggested that the speech-language pathologist
may be helpful in assessing communicative abilities and facilitating improved
communication between the patient and other persons. That is, the
individual can be helped to be more comfortable at his or her stage of the
disease. In some cases, with repeated stimulation and emotional support, the
progressive trend might be slowed. Individuals with mild dementia may be
enlivened with group sessions involving reminiscence about the past.
Strategies for compensated intelligibility of speech production may be valuable
for persons with Parkinson's disease (see next section on speech disorders).
Bayles added that it may be more appropriate to provide counseling for the
family (see Mace & Rabins, 1981). Although direct treatment of language
function has not been show to be efficacious, the speech-language clinician can
play a less direct role by advising on communicative strategies, assisting in
group sessions, and referring to counselors and others trained in helping
elderly persons with cognitive and psychological problems.

Treatment of Speech Disorders

Treatment of speech disorders is directed toward improving the mechanics
involved in all levels of speech production, teaching speech behaviors that
compensate for mechanical inadequacies, and, in the more severely impaired
cases, teaching augmentative or substitutive strategies for communication.

Apraxia of Speech

Treatment of apraxia of speech is often a successful enterprise. "Apraxic
talkers have a _good_ prognosis for recovery of functional communication _without_
treatment and they have an _excellent_ prognosis with it" (Rosenbek, 1983, p.
49). Optimism increases as the amount of accompanying aphasia decreases.

Direct treatment of verbal apraxia is basically aimed toward assisting the
client in achieving conscious control of articulatory programming. Once
volitional control is achieved, repetitive practice is instituted so that
accurate articulation may become more automatic. The intense drill of apraxia

treatment is hard work, and the elderly, especially those with multiple medical problems, will require practice that is carefully paced with ample periods of rest. When the setting permits, several short sessions per week (15-30 min) would be preferred over two 1-hr sessions per week.

Rosenbek (1978) outlined two general stages of apraxia treatment: (a) acute stage, in which the clinician, as a facilitator, attempts to elicit speech in any way possible, and in which the clinician counsels patient and family as to creating a positive environment for improvement to occur; and (b) chronic stage, in which the early procedures are continued but are supplemented with reorganizational efforts to improve the speech programmer. The development of conscious control begins in earnest during the chronic stage.

Imitation of the clinician is the primary procedure early in the treatment (Rosenbek, 1983). Imitation is valuable, because the clinician has complete control over what the client is expected to say. Therefore, words or phrases are carefully selected to be useful to the patient and, yet, also be programmed as to sound structure to maximize the possibility of successful production. The auditory stimulus in imitation is usually accompanied by visual stimuli, such as "watch me," so that the client can see the clinicians production. Simultaneous auditory and visual stimulation has been called integral stimulation, and at a later stage the visual stimulus may be a printed version of the auditory stimulus. Stages of stimulation lead the patient to greater independence in reproduction, as in the eight-step program suggested by Rosenbek, Lemme, Ahern, Harris, and Wertz (1973). This is achieved by gradually fading cues, and such programs can be enhanced by varying temporal relationships between stimulus and response, as described by Rosenbek (1978). Slight modifications of such task continua have been successfully applied to apraxic speakers between ages 61-65 (Deal & Florance, 1970).

Two common methodologies were derived from Luria (1970). Facilitation is often achieved through intrasystemic reorganization, in which the level of response is lowered to achieve production; and then the level is gradually raised so that the response might be produced more volitionally for more natural communicative purposes. For example, particular sound combinations might only be achieved initially through counting to 10 or under the pretense of making a particular nonverbal noise, such as the sound of a cough. Practice of these sounds becomes a matter of increasing the volitional demands of sound

218

production. Intersystemic reorganization may be introduced within the progression of intrasystemic reorganization; or it can be the primary means of facilitating articulatory programming, especially for clients who have little trouble initiating speech. Intersystemic reorganization consists of the introduction into an impaired act of a function that is not normally used in the impaired act. The newly introduced function, called a "reorganizer," acts as a facilitator for the production of impaired speech. Common reorganizers have been used to help the patient slow down the rate of speech production, including timing gestures such as finger-tapping and pacing boards.

A crucial challenge in the treatment of apraxia of speech, or any other motor speech disorder, is achieving generalization of improved skill and of the use of reorganizers to natural communicative situations. Generalization is achieved in part by training that results in the client's becoming more automatic and natural in the production of reprogrammed articulatory behavior. Tasks that permit practice under varied conditions requiring volitional production with increasing external pressures (such as less time to respond) go a long way toward maximizing carry-over. Some of the pragmatic concerns mentioned previously for aphasia apply equally to treatment of elderly persons with apraxia. This is especially true for the selection of verbal units to be practiced. The elderly may have little patience for drill, and motivation can be maximized with the use of stimuli that are pertinent to the patient's daily life. In a nursing home, for example, stimuli should reflect what the client is likely to need to say in that setting. Also, pragmatic activities employed in aphasia treatment, such as PACE and role-playing, provide opportunities for the patient to practice improved articulation in more natural communicative situations, before being sent out to fend for himself or herself.

Dysarthrias

Specific goals and procedures may vary depending on the type of dysarthria (Perkins, 1983). However, the basic goals for treating any dysarthria are (a) to improve and/or increase physiologic support for speech and (b) to achieve "compensated intelligibility" of speech (Rosenbek & LaPointe, 1978). A return to normal function is extremely rare, and elderly clients may possess the additional reductions of physiologic support due to aging that were outlined previously. Therefore, compensated intelligibility is a necessity born from making the best use of remaining physiologic support. Hopefully, the end result is a production that is intelligible to the listener (a perceptual standard of success), but that has been achieved by using modified or different means to achieve that end (by physiologic adjustments). For the most severely impaired cases in which these goals are difficult to achieve, various augmentative and substitutive means of communicating have been developed.

Increasing physiologic support is one of the principal differences between treatment of dysarthria and treatment of verbal apraxia, because dysarthria involves impairment of the neurosmuscular system whereas verbal apraxia does not include such impairment. Treatment is usually directed at all "points" of the system: respiration, phonation, resonance, and the several mechanisms of articulation (Netsell & Daniel, 1979). Simple postural adjustments and bracing may improve some of these systems, especially respiration an phonation. Repetition drill with nonspeech (isometric and isotonic) and speech exercises may improve strength and accuracy of movement. However, speech exercises are sometimes preferred, because the dynamics of movement for speech purposes are different from the dynamics for nonspeech sounds (Netsell, 1983). In addition, intraoral breath support has been improved with prosthetic devices designed to achieve better velopharyngeal closure (Aten, McDonald, Simpson, & Gutierrez, 1984). A few of the successful cases in Aten's study were in their 60s, with none older than 69.

Feedback is an important consideration for improving physiologic support. Self-monitoring avenues include proprioceptive sensory feedback (touching and direct manipulation), perceptual feedback (listening), and biofeedback (visual representations of EMG response or nasal air emission, as two examples). Delayed auditory feedback has been used to reduce speech rate in Parkinson's disease (Hanson & Metter, 1983). Hypertonicity has been reduced through relaxation with EMG feedback (Nemec & Cohen, 1984; Netsell & Cleeland, 1973; Rubow, Rosenbek, Collins, & Celesia, 1984). Even in patients who do not have the perceptual complications of old age, one feedback system at a time increases success over combined auditory and visual feedback channels (Rubow, 1984). Some elderly clients with reduced cognitive skill or speed may have difficulty understanding such tasks in which feedback must be interpreted and then related to target behavior. The equipment itself may be frightening, and so elderly clients may benefit from such procedures only when given substantial preparation including explanation of the purpose of the procedure and familiarization with the equipment and tasks. In a rare report of treatment for a person over age 65, Caligiuri and Murry (1983) found success in using an oscilloscope as visual feedback for treatment of prosody in a patient 75 years of age.

Compensated intelligibility is maximized through a variety of adjustments depending on the nature of interference. When speech rate is too fast, as in Parkinson's disease, the patient learns to slow down. When respiratory support is insufficient, as in flaccid dysarthria, the patient learns to adjust phrase length so that the weakened respiratory system can better support speech. When this type of patient is elderly, there may be even less physiologic support and more pausing. Compensation is even more mandatory, such as use of shorter phrases and sentences that include more semantically potent words. The patient may need to make certain adjustments in articulation to compensate for inadequate velopharyngeal closure. The patient with ataxic dysarthria must pay particular attention to rate of articulation in order to bring the mechanisms under control Yorkston & Beukelman, 1981).

Although nonvocal communication aids may be mandatory for severely impaired individuals as the only means of achieving maximally effective communication, the clinician may have to resort to these procedures for elderly adults who simply reject participation in repetitive speech drill. Beukelman and Yorkston (1977, 1978, 1980) have evaluated numerous augmentative nonvocal communication aids for the individual with severe motor speech disturbance. These devices have included simple to complex communication boards with letters and words, typewriting devices that include printout capability, and electronic communication boards, some of which are equipped to produce synthesized speech. The clinician should be careful to match a device with the motoric and linguistic capabilities of each individual. Devices requiring fine motor control, such as typewriter devices, may pose problems for elderly clients because of slower motor function and movement difficulties with arthritis. Some devices are more efficient than others, especially when the communicative situation includes time constraints. Also, the elderly individual with a hearing loss may not be able to tolerate the sound of synthesized speech. The vast array of possibilities in communication aids have been reviewed recently in several books (see Musselwhite & St. Louis, 1982; Silverman, 1980).

Laryngectomy

Removal of one's larynx, in spite of its necessity to save life, is a frightening prospect to anyone. While the speech-language pathologist becomes involved in assisting the person to adjust psychologically before and after surgery, the primary role of the clinician is to help the individual develop new ways of communicating. Traditionally, the clinician has been able to provide compensatory options for vocalization in the absence of an internal vocal mechanism. These options are esophageal speech and an artificial larynx (Boone, 1983; Keith & Shanks, 1983). Innovative surgical procedures may also provide some individuals with a new vocal energy source that is driven by natural exhalation.

Esophageal speech involves using existing structures in order to create a new sound source. The sound initially is a burping noise from the compression of air within the oropharynx and then the injection of this air into the esophageal space. The basic task of treatment entails developing voluntary control over the initiation of this sound and developing an ability to maintain this sound long enough to support a few syllables of speech. Three methods have been employed: (a) The injection method involves using certain consonant sounds, such as plosives, to facilitate the injection of air back into the esophagus; (b) The inhalation method takes advantage of certain changes in air pressure created by normal inhalation during respiration; and (c) The swallow method, usually introduced when the other methods for initiation are unsuccessful, involves backward movement of the tongue as in normal swallowing. Once sound is achieved, treatment proceeds by gradually increasing the duration of sound in increasing lengths of speech production.

Learning esophageal speech is a physically demanding process, and a body that is generally weakened by aging may have difficulty achieving the physical strength necessary to sustain training. Using esophageal speech can also be fatiguing. Its low pitch is difficult for others to hear, especially when there is competing sound. In the elderly population, there is an increased likelihood that listeners will be hearing-impaired and this increases the demands on an esophageal speaker. A laryngectomee in a nursing home may find it less tiring to use an artificial larynx on some occasions.

An artificial larynx is an external source of sound. There are two types of instruments according to their source of power. The pneumatic type involves connecting an air supply tube to the stoma and then exhaling air through a vibrator contained in the device. A tube, placed between the lips, directs the sound into the oral cavity. The battery-powered electronic type of device is more common, and generates a buzzing sound. One type of device involves pressing the head of the device against the neck allowing the sound to pass through the skin. Another type of electronic device is similar to the pneumatic one in that a small tube is used to direct sound into the mouth. There has been much concern about the use of these devices, as speech-language pathologists have feared that they may become an easy substitute for learning esophageal speech. However, Boone (1983) noted that use of an artificial larynx can be programmed into a total training program and actually becomes supportive in the teaching of esophageal speech. He considered it advantageous for the laryngectomee to have alternative ways of generating voice, especially when the situation turns esophageal speaking into a physically demanding exercise.

The third option is surgical reconstruction that creates a new sound source within the patient. There are different types of surgery involving the use of tissue as a vibrating source or the attachment of an external prosthetic device. Surgery has met with mixed success depending on reactions of the individual patient. Of course, the older the patient, there is more risk with any type of surgical intervention depending on the existence of other complicating medical problems and reduced resistance to infection.

Postscript on Treatment of the Elderly

In our general comment introducing this discussion of language and speech treatment, we presented the idea that reduced physical working capacity in old age should be considered in the scheduling and pacing of treatment sessions. This has been a consistent concern across our discussions of each disorder. We would like to close this discussion with a consideration of the impact of subtle cognitive changes on the efficacy of treatment. Changes in cognitive capabilities (e.g., reduced encoding of new information) may lead to stimulation procedures that are less effective than they would be for younger adults. However, the elderly retain a great deal of cognitive capacity, often being as accurate as young adults but needing more time. Smith and Fullerton (1981) concluded that "there is no strong evidence to suggest that memory changes that occur with age are detrimental to the ability to use language effectively..." (p. 152). The clinician should be prepared simply to give elderly clients more time to respond or to complete a task.

Moreover, several treatment methods involve problem solving and new learning, such as the use of new modes of communicating, utilization of biofeedback, and maintenance of mechanical communication devices. As discussed in our final section, elderly patients must learn to adjust to a new life situation. Studies of intervention with normal elderly persons indicate that older people may have difficulty in benefitting from being shown how to do something (modeling), being told how to do something (instruction), or using feedback (Denny, 1981). Results on the effect of practice have been contradictory. More research is needed, because the elderly are capable of learning new behaviors, but may need more time.

Walker and Williams (1980) wrote an article with the promising title of "The response of a disabled elderly population to speech therapy." Their study of patients in the Geriatric Medicine Department of a hospital provided an unusual focus on persons primarily over age 65. These subjects, with a mean age of 69, had aphasia, apraxia of speech, or dysarthria. The informal nature of testing left a precise description of cases (i.e., as to type of aphasia or dysarthria) unclear; and controls were not instituted so that improvements could be attributed to treatment per se. Nevertheless, over a maximum treatment period of 24 months, 5 of 18 purely aphasic subjects improved their communicative levels, while 22 of 24 purely dysarthric subjects improved their levels. Walker and Williams concluded that aging may have affected improvement from aphasia more than it affected improvement from dysarthria. Although this study suffers from lack of precise measurement and control over factors such as time post-onset, etiology, and so on, it does raise some questions that have not been clearly answered through clinical reports or formal research.

A good deal of attention has been given to aging per se and to the possible effects of old age on rehabilitation. Relatively little attention has been given to its actual role in rehabilitation.

Management of Psychosocial Conditions

The psychosocial environment of the communication-disordered adult has had different meanings for different clinicians as the speech-language pathology profession has developed a concept of its role in rehabilitation. The different meanings add up to a fairly comprehensive approach to factors and variables that are important to a successful speech and language treatment plan. Motivation to improve communication skills and achieving generalization demand the clinician's attention to the client's psychological state, and to people and settings in the client's everyday environment. Lubinski (1981) discussed these as the client's internal and external environments. Consideration of people and settings, in a family home or nursing home, involves achieving an environment that is supportive of the goals for treatment. It also involves dealing with family members' adjustments to drastic changes in their own lives (Davis, 1983).

Communication Disorder as a Life Crises

"Crises can be defined as highly demanding situations in which the individual must adjust his behavior to a new set of circumstances" (Lieberman, 1975, p. 139). Adulthood is a series of adaptations to new circumstances or change. Many of these new circumstances represent standard milestones such as marriage, birth of a child, death of a relative, illness, and children's leaving home. These events bring sadness or joy, and are generally expected. Some people adjust better than others to the changes precipitated by these events. Lieberman (1975) identified two kinds of crises: (a)"events associated with loss, a subjective experience associated with a break in previous attachments to persons, places, or things;" and (b) "situations that disrupt the customary modes of behavior of the people concerned, which alter both their circumstances and their plans and impose a need for strenuous psychological work" (p. 139). Communication disorders belong to both of these categories as a loss of function and a change of customary modes of behavior. At any age, a person's adjustment to these unusual changes will be determined in part by his or her strategies for adjusting to the usual changes.

Our concern here is whether there are attributes of old age that modulate an individual's lifelong strategies for coping with crisis, and whether there are attributes of communication disorders that pose unique challenges in adjustment to crisis.

Communication disorders have been described as forms of loss for the patient and family (Tanner, 1980) and as crises disrupting states of equilibrium or homeostasis in patient and family (Lubinski, 1981a; Webster & Newhoff, 1981). Thurston (1980) characterized stroke in general as being a

225

particularly catastrophic crisis for patient and family. It is at least perceived as being a threat to life. In focusing Thurston's thoughts more specifically on the communication disorders resulting from stroke, Shadden (1983) has described the "communication crisis." A unique feature of many communication disorders is that they are unexpected and sudden. Adjustment is immediately constrained by the relative lack of general understanding of the nature of some of these disorders. They cut at the core of interaction patterns within a family. Accompanying physical and psychological limitations strike out at self-image and ability to continue in standard familial and social roles (Davis, 1983).

Analysis of the ability of elderly persons to cope with stress or adjust to crisis has been aided with the development of models that define the ingredients of adaptation (see Cone, 1975; Lieberman, 1975). Lieberman (1975) instructed that such a model begins with the psychological and biological resources that a person brings to the adaptive effort. First, the individual must possess the cognitive resources required to appraise the situation. Lieberman (1975) carved out three resource areas for his studies of the elderly: "the cognitive, physical, and energy outputs of the individual" (p. 145). Physical and energy reductions have already been discussed relative to normal aging; and cognitive reductions become pronounced in pathological aging. Nevertheless, Lieberman found that some elderly persons are able to cope successfully with crises while others are not so able.

In an effort to determine psychological factors that predict adaptation Lieberman's central finding was that coping processes found in young adults (i.e., ego strength and impulse control) were not predictive of adaptation by elderly adults. The elderly that remained intact in the face of crises were those who were able "to support consistent and coherent self-images." Predictive personality processes included the person's level of hope and his or her ability to introspect. Of particular interest is Lieberman's (1975) characterization of personality traits associated with successful coping by the elderly:

> Those who are aggressive, irritating, narcissistic, and demanding were the individuals we found to be most likely to survive crisis...A certain amount of magical thinking and perceiving oneself as the center of the universe, with a pugnacious stance

toward the world--even a highly suspicious one--seemed more
likely to insure homeostasis in the face of a severe crisis (pp.
155-156).

The young adult clinician may need to be prepared to be comfortable with and
supportive of such personality traits, if he or she is to help the elderly cope
with communication disorders. Several clinicians have discussed strategies for
helping communicatively impaired persons adjust to crisis. Although Lubinski,
Tanner, Webster, and other have discussed different approaches after the crisis
has occurred, Shadden has been dealing with preparation before the crisis
occurs.

Pre-Crisis Intervention

Shadden, Raiford, and Shadden (1983) have developed a rationale and
mechanism for providing Pre-Crisis Intervention (PCI) to people who are at-risk
when it comes to the likelihood of suffering from a communication disorder,
especially as the result of stroke. Elderly persons are considered to be at
much higher risk than younger adults; and the risk increases for those with
familial history of such diseases or with a prior occurrence of a stroke that
did not significantly impair function. In an article summarizing PCI, Shadden
(1983) described the basic goal as improving the resources that a person might
bring to a communication crisis so that the patient and family might be better
able to cope. The mechanism for accomplishing this goal is a PCI workshop that
provides information about communication disorders and provides attitude-
changing experiences. Curriculum and materials for conducting a PCI workshop
were made available by Shadden, et al. (1983). Although speech-language
pathologists are encouraged to offer these workshops in their community,
Shadden (1983) felt that PCI programming can be offered by social service
personnel, psychologists, and education specialists, as well as others
concerned about the elderly population.

Of the disorders discussed here, the only one that can be anticipated with
accuracy is speech without a larynx subsequent to laryngectomy. As Boone
(1983) notes, the decision as to the appropriateness of preoperative visit by a
speech-language pathologist is left to the surgeon, who must decide whether the
patient is psychologically prepared for information about consequences of the
surgery. Often such visits are made by the clinician and a well-adjusted

laryngectomee, and the nature of these visits usually varies depending on the patient's psychological condition and prognosis with the surgery. A primary consideration is the avoidance of creating unrealistic expectations in the patient. Therefore, preoperative visits may be light on information about speaking and heavy on emotional support and general information, or these visits may show that patient the possibilities in speech rehabilitation. An additional advantage for the clinician is that preoperative speaking patterns can be observed, so that treatment will correspond to the patient's natural ability and style.

Counseling after Onset

One of the most helpful recent advances in providing support for the patient and family during a communication crisis has been the viewing of any communicative disorder as a "loss" (of normal function) and the understanding of adjustment as a "grieving process" or adjustment to loss (Tanner, 1980, 1984; Webster & Newhoff, 1981). This process which applies to the family (i.e., in loss of a normal member; loss of homeostasis) as well as to the patient, should be experienced naturally and be allowed to run its course. Various suggestions have been made so that clinicians do not interfere with the process and can facilitate its progression (see Davis, 1983; Tanner, 1980).

The Patient

Although adults with communication disorders may require special assistance for psychological problems that impede the rehabilitation process (e.g., counselor specializing in the elderly), the speech-language pathologist should be prepared to assist with normal adjustments to the communication disorder and to the treatment process. A valuable source of emotional support comes from other persons with a similar disorder. In this sense, group treatment can be a valuable adjunct to individual treatment. Also, many communities have support groups such as local chapters of the National Head Injury Foundation or the American Heart Association's Stroke Clubs. A new publication by Sanders, Hamby, and Nelson (1984) is a manual for how to organize a new stroke club. For the laryngectomees, the American Cancer Society sponsored development of the International Association of

228

Laryngectomies (IAL). Also, local organizations of Lost Chord Clubs provide peer support for the laryngectomee.

Typical counseling problems for the speech-language pathologist include unrealistic expectations about recovery, lack of motivation to work in treatment, and negative reactions to alternative communication modes or devices. Assistance is needed from the family so that these feelings are not reinforced at home. These problems can be minimized with forthright and complete information about the disorder, permission to communicate freely about natural feelings, a treatment program that is truly tuned into the patient's communicative interests and needs, and the gradual introduction of alternative strategies in the clinical setting. Time should be spent explaining treatment to the patient and the family.

Some elderly persons may present special problems relative to the aforementioned standard considerations. An elderly person may have been happily living alone, suffered a stroke, and then was forced to move into a nursing home. Motivation to communicate may be difficult to achieve until adjustment to new surroundings and interpersonal contacts is achieved. An individual who had retired, in order to find respite from social contact and responsibility, may have a difficult time dealing with a clinician who wants the patient to want to talk to people and work hard in treatment. Some elderly persons just want to be left alone and just may not want clinical services. This may be considered to be their right.

One problem faced by a relatively small proportion of the elderly is what Lubinski (1981a, 1981b) called the "communication-impaired environment." Often found in even the best of nursing homes, this environment consists of rigid rules governing communication, few places for a private conversation, minimal communication between staff and residents, and physical constraints in the setting. Lubinski recommended "environmental language intervention" which includes in-service educational programs for the staff and modifications in seating arrangements, lighting, and acoustics that would facilitate communication. With respect to dysarthria, Berry and Sanders (1983) wrote about "environmental education" which consists of similar adjustments to people and settings that would facilitate communication. Too much ambient noise, for example, can reduce intelligibility of a dysarthric speaker and can make an esophageal speaker difficult to hear.

Patient's Family

The family may be involved in the rehabilitation process in several ways. When family members are an available support system for the client, they may be variables in the pragmatic dimension of speech and language treatment by participating in activities such as PACE therapy. They may be extensions of the clinician by monitoring or providing additional speech and language practice. Perhaps most importantly, the family may provide emotional support and encouragement that can sustain the client's motivation to recover impaired functions and to learn new communicative strategies. In fulfilling this role, family support may be best achieved when the adjustment problems of the family members themselves are considered to be important and receive some attention. Several family programs have been reviewed elsewhere (Davis, 1983; Webster & Newhoff, 1981).

The most typical form of family intervention is the regular meeting of family members in a group. Some of these are conducted by a psychologist or psychiatrist, which is advantageous for dealing with serious psychological problems that family members may be experiencing. However, family support groups can be organized and conducted by a speech-language pathologist for the purpose of facilitating natural adjustments to changes in communication patterns within the family. In a sense, these groups serve the function of a Stroke Club, for example, on a more regular basis. Whereas the clinician may focus the group on a particular topic, the therapeutic value of such a group comes from the family members advising and supporting each other. The more experienced members, who have successfully dealt with problems of the first few months post-onset, assist those who are struggling with the issues of early post-onset. The clinician may carry out the four basic counselor functions described by Webster and Newhoff (1981) of giving and receiving information, clarifying feelings, and attitudes, and discussing changes in behavior that may facilitate communication and be more supportive of the patient.

As noted in a previous section, the family support system of the elderly client is likely to differ from that of the middle-aged adult. Instead of dealing with a spouse, the clinician is more likely to be dealing with a son or daughter or, in some cases, with a brother or sister. In a nursing home setting, there is an increased likelihood that there is no family member readily available to support treatment. In this situation, the patient's communicative environment does not involve the family on a regular basis anyway. The support system is now the other residents and the staff of the institutional facility.

There are several interacting implications for this change in support system as a function of age. The most basic implication is that the clinician should be prepared for a greater variety of support systems with different clients. It is more difficult to discuss family intervention with broad generalizations. The need for support may be greater with the elderly, who already may be experiencing a sense of isolation that often accompanies aging. The disorder only compounds the problem of isolation. In this context, there is a greater likelihood of depression which drains energy for pursuing the tasks of treatment. This increases the challenge for the clinician to enhance the support systems that are available. Encouraging the maintenance of support systems may be one feature of a pre-crisis intervention (PCI) workshop. Furthermore, treatment of communication disorders in the elderly requires a team approach involving counselors, nurses, activities personnel, social workers, dieticians, and aides. There may be a greater need for group treatment of the communication problem, whereby other elderly persons may fuel the treatment process with empathic understanding of not only the communication disorder but also the occasional anxieties and loneliness of old age.

Treatment of the elderly can be a delightful experience for the clinician, because many elderly persons bring with them a need for human contact, a raucous sense of humor, and fascinating experiences. It requires understanding, patience, and resultant adjustments to their needs and capabilities, and also involves occasional pats on the back and hand holding. The elderly tend to need a little more consistent structure and general assistance than middle-aged adults. Yet, they should not be dealt with as if they were children; there should be no condescending. They are adults to be treated with respect. While some patients will have a low tolerance for unusual human interaction, many others will relish the opportunity to work regularly with an empathic clinician and will come to appreciate the clinician's efforts with a depth not often found in younger clients.

Self-Study Questions

1. Which of the adult speech and language disorders are most likely to begin after age 60?

231

2. Why has it been difficult to prove that age is related to recovery from aphasia?

3. Explain why language changes in Alzheimers dementia may be thought of as secondary to a primary deficit?

4. What are some general influences of normal aging on the treatment of speech and language disorders?

5. What is the difference between normal and pathological aging?

6. What is precrises intervention? Why is it important?

REFERENCES

Adamovitch, B. L, Henderson, J. A., & Auerbach, S. (1984). Cognitive retraining of the head injured patient: A dynamic approach. San Diego, CA: College-Hill Press.

Albert, M. L. (1978). Subcortical dementia. In R. Katzman, R. D. Terry, & K. L. Dick (Eds.), Alzheimer's disease: Senile dementia & related disorders. Vol. 7, New York: Raven Press.

American Cancer Society, (1984). Cancer facts and figures 1984. New York: American Cancer Society.

Appel, S. H. (1981). A unifying hypothesis for the cause of Amyotrophic Lateral Sclerosis, Parkinsonism, and Alzheimer's disease. Annals of Neurology, 10, 499-505.

Aten, J. L., McDonald, A., Simpson, M., & Gutierrex, R. (1984). Efficacy of modified palatal lifts for improving resonance. In M. R. McNeil, L. C. Rosenbeck, & A. E. Aronson (Eds.), The pysarthrias: Physiology, acoustics, perception, management. San Diego: College-Hill Press.

Barns, E. K., Sac, A., & Shore, H. (1973). Guidelines to treatment approaches: Modalities and methods for use with the aged. Gerontologist, 13, 513-527.

Basso, A., Capitani, E., & Vignolo, L. A. (1979). Influence of rehabilitation on language skills in aphasic patients: A controlled study. Archives of Neurology, 36, 190-196.

Bayles, K. A. (1984). Language and dementia. In A. L. Holland (Ed.), Language disorders in adults: Recent advances. San Diego: College-Hill Press.

Bayles, K. A., & Tomoada, C. K. (1983). Confrontation naming impairment in dementia. Brain and Language, 19, 98-114.

Benjamin, B. J. (1982). Phonological performance in gerontological speech. Journal of Psycholinguistic Research, 11, 159-167.

Ben-Yishay, Y., & Diller, L. (1983). Cognitive remediation. In M. Rosenthal, E. R. Griffith, M. R. Bend, & J. D. Miller (Eds.), Rehabilitation of the head injured adult. Philadelphia: F. A. Davis.

Berry, W. R., & Sanders, S. B., (1983). Environmental education: The universal management approach for adults with dysarthria. In W. R. Berry (Ed.), Clinical dysarthria. San Diego: College-Hill Press.

Beukelman, D. R., & Yorkston, K. M. (1977). A communication system for the severely dysarthric speaker with an intact language system. Journal of Speech and Hearing Disorders, 42, 265-270.

Beukelman, D. R., & Yorkston, K. M. (1978). Communications options for patients with brain stem lesions. Archives of Physical Medicine and Rehabilitation, 59, 337-340.

Beukelman, D. R., & Yorkston, K. M. (1980). Nonvocal communication: Performance evaluation. Archives of Physical Medicine and Rehabilitation, 61, 272-275.

Boone, D. R. (1983). The voice and voice therapy. (3rd ed.). Englewood Cliffs, NJ: Prentice-Hall.

Borod, J. C., Goodglass, H., & Kaplan, E. (1980a). Normative data on the Boston Diagnostic Aphasia Examination, Parietal Lobe Battery, and the Boston Naming Test. Journal of Clinical Neuropsychology, 2, 209-215.

Borod, J. C., Goodglass, H., & Kaplan, E. (1980b). Normative data on neuropsychological test. Boston: Unpublished manuscript.

Brown, J. R., Darley, F. L., & Aronson, A. E. (1970). Ataxic dysarthria. International Journal of Neurology, 7, 302-318.

Brown, J. W., & Jaffe, J. (1975). Hypothesis on cerebral dominance. Neuropsychologia, 13, 107-110.

Caligiuri, M. P., & Murry, T. (1983). The use of visual feedback to enhance prosodic control in dysarthria. In W. R. Berry (Ed.), Clinical dysarthria. San Diego: College-Hill Press.

Chapey, R. (1981). Divergent language intervention. In R. Chapey (Ed.), Language intervention strategies in adult aphasia. Baltimore, MD: Williams & Wilkins.

Clifford, S., & Gregg, J. B. (1981). Considerations for the laryngectomized elderly patient. Seminars in Speech, Language, and Hearing, 2, 157-165.

Cone, J. W. (1975). Formal models of ego development: A practitioner's response. In N. Datan & L. H. Ginsberg (Eds.), Life-span developmental psychology: Normative life crises. New York: Academic Press.

Curtis, A. P., & Fucci, D. (1983). Sensory and motor changes during development and aging. In N. J. Lass (Ed.), Speech and language: Advances in basic research and practice. Vol. 9. New York: Academic Press.

Darley, F. L. (1982). Aphasia. Philadelphia: W. B. Saunders.

Darley, F. L., Aronson, A. E., & Brown, J. R. (1969). Differential diagnostic patterns of dysarthria. Journal of Speech and Hearing Research, 12, 246-249.

Darley, F. L., Aronson, A. E., & Brown, J. R. (1975). Motor speech disorders. Philadelphia: W. B. Saunders.

Darley, F. L., Brown, J. R., & Goldstein, N. P. (1972). Dysarthria in multiple sclerosis. Journal of Speech and Hearing Research, 15, 229-245.

Davis, G. A. (1983). A survey of adult aphasia. Englewood Cliffs, NJ: Prentice-Hall.

Davis, G. A. (1984). Effects of aging on normal language. In A. L. Holland (Ed.), Language disorders in adults: Recent advances. San Diego: College-Hill Press.

Davis, G. A., & Holland, A. L. (1981). Age in understanding aphasia. In D. S. Beasley & G. A. Davis (Eds.), Aging communication processes and disorders. New York: Grune & Stratton.

Davis, G. A., & Wilcox, M. J. (1981). Incorporating parameters of natural conversation in aphasia treatment. In R. Chapey (Ed.), Language intervention strategies in adult aphasia. Baltimore, MD: Williams & Wilkins.

Deal, J. L., & Florance, C. L. (1978). Modification of the eight-step continuum for treatment of apraxia of speech in adults. Journal of Speech and Hearing Disorders, 43, 89-95.

Deming, M. B., & Cutler, N. E. (1983). Demography of the aged. In D. S. Woodruff & J. E. Birren (Eds.), Aging: Scientific perspectives and social issues. Monterey, CA: Brooks/Cole.

Danny, N. W. (1981). Adult cognitive development. In D. S. Beasley & G. A. Davis (Eds.), Aging: Communication processes and disorders. New York: Grune & Stratton.

deVries, H. A. (1983). Physiology of exercise and aging. In D. S. Woodruff & J. E. Birren (Eds.), Aging: Scientific perspectives and social issues (2nd ed.). Monterey, CA: Brooks/Cole.

Diller, L. (1976). A model for cognitive retraining in rehabilitation. Clinical Psychologist, 29, 13.

Eslinger, P. J., & Damasio, A. R. (1981). Age and type of aphasia in patients stroke. Journal of Neurology, Neurosurgery, and Psychiatry, 44, 377-381.

Fernandez R. J., & Samuels, M. A. (1982). Intellectual dysfunction: Mental retardation and dementia. In M. A. Samuels (Ed.), Manual of neurologic therapeutics. Boston: Little, Brown.

Fitch, J. L., & Cross, S. T. (1983). Telecomputer treatment for aphasia. Journal of Speech and Hearing Disorders, 48, 335-336.

Fitch-West, J. (1983). Heightening visual imagery: A new approach to aphasia therapy. In E. Perecman (Ed.), Cognitive processing in the right hemisphere. New York: Academic Press.

Foldi, N. S., Cicone, M., & Gardner, H. (1983). Pragmatic aspects of communication in brain-damaged patients. In S. J. Segalowitz (Ed.), Language functions and brain organization. New York: Academic Press.

Freal, J. E., Kraft, G. H., & Coryell, J. K. (1984). Symptomatic fatigue in multiple sclerosis. Archives of Physical Medicine and Rehabilitation, 65, 135-138.

Gardner, H., Brownell, H. H., Wapner, W., & Michelow, D. (1983). Missing the point: The role of the right hemisphere in the processing of complex linguistic materials. In E. Perecman (Ed.), Cognitive processing in the right hemisphere. New York: Academic Press.

Gardner, W. H. (1966). Adjustment problems of laryngectomized women. Archives of Otolaryngology, 83, 31-42.

Gewirth, L. R., Shindler, A. G., & Hier, D. B. (1984). Altered patterns of word associations in dementia and aphasia. Brain and Language, 21, 307-317.

Goodglass, H., & Kaplan, E. (1983). The assessment of aphasia and related disorders (2nd ed.). Philadelphia: Lea & Febiger.

Hanson, W. R., & Metter, E. J. (1983). DAF speech rate modification in Parkinson's disease: A report of two cases. In W. R. Berry (Ed.), Clinical dysarthria, San Diego, CA: College-Hill Press.

Harasymiw, S. J., Halper, A., & Sutherland, B. (1981). Sex, age, and aphasia type. Brain and Language, 12, 190-198.

Hartman, D. E., & Danhauer, J. L. (1976). Perceptual features of speech for males in four perceived age decades. Journal of the Acoustical Society of America, 59, 713-715.

Helm-Estabrooks, N. (1983). Exploiting the right hemisphere for language rehabilitation: Melodic intonation therapy. In E. Perecman (Ed.), Cognitive processing in the right hemisphere. New York: Academic Press.

Helm-Estabrooks, N., Fitzpatrick, P. M., & Barresi, B. (1982). Visual action therapy for global aphasia. Journal of Speech and Hearing Disorders, 47, 385-389.

Hildick-Smith, M. (1983). Parkinson's disease in the elderly. Journal of the Royal Society of Health, 103, 166-169.

Holland, A. L. (1980). Communicative abilities in daily living. Baltimore: University Park Press.

Hunker, C. J., & Abbs, J. H., (1984). Physiological analyses of Parkinsonian tremors in the orofacial system. In M. R. McNeil, J. C. Rosenbek, & A. E. Aronson (Eds.), The dysarthrias: Physiology, acoustics, perception, management. San Diego: College-Hill Press.

Janiszewski, D. W., Caroscio, J. T., & Wisham, L. H. (1983). Amyotrophic lateral sclerosis: A comprehensive rehabilitation approach. Archives of Physical Medicine and Rehabilitation, 64, 304-307.

Johnson, R. C., Cole, R. E., Bowers, J. K., Foiles, S. V., Nikaido, A. M., Patrick, J. W., & Woliver, R. E. (1979). Hemispheric efficiency in middle and later adulthood. Cortex, 15, 109-119.

Kahane, J. C. (1981). Anatomic and physiologic changes in the aging peripheral speech mechanism. In D. S. Beasley & G. A. Davis (Eds.), Aging: Communication processes and disorders. New York: Grune & Stratton.

Kahane, J. C. (1983). A survey of age-related changes in the connective tissues of the human adult larynx. In D. M. Bless & J. H. Abbs (Eds.), Vocal fold physiology: Contemporary research and clinical issues. San Diego: College-Hill Press.

Katz, R. C. (1984). Understanding questions. Los Angeles: Sunset Software.

Keenan, J. S., & Brassell, E. G. (1975). Aphasia Language Performance Scales. Murfreesboro, TN: Pinnacle Press.

Kertesz, A., & McCabe, P. (1977). Recovery patterns and prognosis in aphasia. Brain, 100, 1-18.

Kertesz, A., & Sheppard, A. (1981). The epidemiology of aphasic and cognitive impairment in stroke: Age, sex, aphasia type and laterality differences. Brain, 104, 117-128.

Kocel, K. M. (1980). Age-related changes in cognitive abilities and hemispheric specialization. In J. Herron (Ed.), Neuropsychology of left-handedness. New York: Academic Press.

Kreul, E. (1972). Neuromuscular control examination (NMC) for parkinsonism: Vowel prolongations and diadochokinetic and reading rates. Journal of Speech and Hearing Research, 15, 72-83.

LaPointe, L. L. (1983). Aphasia intervention with adults: Historical, present, and future approaches. In J. Miller, D. E. Yoder, & R. Schiefelbusch (Eds.), Contemporary issues in language intervention. Rockville, MD: American-Speech-Language-Hearing Association.

236

Lezak, M. D., (1983). Neuropsychological assessment. (2nd ed.). New York: Oxford University Press.

Lieberman, M. A., (1975). Adaptive processes in late life. In N. Datan & L. H. Ginsberg (Eds.), Life span developmental psychology: Normative life crises. New York: Academic Press.

Lubinski, R. (1981a). Environmental language intervention. In R. Chapey (Ed.), Language intervention strategies in adult aphasia. Baltimore: Williams & Wilkins.

Lubinski, R. (1981b). Speech, language and audiology programs in home health care agencies and nurses homes. In D. S. Beasley & G. A. Davis (Eds.), Aging: Communication processes and disorders. New York: Grune & Stratton.

Ludlow, C. L., & Bassich, C. J. (1984). Relationships between perceptual ratings and acoustic measures of hypokinetic speech. In M. R. McNeil, J. C. Rosenbek, & A. E. Aronson (Eds.), The dysarthrias: Physiology, acoustic, perception, management. San Diego: College-Hill Press.

Luria, A. R. (1970). Traumatic aphasia. The Hague, Netherlands: Mouton.

Mace, N. L., & Rabins, P. V. (1981). The 36-hour day. Baltimore: Johns Hopkins University Press.

Mandleberg, I. A., & Brooks, D. N. (1975). Cognitive recovery after severe head injury I. Serial testing on the Wechsler Adult Intelligence Scale. Journal of Neurology, Neurosurgery, and Psychiatry, 38, 1121-1126.

Marshall, R. C., & Phillips, D. S. (1983). Prognosis for improved verbal communication in aphasic stroke patients. Archives of Physical Medicine and Rehabilitation, 64, 497-600.

Martin, A., & Fedio, P. (1983). Word production and comprehension in Alzheimer's disease: The breakdown of semantic knowledge. Brain and Language, 19, 124-141.

Meyer, J. S., Kanda, T., Fukuuchi, Y., Shimazu, K., Dennis, E. W., & Ericsson, A. D. (1971). Clinical prognosis correlated with hemispheric blood flow in cerebral infarction. Stroke, 2, 383-394.

Millar, J. M., & Whitaker, H. A. (1983). The right hemisphere's contribution to language: A review of the evidence form brain-damaged subjects. In S. J. Segalowitz (Ed.), Language functions and brain organization. New York: Academic Press.

Mills, R. H., & Thomas, R. P. (1983). Word recognition programs. Ann Arbor, MI: Brain-Link Software.

Musselwhite, C. R., & St. Louis, K. W. (1982). Communication programming for the severely handicapped: Vocal and non-vocal strategies. San Diego: College-Hill Press.

Myers, P. S. (1984). Right hemisphere impairment. In A. L. Holland (Ed.), Language disorders in adults: Recent advances. San Diego: College-Hill Press.

Nemec, R. E., & Cohen, K. (1984). EMG biofeedback in the modification of hypertonia in spastic dysarthria: Case report. Archives of Physical Medicine and Rehabilitation, 65, 103-104.

Netsell, R., & Cleeland, C. S. (1973). Modification of lip hypertonia in dysarthria using EMG feedback. Journal of Speech and Hearing Disorders, 38, 131-140.

Netsell, R. (1983). Speech motor control: Theoretical issues with clinical impact. In W. R. Berry (Ed.), Clinical dysarthria. San Diego: College-Hill Press.

Netsell, R., & Daniel, B. (1979). Dysarthria in adults: Physiologic approach to rehabilitation. Archives of Physical Medicine and Rehabilitation, 60, 502-508.

Obler, L. K., & Albert, M. L. (1981). Language in the elderly aphasic and in the dementing patient. In M. T. Sarno (Ed.), Acquired aphasia. New York: Academic Press.

Obler, L. K. & Albert, M. L., Goodglass, H., & Benson, D. F. (1978). Aging and aphasia type. Brain and Language, 6, 318-322.

Perkins, W. H. (Ed.). (1983). Dysarthria and apraxia. New York: Thieme-Stratton.

Pickersgill, M. J., & Lincoln, N. B. (1983). Prognostic indicators and the pattern of recovery of communication in aphasic stroke patients. Journal of Neurology, Neurosurgery, and Psychiatry, 46, 130-139.

Porch, B. E. (1967). Porch index of communicative ability, Volume I: Theory and development. Palo Alto, CA: Consulting Psychologists Press.

Porch, B. E. (1981). Porch index of communicative ability, Volume II: Administration, scoring, and interpretation (3rd ed.). Palo Alto, CA: Consulting Psychologists Press.

Prescott, T., Selinger, M., & Loverso, F. (1982). An analysis of learning, generalization, and maintenance of verbs by an aphasic patient. In R. H. Brookshire (Ed.), Clinical aphasiology conference proceedings. Minneapolis: BRK.

Ramig, L. A. Effects of physiological aging on speaking and reading rates. Journal of Communication Disorders, 16, 217-226.

Ramig, L. A., & Ringel, R. L. (1983). Effects of physiological aging on selected acoustic characteristics of voice. Journal of Speech and Hearing Research, 26, 22-30.

Ronch, J. L. (1981). Considerations in counseling elderly person. Seminars in Speech, Language, and Hearing, 2, 219-225.

Rosenbek, J. C. (1978). Treating apraxia of speech. In D. F. Johns (Ed.), Clinical management of neurogenic communicative disorders. Boston: Little, Brown.

Rosenbek, J. C. (1978). Treating apraxia of speech in adults. In W. H. Perkins (Ed.), Dysarthria and apraxia. New York: Thieme-Stratton.

Rosenbek, J. C., & LaPointe, L. L. (1978). The dysarthrias: Description, diagnosis, and treatment. In D. F. Johns (Ed.) Clinical management of neurogenic communicative disorders. Boston: Little, Brown.

Rosenbek, J. C., Lemme, M. L., Ahern, M. B., Harris, E. H., & Wertz, R. T. (1973). A treatment for apraxia of speech in adults. Journal of Speech and Hearing Disorders, 38, 462-472.

Rubow, R. (1984). Role of feedback, reinforcement, and compliance training in biofeedback-based rehabilitation of motor speech disorders. In M. R. McNeil, J. C. Rosenbek, and A. E. Aronson (Eds.), The dysarthrias: Physiology, acoustics, perception, management. San Diego: College-Hill.

Rubow, R., Rosenbek, J. C., Collins, M. J., & Celesia, G. G. (1984). Reduction of hemifacial spasm and dysarthria following EMG biofeedback. Journal of Speech and Hearing Disorders, 49, 20-33.

Ryan, W., & Burk, K. (1974). Perceptual and acoustic correlates of aging in the speech of males. Journal of Communication Disorders, 7, 181-192.

Sahs, A. L., Hartman, E. C., & Aronson, S. M. (Eds.). (1976). Guidelines for stroke care (DHEW Publication No. [HRA] 76-14017). Washington, DC: U.S. Government Printing Office.

Salvatore, A. (1982). Artificial language learning in brain damaged adults using a matrix training program. In R. H. Brookshire (Ed.), Clinical aphasiology conference proceedings. Minneapolis: BRK.

Sanders, S., Hamby, E. I., & Nelson, M. (1984). You are not alone. Nashville, TN: American Heart Association-Tennessee Affiliate.

Sarno, M. T. (1981). Recovery and rehabilitation in aphasia. In M. T. Sarno (Ed.), Acquired aphasia. New York: Academic Press.

Schaie, K. W. (1980). Intelligence and problem solving. In J. E. Birren & R. B. Sloane (Eds.), Handbook of mental health and aging. Englewood Cliffs, NJ: Prentice-Hall.

Schuell, H. M. (1972). Minnesota Test for Differential Diagnosis of Aphasia. (rev. ed.). Minneapolis: University of Minnesota Press.

Schuell, H. M., Jenkins, J. J., & Jimenez-Pabon, E. (1964). Aphasia in adults. New York: Harper & Row.

Shadden, B. B. (1983). Pre-crisis intervention: A tool for reducing the impact of stroke-related personal and family crisis. Journal of Gerontological Social Work, 6, 61-74.

Shadden, B. B., Raiford, C. A., & Shadden, H. S. (1983). Coping with communication disorders in aging. Tigaard, OR: C. C. Publications.

Shames, G. H., Font, J., & Matthews, J. (1963). Factors relating to speech proficiency of the laryngectomized. Journal of Speech and Hearing Disorders, 28, 273-287.

Shanks, S. (1970). Effects of aging upon rapid syllable repetition. Perceptual and Motor Skills, 30, 687-690.

Silverman, F. H. (1980). Communication for the speechless. Englewood Cliffs, NJ: Prentice-Hall.

Sklar, M. (1983). Sklar Aphasia Scale. Los Angeles: Western Psychological Services.

Smith, A. D., & Fullerton, A. M. (1981). Age differences in episodic and semantic memory: Implications for language and cognition. In D. S. Beasley & G. A. Davis (Eds.), Aging: Communication processes and disorders. New York: Grune & Stratton.

Sparks, R. W. (1981). Melodic intonation therapy. In R. Chapey (Ed.), Language intervention strategies in adult aphasia. Baltimore: Williams & Wilkins.

Spradlin, J. E., & Siegel, G. M. (1982). Language training in natural and clinical environments. Journal of Speech and Hearing Disorders, 47, 2-6.

Stoicheff, M. L. (1981). Speaking fundamental frequency characteristics of nonsmoking female adults. Journal of Speech and Hearing Research, 24, 437-441.

Tanner, D. C. (1980). Loss and grief: Implications for the speech-language pathologist and audiologist. Asha, 22, 916-928.

Tanner, D. C. (1984). Aphasia: The family's guide to the psychology of loss, grief and adjustment. Tulsa, OK: Modern Education corporation.

Thompson, C., & Kearns, K. (1981). An experimental analysis of acquisition, generalization, and maintenance of naming behavior in a patient with anomia. In R. H. Brookshire (Ed.), Clinical Aphasiology Conference Proceedings. Minneapolis: BRK.

Thompson, C., McReynolds, L., & Vance, C. (1982). Generative use of locatives in multiword utterances in agrammatism: A matrix training approach. In R. H. Brookshire (Ed.), Clinical aphasiology conference proceedings. Minneapolis: BRK.

Thurston, F. D. (1980). Stroke: A catastrophic event. Journal of Gerontological Social Work, 3, 53-61.

Valenstein, E., (1981). Age-related changes in the human central nervous system. In D. S. Beasley & G. A. Davis (Eds.), Aging: Communication processes and disorders. New York: Grune & Stratton.

Walker, S. A., & Williams, B. O. (1980). The response of a disabled elderly population to speech therapy. British Journal of Disorders of Communication, 15, 19-29.

Webster, E. J., & Newhoff, M. (1981). Intervention with families of communicatively impaired adults. In D. S. Beasley & G. A. Davis (Eds.), Aging: Communication processes and disorders. New York: Grune & Stratton.

Weigl, E., & Bierwisch, M. (1970). Neuropsychology and linguistics: Topics of common research. Foundations of Language, 6, 1-18.

Weiner, F. F. (1984). Aphasia I, II, III. Baltimore: University Park Press.

Weismer, G. (1984). Articulatory characteristics of Parkinsonian dysarthria: Segmental and phrase-level timing, spirantization, and glottal-supraglottal coordination. In M. R. McNeil, J. C. Rosenbek, & A. E. Aronson (Eds.), The dysarthrias: Physiology, acoustics, perception, management. San Diego: College-Hill Press.

Weismer, G., & Fromm, D. (1983). Acoustic analysis of geriatric utterances: Segmental and nonsegmental characteristics that relate to laryngeal function. In D. M. Bless & J. H. Abbs (Eds.), Vocal fold physiology: Contemporary research and clinical issues. San Diego: College-Hill Press

Wepman, J. M. (1951). Recovery from aphasia. New York: Ronald Press.

Wepman, J. M. (1976). Aphasia: Language without thought or thought without language. Asha, 18, 131-136.

Wertz, R. T. (1983). Language intervention context and setting for the aphasic adult: When? In J. Miller, D. E. Yoder, & R. Schiefelbusch (Eds.), Contemporary issues in language intervention. Rockville, MD: American Speech-Language-Hearing Association.

Wertz, R. T., Lapointe, L. L., & Rosenbek, J. C. (1984). Apraxia of speech in adults. New York: Grune & Stratton.

Wilcox, M. J., & Davis, G. A. (in press). Pragmatics, PACE, and Adult Aphasia. San Diego: College-Hill Press

Yorkston, K. M., & Beukelman, D. R. (1980). An analysis of connected speech samples of aphasic and normal speakers. Journal of Speech and Hearing Disorders, 45, 27-36.

Yorkston, K. M., & Beukelman, D. R. (1981). Ataxic dysarthria: Treatment sequences based on intelligibility and prosodic considerations. Journal of Speech and Hearing Disorders, 46, 398-404.

Young, J. L., Percy, C. L., & Asire, A. J. (Eds.). (1981). Surveillance, epidemiology, and end results: Incidence and mortality data, 1973-1977 (NCI Monograph No. 57, NIH Publication No. 81-2330). Washington, DC: U.S. Government Printing Office.

Suggested Readings

Normal Aging

Beasley, D. S., & Davis, G. A. (Eds.). (1981). Aging: Communication processes and disorders. New York: Grune & Stratton.

Birren, J. E., & Sloane, R. B. (Eds.). (1980). Handbook of mental health and aging. Englewood Cliffs, NJ: Prentice-Hall.

Datan, N., & Ginsberg, L. H. (Eds.). (1975). Life-span developmental psychology: Normative life crises. New York: Academic Press.

Davis, G. A. (1984). Effects of aging on normal language. In A. L. Holland (Eds.), Language disorders in adults: Recent advance. San Diego: College-Hill Press.

Woodruff, D. S., & Birren, J. E. (Eds.). (1983). Aging: Scientific perspectives and social issues (2nd ed.). Monterey, CA: Brooks/Cole.

Aphasia

Albert, M. L., Goodglass, H., Helm, N. A., Rubens, A. B., & Alexander, M. P. (1981). Clinical aspects of dysphasia. New York: Springer-Verlag.

Chapey, R. (Eds.). (1981). Language intervention strategies in adult aphasia. Baltimore: Williams & Wilkins.

Davis, G. A. (1983). A survey of adult aphasis. Englewood Cliffs, NJ: Prentice-Hall.

Holland, A. L. (Eds.). (1984). Language disorders in adults: Recent advances. San Diego: College-Hill Press.

Secondary Language Impairments

Adamavitch, B. L., Henderson, J. A., & Auerbach, S. (in press). Cognitive retraining of the head injured patient: A dynamic approach. San Diego: College-Hill Press.

Mace, N. L., & Rabins, P. V. (1981). The 36-hour day. Baltimore: Johns Hopkins University Press.

Motor Speech Disorders

Costello, J. M. (Eds.). (1984). Speech disorders in adults: Recent advances. San Diego: College-Hill Press.

Perkins, W. H. (Eds.). (1983). Dysarthria and apraxia. New York: Thieme-Stratton.

Rosenbek, J. C., & LaPointe, L. L. (1978). The dysarthrias: Description, diagnosis, and treatment. In D. F. Johns (Eds.), Clinical management of neurogenic communicative disorders. Boston: Little, Brown.

Wertz, R. T., La Pointe, L. L., & Rosenbek, J. C. (1984). Apraxia of speech in adults: The disorder and its management. New York: Grune & Stratton.

Laryngectomy

Boone, D. R. (1983). The voice and voice therapy. (3rd ed.). Englewood Cliffs, NJ: Prentice-Hall.

Keith, R. L., & Shanks, J. C. (1983). Laryngectomee rehabilitation: Past and present. In N. J. Lass (Ed.), Speech and language: Advances in basic research and practice. (Vol. 9). New York: Academic Press.

Weinberg, B. (Ed.). (1980). Readings in speech following total laryngectomy. Baltimore: University Park Press.

Counseling and Other Rehabilitation Issues

Brubaker, S. H. (1981). Aphasia: A guide to family resources and activities. Detroit, MI: Wayne State University Press.

Hale, G. (1979). The source book for the disabled. New York: Bantam Books.

Sanders, S., Hamby, E. I., & Nelson, M. (1984). You are not alone. Nashville, TN: American Heart Association-Tennessee Affiliate.

Sarno, J. E., & Sarno, M. T. (1979). Stroke: A guide for patients and their families (rev. ed.). New York: McGraw-Hill.

Shadden, B. B., Raiford, C. A., & Shadden, H. S. (1983). Coping with communication disorders in aging. Tigaard, OR: C. C. Publications.

Tanner, D. C. (1984). Aphasia: The family's guide to the psychology of loss, grief, and adjustment. Tulsa, OK: Modern Education Corporation.

Management of the Hearing Impaired Elderly

Barbara E. Weinstein
Columbia University, New York

The rehabilitation literature is replete with definitions of the rehabilitation process. A particularly descriptive definition is the application of techniques to "enable a handicapped person to live as full a life as remaining abilities and degree of health will allow" (Encyclopedia Britannica, 1978, p. 484; Loebel & Eisdorfer, 1984, p. 41). Depending on the nature of the disorder, Loebel & Eisdorfer (1984) emphasize that the goal should be to maximize remaining function or to restore one to an optimal level of function. Implicit in the above definition is that rehabilitation efforts are comprehensive in scope, individualized in approach, focusing at all times on the complex interplay between the disease entity and the handicapped individual (Clark & Bray, 1984). Hull's (1982) conception of aural rehabilitation as "an attempt at reducing barriers to communication resulting from hearing impairment and facilitating adjustment relative to the possible psychosocial, occupational and educational impact of the auditory deficit" (p. 6) goes beyond the more traditional approach to aural rehabilitation and is therefore in keeping with the holistic/multifaceted philosophy advanced by the Encyclopedia Britannica (1978) (Loebel & Eisdorfer 1984). Thus while in the 1960s aural rehabilitation implied lipreading, auditory training, and training in the use of hearing aids, aural rehabilitation now encompasses some or all of the following techniques:

1. hearing aid selection and hearing aid orientation/auditory training;
2. motivational, informational, and personal adjustment counseling;
3. visual communication training, and
4. family counseling.

Before discussing each of these components, the factors which may impact on the decision to intervene and the outcome of rehabilitation efforts will be reviewed.

Aural Rehabilitation Candidacy

The audiologist must have a set of criteria for determining the
appropriateness of aural rehabilitation, the form it should take and the
techniques to be adopted for each individual. For example, a hearing aid and
hearing aid orientation may be recommended for some, whereas motivational and
family counseling may be appropriate for others. Although there is a dirth of
audiologic research defining the preselection criteria highly predictive of a
successful rehabilitation outcome, psychiatrists, psychologists, and
sociologists with a specialization in geriatrics have identified factors which
impact on the outcome of rehabilitation with the elderly. Loebel and Eisdorfer
(1984) identified a host of intrinsic and extrinsic factors which influence the
potential of rehabilitation and should thus enter into one's decision-making
process.

The intrinsic factors which reside within the individual include:
(a) physical status, (b) motivation, and (c) self-perceived effects of the
disorder (i.e., handicap). The extrinsic variables which arise outside the
individual include: (a) the environment, (b) life-style, (c) social support
system, and (d) financial status (Loebel & Eisdorfer, 1984). The discussion
below details how each of these factors may influence the audiologist's
decision regarding candidacy for rehabilitation, the needs of the individual,
or the efficacy of rehabilitation.

Intrinsic Factors

Physical Impairments

The audiogram. The evidence to date is equivocal regarding hearing aid
satisfaction and audiometric variables. Whereas Ewertsen (1974) and Surr,
Schuchman, and Montgomery (1978) reported that frequency of hearing aid use
varies directly with hearing loss severity, Kapetyn (1977) found no substantial
relationship between use of amplification and degree of loss. Despite the lack
of agreement, it is clear that the severity of the hearing loss and speech
recognition ability should not be the primary determinants of need or candidacy
for amplification and after care. Audiometric data (e.g., uncomfortable
listening level, speech recognition ability, dynamic range) should, however,

guide in decisions regarding the sensory aid (e.g., hearing aid, vibrotactile aid) and the electroacoustic characteristics to be recommended. Additionally, audiometric data may provide a gross estimate of benefits to be derived from amplification. For example, whereas a hearing aid may help individuals with a profound hearing loss hear environmental sounds primarily, it may make speech louder, more audible, and possibly clearer for those with mild to moderate losses (Davis & Hardick, 1981). A general rule to be kept in mind is that irrespective of severity, any hearing-impaired person who reportedly has difficulty communicating should consider a hearing aid.

Upper limb function. Limitations in the range of motion caused by some forms of arthritis involving the hands and shoulders is quite common in the elderly. Similarly, many elderly persons suffer from manual dexterity problems, a decline in hand function and decreased tactile sensation (Baum, 1984). Each of these physiological changes may interfere with the ability to grasp, manipulate, or release a device as small as a hearing aid. Similarly, the clumsiness or shakiness that may result from loss of manual dexterity, the inability to perform fine motor acts resulting from diminished tactile sense, and the difficulty in reaching resulting from limitation in range of motion can interfere with the manipulation of a hearing aid (Itoh, Lee, & Shapiro, 1984). The audiologist must carefully assess the ability to perform the gross and fine motoric acts necessary to independent hearing aid use. Also deserving of careful assessment are other factors (i.e., client limitations, role of significant others) which may influence the recommendation of, and adjustment to, amplification devices.

Vision. In addition to reduction in hearing sensitivity, declines in visual acuity (ability to see objects at a distance) are quite prevalent in the elderly. According to the National Center for Health Statistics (1981), 14% of elderly individuals suffer from visual impairment, which may include blurred vision due to cataracts or macular degeneration, a reduced capacity to see fine detail, and reduced ability to focus on objects at a close distance (Karp, 1983). In that visual acuity can influence auditory-visual speech recognition and benefits to be derived from amplification, the communication specialist must assess the visual status of the hearing-impaired (e.g., screen for binocular far-visual acuity using the Snellen Eye Chart American Optical No. 1930 (Garstecki, 1983). In addition, the patients should be queried regarding visual status and the use of corrective lenses or low visual aids such as magnifiers (Karp, 1983).[1] It should be emphasized that although the presence of a visual impairment will not contraindicate rehabilitative intervention, the severity of the problem may influence the rehabilitation techniques employed, and the achievement of certain rehabilitation goals.

Age. The literature on the effects of chronological age on hearing aid use/satisfaction is equivocal. Although Kapetyn (1977), Tyler, Baker, and Bednell (1983), and Ewertsen (1974) found little or no effect of age on hours of use, Jerger and Hayes (1976) and Alberti (1977) reported a slight age effect. Given the inconclusiveness of the data, chronological age in and of itself should not contraindicate hearing aid use. In fact, until proven otherwise, Kasten's (1979) philosophy "aging individuals can and should be hearing aid users" should apply (p. 81). It should be noted, that the concomitants of age (mobility limitation, physical impairments, reduced adaptability, and feelings of loneliness and powerlessness) will undoubtedly influence the acclimation process, patient motivation, and the extent of satisfaction. Therefore, the young-old should be encouraged to consider a hearing aid before the "concomitants of old age turn a previously manageable hearing loss into an intolerable burden" (Alberti, 1977, p. 421).

Mental status. In that declines in memory and orientation are hallmarks of certain disease states associated with advancing age (e.g., organic mental syndrome), these cognitive functions should be assessed prior to initiating intervention. One should not use a medical diagnosis of "organic mental syndrome (OMS)," "senility," or "Alzheimer's disease" as a mitigating factor in a hearing aid recommendation. In many cases, clients with moderately-severe to profound hearing levels are inappropriately labeled senile, because they are unable to hear or understand the questions typically asked by psychologists and psychiatrists to assist in a diagnosis of "OMS." Accordingly, the audiologist should informally assess the candidate's "mental status" using a modified

---

[1]Sample questions to be asked to identify possible visual impairments (modified from Karp, 1983):

1. Do you have problems with your vision? What kind?
2. Do you wear eyeglasses? Do you use low vision aids? Do they help you see?
3. Can you see my mouth clearly?
4. What environmental conditions interfere with your ability to see? (e.g., glare, poor lighting)

version of the Mental Status Questionnaire (MSQ) (if applicable) or by asking simple questions which will yield information regarding memory and orientation. An auditory trainer, hearing aid or the speech circuit of the audiometer should be used to insure that the patient hears/understands the questions being asked.

If memory loss and disorientation is confirmed, a significant other or caregiver must be willing to assume responsibility for the hearing aid before it is recommended. In view of the behavioral manifestations of "OMS" the potential candidate should be monitored closely to determine if the hearing aid is beneficial or if it is appropriate--oftentimes an alternative listening device placed at the bedside will be preferable.

Motivation

Motivation is a key factor in the outcome of rehabilitation with the older adult. Therefore, the patient's attitude toward hearing aid use and rehabilitation must be explored prior to making a recommendation. If motivation is lacking, it is incumbent on the audiologist to probe the reasons contributing to this. If lack of motivation is due to misconceptions about intervention options and limitations inherent in hearing aids, the audiologist should clarify the client's concerns and help them to "self-discover" the fallacies in their reasoning. An aggressive approach to motivating the client to participate in rehabilitation should be avoided. This tends to reinforce negative attitudes (Kasten, 1982), and is thus counterproductive. It is important to emphasize that regardless of one's professional opinion, the decision to intervene audiologically must ultimately come from the patient.

Psychosocial Factors

The findings of Garstecki (1984), Hutton (1980), Kapetyn (1977), and Stephens and Goldstein (1983) suggest that hearing aid satisfaction is contingent to a large extent on psychosocial factors (e.g., social interaction, family attitude, acceptance of the hearing loss). These psychosocial factors can be surveyed by using a communication profile or a hearing handicap scale. In that successful hearing aid use varies considerably with psychosocial factors and bears an imperfect relation to hearing impairment (i.e., two individuals with similar degrees of impairment differ in their perception of the handicap) (Weinstein & Ventry, 1983), it is imperative that the handicap be assessed directly using a reliable and valid scale. The direct assessment of hearing handicap is of utmost importance in the elderly due to the numerous nonaudiologic factors (e.g., declining health, financial status, lifestyle) which condition the extent to which an impairment will pose a handicap. Several self-assessment scales including the Hearing Handicap Inventory for the Elderly (Appendix A) and the Self-Assessment of Communication (SAC) (Appendix B) reliably measure self-assessed handicap in the elderly (Schow & Nerbonne, 1982; Ventry & Weinstein, 1982). Information gleaned from self-report data should be used in conjunction with audiometric findings to make recommendations regarding intervention. Similarly, hearing handicap data can be used to quantify the perceived benefit from hearing aid use (Walden, Demorest, & Hepler, 1984).

External Factors

Social Support Systems

The presence of a significant other (e.g., spouse, child) or in the case of the institutionalized, a caregiver (e.g., nurse's aid) will influence the outcome of rehabilitation efforts. These individuals can influence both adjustment to the disorder and the effectiveness of rehabilitative efforts (Loebel & Eisdorfer, 1984). In the case of the noninstitutionalized, the audiologist must determine the actual presence, the availability, and the attitudes of the members of the client's support system (Silverstone, 1984). On the other hand, the structure of the long-term care facility, the staff's willingness to learn and assist the patient, and the belief systems held by caregivers must be taken into consideration when deciding on the appropriateness of a hearing aid or intervention for an institutionalized patient (Loebel & Eisdorfer, 1984). In sum, the audiologist must assess the commitment, attitudes, and availability of significant others who must participate in the rehabilitation process if it is to be successful (Loebel & Eisdorfer, 1984).

Environment

The emotional climate, the physical and social environment in which intervention takes place will have a psychological impact on rehabilitation and thus should influence one's decision to intervene (Loebel & Eisdorfer, 1984).

For example, if family members or staff (e.g., nurses, doctors) view communication as important, they will enthusiastically endorse rehabilitative efforts to promote and facilitate carryover of newly acquired skills into daily life. Similarly, if the acoustic environmment (e.g., lighting, furniture arrangement) is conducive to interactions among individuals, rehabilitation efforts are more likely to succeed. Conversely, if the staff or significant others are not sensitive to the importance of communication, the opportunity for interactions will be diminished, level of motivation will decline, and rehabilitative efforts stifled (Silverstone, 1984). It is imperative that prior to instituting aural rehabilitation, a careful analysis of the attitudes of individuals in the environment and the physical characteristics of the environment be assessed. This is especially true in institutions where the nature of institutional care is typically custodial rather than therapeutic (Loebel & Eisdorfer, 1984).

Financial Factors

The willingness and ability of a client to pay for audiological services must be explored as this is a paramount issue in the decision to intervene (Silverstone, 1984). The majority of older persons are reluctant to "pay money to restore hearing" even if the ability exists. It is, thus, incumbent on the audiologist to explore every avenue to enable financial accessibility to audiological and aural rehabilitation services. Although most private insurance carriers and Medicare exclude rehabilitation services, economic factors do not have to inhibit our efforts. The policies of the following agencies should be explored when financial constraints threaten accessibility of services:

1. The Veterans Administration (all World War I veterans are eligible for hearing aids);
2. vocational rehabilitation agencies;
3. state Medicaid programs;
4. community organizations (e.g., Lion's Club is often responsive to requests for financial assistance for the elderly); and
5. worker's compensation.

If the above programs cannot meet the needs of the hearing-impaired elderly, mechanisms for obtaining less costly services can be explored. For example:

1. A stock of donated hearing aids from a variety of sources can be maintained (the electroacoustic characteristics should conform to manufacturer specifications) and dispensed at a reduced cost;.

2. reconditioned hearing aids can be sold at less than the cost of a new hearing aid;

3. alternative listening devices which are less expensive, and

4. economy hearing aids can be ordered from some hearing aid manufacturers.

Given the variety of mechanisms available, hearing-impaired elderly individuals should not be denied access to services for financial reasons.

In sum, financial, institutional, and patient variables (e.g., personality) can pose a significant barrier to the implementation of an effective rehabilitation plan (Silverstone, 1984). It behooves the communication specialist to investigate these intrinsic and extrinsic factors, and direct efforts at overcoming these obstacles. The discussion that follows offers approaches to overcoming the conditions which may impinge on the potential outcome of rehabilitation.

The Hearing Aid Evaluation

The selection of an appropriate hearing aid and earmold is the most important component of the aural rehabilitation process. This is especially true in the hearing-impaired elderly where rehabilitation efforts will primarily be directed toward promoting the use of amplification to maximize residual hearing in a variety of listening situations (Davis & Hardick, 1981; Hull, 1982).

The components of the hearing aid evaluation include the preselection and selection process. During the preselection process the audiologist determines candidacy for amplification and the type and style of sensory aid which will best meet the client's needs. During the selection process warble tones, speech materials, and quality judgments are used to decide on the electroacoustic characteristics of the specific unit to be recommended. At each stage of the preselection/selection process, the client should be actively involved in the decision-making process. Although time does not permit a lengthy discussion of the hearing aid evaluation, a few variables to be kept in mind during the preselection process (e.g., choice of a particular style hearing aid) will be discussed.

The aforementioned intrinsic and extrinsic factors should be considered during the preselection process, since they will influence the style of hearing aid to be recommended (e.g., body aid vs. canal aid). In deciding on the style of device to be assessed, high priority should be given to the patient's preference as one is unlikely to use a hearing aid with which one is uncomfortable. Similarly, preference should be given to the style unit which the patient will be likely to manipulate independently. These twoconsiderations will often be in conflict as the hearing aid having the greatest cosmetic appeal (e.g., canal aid) often cannot be manipulated independently nor is it appropriate to the hearing levels characteristic of many hearing-impaired elderly individuals. Similarly, the hearing aid which can be manipulated most easily (i.e., body aid) is cosmetically obtrusive and undesirable. Priority should always be given to the unit which will allow the individual to function as independently as physical and mental status will allow. Self-mastery and self-reliance will be critical to the new hearing aid user who is increasingly dependent on significant others to function in everyday life (Friedman & Capulong, 1984). In short, as Friedman and Capulong (1984) so aptly suggested, "relying on an assistive device to help one function is nowhere near as demeaning as the need to ask someone else to help with a simple task."

Before proceeding to the hearing aid orientation, it should be noted that whenever a hearing aid is recommended, a 30-day trial period with amplification should be arranged. If the audiologist remains undecided about recommending a particular unit, performance with the consignment hearing aid should be monitored for a few weeks. For example, with the noninstitutionalized the clinic aid can be used during the orientation and auditory-visual communication training sessions; after a few weeks a decision can usually be reached. In the case of the institutionalized, the consignment aid can be used during therapy, and can be worn on the floors under the close supervision of a nurse (who is acquainted with hearing aids and hearing loss) or a volunteer. Feedback from a staff person and/or the patient can often assist the audiologist in reaching a final decision. Using the 30-day trial period to assist in making a final decision, can prove quite helpful with borderline hearing aid candidates.

The Hearing Aid Orientation Informational Counseling

The hearing aid orientation which begins during the hearing aid evaluation is an ongoing process which should continue into the auditory and visual communication training sessions. In general, the purpose of hearing aid orientation is to assist the patient to derive maximum benefit from the hearing aid. Therefore, providing a thorough understanding of the hearing aid, its operation, maintenance, advantages, and limitations is the goal of the hearing aid orientation. Although there is little evidence attesting to the most effective form the hearing aid orientation should take, it is clear that orientation/counseling increases the hours of use (Brooks, 1979; Surr et al., 1978), reduces the hearing handicap associated with the impairment (Birk-Nielsen & Ewersten, 1974; Brooks, 1979) and promotes hearing aid satisfaction.

The approach to the hearing aid orientation/counseling must be individualized and client-centered taking physical/mental condition, personality and the milieu into account. Similarly, the goals should be target specific and realistic, depending in large part on the individual's potential. Instruction should proceed in small incremental steps, reinforcement should be provided on a regular basis and small gains in function should be valued as much as dramatic improvements (Silverstone, 1984). It is imperative that the clinician collaborate with the client and a significant other throughout the hearing aid orientation process in deciding on the goals of each session and in the decision to terminate the orientation. To insure carryover, the patient and significant other should be sensitized to the objectives of the hearing aid orientation (Silverstone, 1984).

With regard to scheduling, sessions should be offered on an individual basis (at first), take place regularly (e.g., one twice-a-week), be brief (30-45 minutes in duration depending on motivational level and patient understanding, among other factors), and take place in an environment free of distraction and interference. Each session should conclude with the client or significant other demonstrating mastery of the newly acquired skill(s). Similarly, each session should begin with a discussion of difficulties encountered in daily use of the hearing aid and a review of the client's capabilities vis-a-vis the previous session. A scale such as the one appearing in Appendix C is a useful guide for determining the client's progress and deciding on the objectives of each session. To insure carryover the client should be given written instructions summarizing the material covered in each session. Finally, throughout the rehabilitation process, the clinician must convey a positive and supportive attitude toward the patient and the rehabilitative process (Loebel & Eisdorfer, 1984).

The hearing aid orientation/counseling sessions should proceed from a general overview of hearing aids to a specific discussion of their operation maintenance and situational uses. Although the depth of the discussion will vary with the patient's capabilities and motivational level, the following topics should be discussed:

1. Purpose(s) of a hearing aid (e.g., make sound louder).

2. Advantages and limitations of hearing aids--the psychoacoustic and technological limitations of the unit and the situations in which the hearing aid will be least beneficial (e.g., noise, groups) and most beneficial (e.g., quiet, within 3-6 ft (.99144m-1.8288m) of speaker). The goal in discussing these factors is to set realistic expectations and to dispel the prejudices and misconceptions held by most elderly individuals (Garstecki, 1981).

3. The function/operation of each component (e.g., microphone) and manipulation of the various controls. It is often helpful to use two hearing aids during instruction to insure adequate reception of the information and for demonstration purposes. In addition, patients should be encouraged to use corrective lenses or low vision aids (e.g., magnifiers) during the orientation sessions to insure understanding of the required operations. Table 1 lists each of the controls and offers suggestions for mastering each.

During the hearing aid orientation sessions, begin with the easiest control to instill confidence and to raise the patient's motivational level and gradually proceed to more difficult tasks. Encourage the patient to touch and examine the hearing aid as often as necessary. After the clinician demonstrates proper manipulation, the client should be asked to adjust the control so as to clarify any misunderstanding. The clinician should anticipate potential memory problems and provide liberal repetition of instructions and allow the client the opportunity to demonstrate newly acquired skills at least

Table 1. Strategies for hearing aid orientation.[2]

Component/control	Function	Suggested strategies
Volume control	Makes sound louder/softer; may serve as on/off switch	1. I-T-E—patient can place forefinger on the volume control and twist the wrist in the specified direction. 2. All other styles—tell the patient which direction to move the control (e.g., floor/ceiling; up/down; have the patient adjust volume control while talking and note change in loudness as dial is rotated. 3. If patient has difficulty adjusting control, tape control in place temporarily. 4. Tell patient color or numeral on volume control associated with most comfortable listening level.[2] This will be useful for those patients who find it easier to adjust volume control prior to positioning the unit.
Tone control	Influences quality of amplified sound	1. Show patient position of control and instruct patient not to manipulate. 2. Tape in place so it is not inadvertently shifted to a different setting. 3. To avoid patient interference with setting, order hearing aid with preset tone control.
Input selector switch M/T/MT	Selects type of input; (microphone or environmental sound); telecoil (T) for telephone use; or turns hearing aid on/off	1. Patient should understand the functions of the M/T/MT switch and the setting for daily use or telephone use. Discuss telephone compatibility and practice telephone use. If patient does not need hearing aid for telephone use, order hearing aid without Telecoil or tape switch in "M" position and instruct patient to open and close battery case when turn aid on/off.
Battery B-T-E 13,675 Body-aid-AA 401 CA-312 I-T-E-13	Power source	1. Discuss cost (air cell vs. mercury), battery life, signs of exhausted battery, where to purchase battery, insertion techniques (e.g., positive side flat, negative side round), factors that influence battery life.
Earmold[4]	Couples hearing aid to ear, eliminates feedback when properly inserted, can modify frequency response of hearing aid	1. Use plastic demonstration ears for practice (available from Hal-Hen). 2. Have patient practice inserting and removing mold, from clinician's ear. 3. Break insertion process down into steps (e.g., place earmold into ear and then aid over ear; place aid over ear and then place earmold into ear; separate earmold from hearing aid. 4. Offer techniques for grasping earmold. 5. Remove helix portion.

[2]Hull, 1982; Maurer & Rupp; 1979, Traynor, 1982.
[3]Color code the volume control if necessary.
[4]May need to employ a number of strategies before the new hearing aid user masters the act of inserting and removing the earmold.

2-3 times during the session. If the patient does not grasp the concept after three or four attempts, move on to another task as the frustration can hamper future rehabilitation efforts. The subsequent task should be one that will bring success to the patient.

4. Care and maintenance of the hearing aid and its components. The following points should be made:

> a. hearing aid -- avoid exposure to excessive heat, moisture, dust, hair spray; remove hearing aid when standing on a resilient surface (e.g., carpet); place hearing aid in a safe place when removed (not in pockets); users of body aids should have a supply of cords and receivers; users of in-the-ear aids should have an earmold.
>
> b. earmold -- proper care of the mold (e.g., cleansing, removing wax); how to connect and disconnect the earmold from the hearing aid.
>
> c. battery -- storage (e.g., air cells remain sealed); how to test battery; pricing; tips for preserving battery life (e.g., open battery compartment when removing hearing aid).

Although most authors advocate instruction in troubleshooting techniques, clinical experience suggests that the typical elderly individual will not make the necessary effort to detect malfunction. Perhaps a better solution is to train the significant other in the art of troubleshooting and/or give the patient a handout describing simple troubleshooting procedures. The patient should be encouraged to see the audiologist or hearing aid dispenser if a problem arises which the family member or patient cannot resolve.

5. Suggestions for adjustment to amplification—the audiologist/speech-language pathologist must offer step-by-step procedures for gradually accommodating to the hearing aid. Important points to be addressed include: number of hours per day to wear the hearing aid, the listening situations in which the patient should and should not wear the hearing aid, strategies for coping with difficulties noted in adverse listening situations. At successive sessions, the number of hours of use should be increased (depending on communicative demands) and situational use should be expanded so that ultimately the patient can comfortably use the aid in easy listening situations

(e.g., quiet, close distance) and in situations of increasing difficulty (e.g., groups, noisy situations). Input from the client and significant other should be sought both informally and formally (communication profile/handicap scales) regarding situations where the client has encountered difficulty so that these situations can be attempted and mastered with the hearing aid. Listening activities which are graduated in difficulty (vary distance signal/noise type competition) should be planned to assist the client in communicating in these adverse listening conditions (these auditory training exercises can best be accomplished during group meetings).

Alternative Listening Devices

Although beneficial in quiet, hearing aids are of minimal benefit in the situations in which they are most needed, namely listening to the television, in noisy or reverbant rooms, group situations or large lecture halls (Vaughn & Gibbs, 1982). Similarly, these listening situations may be difficult for individuals with mild hearing impairments which may warrant a hearing aid. Finally, psychosocial factors, financial factors or physical/mental status may militate against a hearing aid in individuals with a significant hearing loss/handicap. Alternative listening devices which enhance speech understanding in suboptimal listening situations are ideal for individuals with any of the above characteristics (Vaughn & Gibbs, 1982). These assistive devices, known as Situational Personal Acoustic Communication Equipment (SPACE AIDS) have proven particularly useful with the institutionalized and noninstitutionalized elderly (Vaughn, 1983).

The SPACE devices provide the following advantages: (a) a favorable signal to noise ratio (S/N) (i.e., allowing the speech to reach the listener's ear at a louder level than the noise), (b) a high-fidelity microphone, and (c) portability, durability, and ease of manipulation at a reasonable cost (Vaughn & Gibbs, 1982; Vaughn, Lightfoot, & Gibbs, 1983). An incidental advantage is that a lengthy orientation process is not necessary for adapting to any of the SPACE devices. Three types of SPACE devices are available: hardwire, FM, or infra-red. Each system is designed to improve the coupling between the listener's ears and the amplified sound. Although each SPACE aid consists of a microphone held close to the sound source, an amplifier and a high-quality transducer (i.e., earphone), each system differs in its transmission properties. The hardwire system relies on a hardwire connection between the microphone, receiver, and amplifier. The infra-red system uses infra-red light waves as the carrier signal while the FM system uses radio frequencies as the carrier signal.

Hardwire System

The parts for the hardwire system, namely the external microphone, a minispeaker amplifier and earphone are available at Radio Shack or other commercial establishments which specialize in audio/communications equipment (Vaughn, Lightfoot, & Gibbs, 1983). The hardwire option which is the least expensive ($60-$160) of all SPACE aids is ideal for individuals with mild to severe hearing loss who have difficulty in one-to-one situations, or interpersonal listening in noise (i.e., indoors/outdoors). In that the microphone can be passed from talker to talker the hardwire system also enhances small group communication and communication in an automobile (Vaughn, Lightfoot, & Gibbs, 1983). In addition to facilitating communication with family and friends, the hardwire system can enhance communication between health professionals (e.g., nurse, social workers, doctors) and the hearing-impaired. It is especially useful in nursing-homes where many of the elderly are hearing-impaired but their physical/mental status contraindicates hearing aid use. Finally, the hardwire system can be connected directly into the television/radio minimizing room noise and enhancing television listening (Vaughn, Lightfoot, & Gibbs, 1983), and can be coupled to a telephone to amplify the conversation.

Infra-red System

Infra-red listening systems consist of a microphone, a transmitter which converts the acoustic signal into infra-red light waves and a receiver (e.g., stethoscope headphone) which converts the light waves into an audio signal. Although not popular for interpersonal communication, infra-red systems are ideal for indoor transmission of music in large areas (e.g., theater, concerts) or lectures (e.g., church auditorium). In addition to large group listening, small infra-red units have been designed for home use with the television/radio. The infra-red transmitter can be plugged directly into the jack of the television or is placed on top of the television (Vaughn, et al. 1983). It is important to emphasize that infra-red systems do not transmit through walls of a room (i.e., transmission is confined to the room which houses the transmitter), that the range of the transmitter is dependent on its size, and that the transmitter generally requires AC power limiting its portability (Vaughn & Gibbs, 1982). Infra-red systems vary widely in price ($280-$1,010) depending on the size of the transmitter and listening area to be served and are available from a number of sources including Sears, Hal-Hen, and Siemens Hearing Instruments.

FM Systems

The wireless FM systems consist of a microphone, an FM radio transmitter, and a receiver (e.g., headphone, neckloop that couples to the telecoil of a hearing aid). Although more costly than the other systems, the FM systems are portable, unobtrusive, compatible with hearing aids, and lend themselves to indoor and outdoor use as well as large and small group situations (Vaughn, et al. 1983). Specifically, FM systems can be used in large areas such as concert or lecture halls, during outdoor recreational activities, and for all types of interpersonal communication (e.g., at parties, family gatherings) (Vaughn, et al. 1983). Finally, the FM listening devices enhance television or radio listening and can be used with the telephone. FM systems which are commercially available from a number of companies including Phonic Ear, Telex, or Com-Tek range in price form $600-$1,200.

In sum, although each assistive device delivers the signal directly to the listener's ears, minimizing the effects of background noise on speech understanding, as is evident from Table 2, the situational applications differ (Vaughn, et al. 1983). Therefore, the audiologist must carefully assess the patient's lifestyle, situational difficulties with and without a hearing aid, and communication demands before recommending a particular style of device. Finally, it should be emphasized that assistive devices can be used as companions to hearing aids or can be used as a substitute for a hearing aid in situations where a hearing aid is of minimal benefit or for individuals who are not hearing aid candidates.

Table 2. Situational applications of assistive devices.[5]

Device	Situations							
	One-One	Telephone	Noise	Large areas	Small areas	Television/ Radio	Indoors	Outdoors
Hardwire (least costly)	•	•	•		•	•	•	•
Infra-red (moderately priced)		•	•	•		•	•	
FM (most expensive)	•	•	•	•	•	•	•	•

[5]See Vaughn & Gibbs (1982), and Vaughn, Lightfoot, & Gibbs, (1983) for sources for devices and descriptions of components of each system.

Personal Adjustment Counseling

An important goal of aural rehabilitation is facilitating adjustment to and acceptance of a hearing loss. The first step in this process is an assessment of the patient's reaction to the hearing loss using a communication profile such as the McCarthy-Alpiner Scale (1983) or a hearing handicap scale such as the Hearing Handicap Inventory for the Elderly or the Self-Assessment of Communication (SAC). A family member's assessment of psychosocial effects of the hearing loss can provide information as well. A systematic psychosocial assessment will acquaint the clinician with the patient's reaction to the hearing loss, the patient's attitude toward the loss, the emotional impact of the hearing loss, and the pattern of adaptation to the hearing loss (Silverstone, 1984). In addition, response to the assessment will assist in developing a plan for intervention with the patient and/or significant others.

In a few cases, the opportunity to talk with an empathetic person about the feelings triggered by a hearing loss may be all that is necessary for the patient to adapt to the hearing loss. Others may need direction and suggestions for coping with the effects of hearing loss (Silverstone, 1984). For example, if responses indicate that the patient is denying the hearing loss efforts should be directed at promoting psychological acceptance of the loss and refraining from nonproductive behaviors such as pretending to understand others (Davis & Hardick, 1981). Similarly, if the major defense mechanism is projection, efforts should be directed at facilitating acceptance of the natural consequences of hearing loss. If the client is avoiding communication situations due to frustration/embarrassment associated with misunderstanding others, strategies for coping with difficult situations, and suggestions for attitude modification should be offered (Stephens & Goldstein, 1983).

The individual can be assisted in working through some of their struggles and difficulties by including family members in the rehabilitation process. Additionally, group meetings with other hearing-impaired individuals who are experiencing similar problems or have resolved their difficulties can be quite productive. Group therapy will promote sociability, will provide an opportunity for participants to express mutual frustrations, feelings and concerns, and will help participants to realize that their problems are not unique (Davis & Hardick, 1981). It is important to emphasize that personal adjustment counseling is an ongoing process which must meet the changing needs of the hearing-impaired elderly. Periodic assessment of the client's attitude toward his impairment/handicap will help guide the communication specialist in selecting strategies and behaviors to be modified.

Auditory-Visual Communication Training

The term auditory-visual communication refers to the reception of the spoken message through the auditory and visual channels (Garstecki, 1981; Hull, 1982). Therefore, the goal of auditory-visual communication training is to assist the individual to improve overall communication function in easy and adverse conditions by maximizing ability to integrate input from auditory and visual channels (Garstecki, 1981; Garstecki, 1984; Hull, 1982; McCarthy & Alpiner, 1982). McCarthy and Alpiner (1982) suggest that although auditory-visual communication training emphasizes the coupling of audition to vision, it should be initiated by introducing strategies for maximizing input from each sensory modality in isolation and then in combination. Training the individual to improve signal perception through vision (e.g., speechreading) and audition will enable the individual to use the two sensory modalities "alternately, independently, and simultaneously" (McCarthy & Alpiner, 1982, p. 108).

Visual communication training/speechreading is the process whereby the individual is trained to make use of nonauditory cues (e.g., facial cues) to supplement audition. In short, remediation efforts should be directed at maximizing the individual's "ability to use combined sensory input in message perception" (Garstecki, 1984, p. 186). Early approaches to visual communication training were analytic. The client was taught how phonemes are produced and subsequently trained to recognize speech on the basis of articulatory movements (e.g., lip movements), using stimuli which increased in complexity from syllables to paragraphs (Davis & Hardick, 1981). To date there is little direct evidence of the value of an analytic approach with the elderly. When speechreading training is adopted with the elderly the synthetic approach is preferable to the analytic. The individual should be trained to synthesize the redundancies of the language and the situation to obtain meaning from the spoken messages (Kaplan, 1979). Specifically, this approach involves training the individual to "anticipate information based on the context, situation and linguistic rules" and ascribe meaning when information is lacking because of poor visibility of phonemes (Davis & Hardick, 1981, p. 75).

According to Ward & Gowers (1981a, 1981b) a synthetic approach to speechreading reduces self-assessed hearing handicap. Similarly Garstecki's (1979) findings suggest that training the elderly in the use of situational cues enhances speechreading ability. Finally, Binnie (1977) noted that although absolute scores on speechreading tests (e.g., Utley Lipreading Test) may not improve following intervention, he found that visual communication training reportedly enhances communication ability and increases confidence in asserting oneself in communication situations.

Visual communication training in the elderly should emphasize the importance of visual attentiveness to linguistic and nonlinguistic cues, specifically, the role of vision in speech understanding. The variables which influence speechreading ability and tactics for improving speechreading proficiency should be discussed (Stephens & Goldstein, 1983). Training can be implemented most effectively on a group basis. Each week specific topics are discussed, communication strategies offered, and activities planned for illustrating use of visual cues to enhance communicative effectiveness (Giolas, 1982).

Most hearing-impaired elderly individuals will report for hearing therapy to "improve lipreading skills." Their expectations regarding the purpose of speechreading training are typically unrealistic. That is, they firmly believe the "speechreading lessons" will enable them to rely on articulatory movements for understanding speech that is inaudible. In that these unrealistic expectations will have a negative impact on the outcome of rehabilitation, the clinician must begin communication training by dispelling their misconceptions. Specifically, the goal should be to clarify the limitations of "lipreading per se" as a substitute for audition and to set realistic goals regarding the contribution of vision to speech understanding (Davis & Hardick, 1981; Hull, 1982; & McCarthy & Alpiner, 1982). With regard to the former, those factors which influence "lipreading" ability should be (a) the visibility of speech sounds; (b) the concept of homophenous phonemes/words; (c) rapidity of speech; (d) changes in visual acuity associated with age, and environmental factors (Berger, 1972; Davis & Hardick, 1981). Relevant group activities should be developed to illustrate how each of these variables may preclude deriving meaning from articulatory movements (Davis & Hardick, 1981; Giolas, 1982;

McCarthy & Alpiner, 1982). Once the limitations of speechreading are understood, the benefits of visual attentiveness should be addressed. Once again, the fact that lipreading is one aspect of visual communication training should be reiterated as well as the importance of attentiveness to and observation of facial cues, expression, gestures and situational environmental cues in speech understanding. In addition, suggestions for reacting to and compensating for auditory failure should be offered (e.g., admitting that they have a hearing loss, asking for repetitions, etc.) (Giolas, 1982). Role-playing can be used effectively to demonstrate the importance of awareness to visual and situational cues. Compensatory strategies and suggestions for taking advantage of the supplemental information derived from visual cues should be enumerated and activities planned for familiarizing group members with ways of maximizing the use of these variables in communication (Giolas, 1982). Table 3 lists and defines each of these redundancies and offers suggestions for promoting the use of contextual, situational, and communication redundancies to supplement audition. At all times the fact that speechreading is an adjunct and not a substitute for audition should be discussed. Activities which provide practice in using visual cues to supplement auditory cues should be planned (see Davis & Hardick, 1981; Giolas, 1982; McCarthy & Alpiner, 1982 for suggested activities). After each demonstration a discussion among group members should highlight the important principles of each activity. As in the hearing aid orientation, activities should be structured so that the group members initially experience success. In other words, begin with familiar and relevant topics/activities in favorable listening conditions and proceed to more difficult tasks and activities which simulate adverse listening experiences and poor environmental conditions.

Table 3. Strategies for promoting speechreading proficiency.[6]

Variables affecting speechreading proficiency	Communication strategies
Facial cues (may substitute for spoken message; offer clue to psychological state and opinions about subject matter)	1) face speaker 2) watch facial expressions (e.g., smile symbolizes satisfaction) 3) position self at an angle which will provide a complete view of speaker's face
Gestural movements (may supplement speakers' words, add emphasis or clarity, may substitute for spoken message)	1) take advantage of head, body, and limb movements (e.g., head shake symbolizes yes/no)
Situational cues (help suggest subject matter)	1) take note of objects in environment, physical location (i.e., context) and participants in communication exchange
Environmental factors (can be manipulated to facilitate understanding	1) concentrate light on speaker's face, not behind speaker 2) maintain a distance from speaker of 3-6 feet (.99144m-1.8288m) at most 10 ft (3.48m) 3) sit toward front of room when in a large area 4) remove visual distractions when speaking with others 5) insure that room is well illuminated but free of glare
Articulatory movements can enhance consonant identification (e.g., bilabials, labiodentals, linguadentals)	1) attend to lip movements/posture 2) ask speaker to speak at a slightly slower rate than normal, not to exaggerate articulatory movements and to speak at normal or slightly raised intensity
Linguistic (enables prediction of message content by reliance on the redundancies of the language)	1) familiarize self with topic 2) keep abreast of current events 3) look for salient ideas rather than concentrating on individual words

[6]Berger (1972); Hull (1982); McCarthy & Alpiner (1982).

Educating Significant Others

The Family

In that communication involves the hearing-impaired person and family members (e.g., spouse, child), these individuals should be meaningfully included in the aural rehabilitation process from the onset. They should be encouraged to attend those individual/group sessions which relate to the client's adjustment to the hearing loss/hearing aid including the hearing aid orientation, as well as environmental manipulation and visual communication training sessions. In some cases the significant other should also be seen on an individual basis for supportive and education counseling. Involvement of family members will be instrumental in adjustment to amplification, will assist the patient to maximize communication skills and will ensure efficient transfer of new information. Finally, carryover of treatment into the client's daily activities will be enhanced as the family member will know the newly acquired behavior to reinforce or to discourage (Hull, 1982; Kaplan, 1979; Maurer & Rupp, 1979; Silverstone, 1984).

The goal of educational counseling with the family should be to establish realistic expectations regarding communication and hearing aid use and to achieve a "close fit between expectation and performance" (Loebel & Eisdorfer, 1984, p. 49). This is critical as unrealistic expectations will inhibit chances for successful rehabilitation. To this end, the audiologist must educate the family member about:

1. hearing loss and its potential impact on communication and psychosocial function,

2. the maintenance and operation of the hearing aid,

3. the limitations and benefits of amplification,

4. environmental modifications which will promote effective communication and successful hearing aid use,

5. the role of vision, gestures, contextual cues, and facial movements in speech understanding,

6. use of communication strategies to facilitate understanding on the part of the hearing-impaired.

Table 4 offers techniques to enhance the speakers' communication expressiveness and effectiveness (Bode, Tweedie, & Hull, 1982).

Table 4. Tips for communicating with the hearing-impaired.[7]

═══

1. Position oneself so that maximal light shines on the speaker's face, not on the hearing-impaired person.

2. Do not shout at the individual—this distorts the message. Speak in an audible voice using clear distinct articulation. Always face the hearing-impaired when speaking; do not speak over a large distance (two different rooms).

3. Use natural, not exaggerated facial gestures.

4. Keep mouth unobstructed and avoid chewing or smoking when speaking.

5. Look for clues of misunderstanding and when necessary, restate what has been said using simple words and short phrases. Do not show annoyance when patient does not understand; this will trigger withdrawal.

6. When conversing, try to position yourself in a noise-free environment. The presence of background noise will make for a frustrating and difficult listening situation. In short, assist patient in creating an ideal situation for communication to take place.

7. Try to be on the same level as the hearing-impaired individual. If he is in a wheelchair, sit down in a chair to talk; if not, it will be difficult for the hearing-impaired to lipread when the speaker's face is too high or too low.

═══

[7]Hull, 1982; Kaplan, 1979; Maurer & Rupp, 1979.

Caregivers

In long-term care facilities the nurse plays a vital role in the management and rehabilitation of the hearing-impaired elderly resident. He/she initiates referrals, interacts with the residents on an ongoing basis, has primary responsibility for the institutional environment as it affects the effectiveness of care and is responsible for carryover of newly acquired techniques into daily life (Hepler, 1982). Hence, the commitment and attitude of the nursing staff (i.e., RNs, LNs, aides) will affect the eventual outcome of the aural rehabilitation process. To insure that the nurse carries out his/her multifaceted responsibilities effectively in-service training programs should:

1. Promote understanding of the structure of the auditory mechanism, the the causes and the effects (e.g., psychosocial) of hearing loss in the elderly;

2. Acquaint staff with the role of the audiologist in the hearing health care of the residents;

3. Provide suggestions for improving communication expressiveness and effectiveness of the staff (e.g., discuss methods for effective communication listed in Table 4);

4. Orient staff to the maintenance, operation, advantages, and disadvantages of hearing aids. Emphasis should be placed on battery placement and volume control adjustment, causes and ways to alleviate feedback, and earmold insertion. The dependence of the residents on the nurse for handling, inserting, and removing the hearing aid should be reiterated throughout the sessions.

5. Offer suggestions for creating/structuring the institutional environment so that it facilitates interpersonal relationships among residents and staff (Bode et al., 1982; Dancer & Keiser, 1980; Davis & Hardick, 1981; Hepler, 1982).[8]

The structure of and approach to in-service training will influence the staff's commitment to rehabilitative efforts and hence continuity of care. Training sessions should be scheduled on a regular basis due to high turnover of personnel) and during each nursing shift (e.g., 8-4, 4-12). Each group of nurses should attend at least three one-hour sessions per year with each

---

[8]Whenever a patient is given a hearing aid, the nurse should be contacted directly and instructed about needs of the patient.

session having a different emphasis. Additional sessions should be scheduled depending on the needs and enthusiasm of the staff. It is imperative that the sessions are (a) geared to the level of understanding of the participants (e.g., RNs vs. nurses' aides); (b) the staff is actively involved in the sessions (e.g., hands-on experience with hearing aids is critical); and (c) auditory and visual aids (e.g., audiotapes, diagrams, handouts) are employed throughout the training (Davis & Hardick, 1981; Kaplan, 1979). Further, the problems and the needs of individual patients should be addressed and the responsibilities of the staff for facilitating carryover outlined. The more basic, individualized, patient, and target-specific the training sessions the more likely the staff will be to implement the suggestions of the communication specialist. Finally, although the communication specialist will often be frustrated in attempts at educating the staff, patience and respect must be maintained at all times. The communication specialist must remain an ally of nursing professionals if these individuals are to assist us in restoring the hearing-impaired institutionalized elderly person to his/her maximum level of communication function (Hepler, 1982).

Considerations in the Remediation Process

A number of variables must be considered in the planning and execution of the aural rehabilitation program. These include the physical environment, materials, scheduling, and format.

Physical Environment

The therapy room should be accessible to those with physical disabilities (e.g., wheelchair-bound), free of ambient noise and visual distractions. The temperature in the room should be maintained at a moderate level and the furniture comfortable and home-like (Loebel & Eisdorfer, 1984). The importance of proper lighting cannot be overemphasized. Fluorescent light should be avoided, and indirect light is preferable to direct light (Hull, 1982). Glare in the therapy room should be reduced (e.g., client should place back toward windows). Because there are numerous etiologies of visual disorders in the elderly the communication specialist should consult with a low vision specialist to determine the type of lighting to be used during rehabilitation (Karp, 1983).

269

Materials

Activities/materials should be practical and relevant to the lifestyle of the hearing-impaired individual. The therapist should consult the client regarding his/her interests to facilitate selection of meaningful materials and promote learning and motivation (Kaplan, 1979).

Scheduling

Fatigue, alertness, and motivational level are three variables to take into account when deciding the time of day for treatment and the length of the remediation process (Davis & Hardick, 1981; Hull, 1982; McCarthy & Alpiner, 1982). Sessions should be scheduled as soon as possible after the initial evaluation, at a time when the elderly are most alert (e.g., morning hours). In the case of the institutionalized, the time of the session should not conflict with other major events or therapies. The length of the session should vary with the nature of the task and the interest and attention span of the client. While 30-60 minutes is ideal for individual therapy, 60-90 minutes is more appropriate for group therapy (Davis & Hardick, 1981; McCarthy & Alpiner, 1982). The rehabilitation program should be short-term approximately 6-12 weeks in duration depending on the form (e.g., individual vs. group) and the goals.

Inasmuch as both an individual and a group approach to treatment has distinct advantages, a combined approach will probably be the most efficacious. Individual treatment allows the therapist to be more responsive to the individual needs of the client and to attend to personality variables (e.g., unwillingness to cooperate, anxiety) which may interfere with the progress of therapy. In that individual therapy is more intensive, fewer sessions are required to achieve the objectives of rehabilitation. Given their unique problems, clients with multiple disabilities (e.g., deaf-blind), severe hearing loss, mental confusion, and significant language problems should be treated on an individual basis (Davis & Hardick, 1981). Finally, in view of the individual variability in acclimation to a hearing aid, hearing aid orientation sessions should be initiated on an individual basis.

Group therapy is important for reinforcement, support, stimulation, and socialization (McCarthy & Alpiner, 1982; Sarno, 1984). Similarly, it provides an opportunity to share and resolve common worries, frustrations, and problems associated with the hearing loss. Finally, by monitoring the interactions among the participants, the therapist can informally assess the client's auditory-visual speech recognition skills. Group therapy treatment which should include at most eight participants is ideal for informational/personal adjustment counseling, and auditory-visual speech recognition training. An effective format for group therapy is to combine formal presentations (e.g., hearing aids, contributions of vision to speech-understanding) with informal discussions of specific situational difficulties encountered by group members; to plan problem solving activities (e.g., who am I, role-playing) which will help illustrate communication strategies for facilitating speech understanding and to set aside time for a coffee break which will allow an opportunity for socialization among the clients (Giolas, 1982).

In sum, given the unique needs of the hearing-impaired elderly, the therapist should work closely with the client to design and implement a program which will best meet his/her needs.

Conclusions

The goal of aural rehabilitation with the elderly is to provide assistance in adjustment to amplification (i.e., hearing aid orientation, auditory training), to promote adjustment to and acceptance of the acquired hearing loss (i.e., personal adjustment counseling, educating significant others), and to develop auditory-visual speech recognition skills (i.e., auditory-visual communication training). Although the components of aural rehabilitation were discussed separately, each is only one integral part of the total aural rehabilitation process. The successful program should incorporate all or some of the components in each session depending on the interest and needs of the patient.

Self-Study Questions

1. Aural rehabilitation encompasses all of the following procedures with the exception of:

    a) hearing aid selection

    b) hearing aid orientation

    c) auditory-visual training

    d) restoration of speech-language function

2. The <u>most</u> important factor influencing hearing aid candidacy is:

    a) pure-tone test results

    b) word recognition ability

    c) patient motivation

    d) financial status

3. An infrared system is <u>most</u> beneficial in which of the following situations?

    a) large concert hall

    b) outdoors

    c) one-to-one communicative situations

    d) telephones

4. The major advantage of a SPACE aid over a hearing aid is:

    a) smaller and less visible

    b) enhances signal-to-noise ratio

    c) higher output

    d) broader frequency response

5. Responses to a handicap scale can be used in all but which of the following situations?

    a) quantify the effect of intervention

    b) provide quantitative information about a hearing impairment

    c) design an individualized rehabilitation program

    d) counselling

6. The goal(s) of auditory visual training is/are to?

    a) train the individual to recognize articulatory postures associated with phoneme production

    b) promote use of non-auditory cues to supplement audition

    c) enhance understanding of speech in adverse listening conditions

    d) all of the above

REFERENCES

Alberti, P. (1977). Hearing aids and aural rehabilitation in a geriatric population. The Journal of Otolaryngology, 6,(4) 1-49.

Baum, J. (1984). Rehabilitation aspects of arthritis in the elderly. In F. Williams, (Ed.), Rehabilitation in the elderly (pp. 345-358). New York: Raven Press.

Berger, K. (1972). Speechreading principles & methods. Baltimore: National Educational Press.

Binnie, C. (1977). Attitude changes following speechreading training. Scandinavian Audiology, 6, 13-19.

Birk-Nielson, H., & Ewertsen, H. (1974). Effective hearing aid treatment. Scandanavian Audiology, 3, 35-38.

Bode, D., Tweedie, D., & Hull, R. (1982). Improving communication through aural rehabilitation. In R. Hull (Ed.), Rehabilitative audiology (pp. 101-117). New York: Grune & Stratton.

Brooks, D. (1979). Counseling and its effects on hearing aid use. Scandinavian Audiology, 8, 101-107.

Clark, G., & Bray, G. (1984). Development of a rehabilitation plan, In T. F. Williams (Ed.), Rehabilitation in the aging. New York: Raven Press.

Dancer, J., & Keiser, H. (1980, February). The hearing impaired elderly: Training others to help. Hearing Aid Journal (pp. 10, 36-37).

Davis, J., & Hardick, E. (1981). Rehabilitative audiology or children and adults. New York: Wiley.

Encyclopedia Britannica: Micropedia, Vol. 8, p. 454, (1978). In: J. Loebel & C. Eisdorfer (Eds.), Psychological and psychiatric factors in the rehabilitation of the elderly (pp. 41-55).

Ewersten, H. (1974). Use of hearing aids. Scandinavian Audiology, 3, 173-176.

Friedman, L., & Capulong, E. (1984). Specific assistive aids. In T. F. Williams (Ed.), Rehabilitation in aging (pp. 315-345). New York: Raven Press.

Garstecki, D. (1981). Aural rehabilitation for the aging adult. In D. S. Beasley & G. A. Davis (Eds.), Aging, communication processes & disorders, New York: Grune & Stratton.

Garstecki, D. (1983). Auditory, visual and combined auditory-visual speech perception. Journal Academy of Rehabilitative Audiology, 16, 221-234.

Garstecki, D. (1984). Rehabilitation of hearing impaired adults. In J. Jerger (Ed.), Hearing disorders in adults (pp. 175-221). San Diego: College-Hill Press.

Giolas T. (1982). Hearing handicapped adults. Englewood Cliffs, NJ: Prentice-Hall.

Hepler, J. (1982). The nurse in the aural rehabilitation process. In R. Hull, (Ed.), Rehabilitation audiology (pp. 445-452). New York: Grune & Stratton.

Hull, R. (1982). Programs in the health care facility. In R. Hull, (Ed.), Rehabilitation audiology (pp. 425-445). New York: Grune & Stratton.

Hull, R. (1982). Techniques for aural rehabilitation treatment for elderly clients. In R. Hull, (Ed.), Rehabilitation audiology (pp. 383-407). New York: Grune & Stratton.

Hull, R. (1980). Responses to a hearing problem inventory. Journal of the Academy of Rehabilitative Audiology, 13, 133-154.

Itoh, M., Lee, M., & Shapiro, J. (1984). Self-help devices of the elderly population living in the community. In S. F. William, (Ed.), Rehabilitation in the elderly (pp. 345-358). New York: Raven Press.

Jerger, J., & Hayes, O. (1976). Hearing aid evaluation: Clinical experience with a new philosophy. Archives of Otolaryngology, 102 214-225.

Kapetyn, T. (1977). Satisfaction with fitted hearing aids: An investigation into the influence of psycho-social factors. Scandinavian Audiology, 6, 171-177.

Kaplan, H. (1979). Development composition and problems with elderly aural rehabilitation groups. In M. Henoch (Ed.), Aural rehabilitation in the elderly (pp. 53-71). New York: Grune & Stratton.

Karp, A. (1983). Aural rehabilitation strategies for the visually and hearing impaired patient. Journal Academy of Rehabilitative Audiology, 16, 23-33.

Kasten, R. (1982). Determination of need for rehabilitation. In R. Hull, (Ed.), Rehabilitation audiology (pp. 35-51). New York: Grune & Stratton.

Kasten, R. (1979). Evaluation and fitting of amplification for the aging population. In M. Henoch, (Ed.), Aural rehabilitation in the elderly (pp. 71-83). New York: Grune & Stratton.

Loebel, J., & Eisdorfer, C. (1984). Psychological and psychiatric factors in the rehabilitation of the elderly. In Williams, T. F. (Ed.), Rehabilitation in the Aging (pp. 41-59). New York: Raven Press.

Maurer, J., & Rupp, R. (1979). Hearing and aging. New York: Grune & Stratton.

McCarthy, P., & Alpiner, J. (1982). The remediation process. In J. Alpiner (Ed.), Handbook of adult rehabilitation audiology, (pp. 99-128). Baltimore: Williams & Wilkins.

McCarthy, P., & Alpiner, J. (1983). An assessment scale of hearing handicap for use in family. Journal of Academy of Rehabilitative Audiology, 16, 256-271.

Sarno, M. (1984). Communication disorders in the elderly. In T. F. Williams (Ed.), Rehabilitation in aging (pp. 161-177). New York: Raven Press.

Schow, R., & Nerbonne, M. (1982). Communication screening profile: Use with elderly clients. Ear and Hearing, 3, 135-148.

Silverstone, B. (1984). Social aspects of rehabilitation. In T. F. Williams, (Ed.), Rehabilitation in aging (pp. 59-81). New York: Raven Press.

Stephens, S., & Goldstein, R. (1983). Auditory rehabilitation in the elderly. In R. Hinchcliffe (Ed.), Hearing and balance in the elderly (pp. 201-227). New York: Churchill Livingstone.

Surr, R., Schuchman, G., & Montgomery, A. (1978). Factors influencing use of hearing aids. Archives of Otolaryngology, 104, 732-737.

Tyler, R., Baker, L., & Bednell, G. (1983). Difficulties experienced by hearing aid candidates and hearing aid users. British Journal of Audiology, 17, 191-201.

Vaughn, G., & Gibbs, S. (1982). Alternative and companion listening devices for the hearing impaired. In R. Hull, (Ed.), Rehabilitation audiology (pp. 107-129). New York: Grune & Stratton.

Vaughn, G. (1983). Large area sound systems. Asha, 25, 25-33.

Vaughn, G., Lightfoot, R., & Gibbs, S. (1983). SPACE. Asha, 25, 33-47.

Ventry, I., & Weinstein, B. (1982). The hearing handicap inventory for the elderly: A new tool. Ear and Hearing, 3, 128-134.

Walden, B., Demorest, M., & Hepler E. (1984). Self-report approach to assessing benefit and derived from amplification. Journal of Speech and Hearing Disorders, 27, 49-56.

Ward, P., & Gowers, J. (1981a). Hearing tactics: The long-term effects of instruction. British Journal of Audiology, 15, 261-262.

Ward, P., & Gowers, J. (1981b). Teaching hearing aid skills to elderly people: Hearing tactics. British Journal of Audiology, 15, 257-259.

Weinstein, B., & Ventry, I. (1983). Audiologic correlates of the hearing handicap inventory for the elderly. Journal of Speech and Hearing Disorders, 26, 148-150.

Appendix A

Instructions:

The purpose of this scale is to identify the problems your hearing loss may be causing you. **Answer YES, SOMETIMES, or NO for each question. Do not skip a question if you avoid a situation because of your hearing problem. If you use a hearing aid,** please answer the way you hear without the aid.

		YES (4)	SOME-TIMES (2)	NO (0)
S-1.	Does a hearing problem cause you to use the phone less often than you would like?	____	____	____
E-2.	Does a hearing problem cause you to feel embarrassed when meeting new people?	____	____	____
S-3.	Does a hearing problem cause you to avoid groups of people?	____	____	____
E-4.	Does a hearing problem make you irritable?	____	____	____
E-5.	Does a hearing problem cause you to feel frustrated when talking to members of your family?	____	____	____
S-6.	Does a hearing problem cause you difficulty when attending a party?	____	____	____
E-7.	Does a hearing problem cause you to feel "stupid" or "dumb"?	____	____	____
S-8.	Do you have difficulty hearing when someone speaks in a whisper?	____	____	____
E-9.	Do you feel handicapped by a hearing problem?	____	____	____
S-10.	Does a hearing problem cause you difficulty when visiting friends, relatives, or neighbors?	____	____	____
S-11.	Does a hearing problem cause you to attend religious services less often than you would like?	____	____	____
E-12.	Does a hearing problem cause you to be nervous?	____	____	____
S-13.	Does a hearing problem cause you to visit friends, relatives, or neighbors less often than you would like?	____	____	____
E-14.	Does a hearing problem cause you to have arguments with your family members?	____	____	____
S-15.	Does a hearing problem cause you difficulty when listening to TV or radio?	____	____	____
S-16.	Does a hearing problem cause you to go shopping less often than you would like?	____	____	____
E-17.	Does any problem or difficulty with your hearing upset you at all?	____	____	____
E-18.	Does a hearing problem cause you to want to be by yourself?	____	____	____
S-19.	Does a hearing problem cause you to talk to family members less often than you would like?	____	____	____
E-20.	Do you feel that any difficulty with your hearing limits or hampers your personal or social life?	____	____	____
S-21.	Does a hearing problem cause you difficulty when in a restaurant with relatives or friends?	____	____	____
S-22.	Does a hearing problem cause you to feel depressed?	____	____	____
S-23.	Does a hearing problem cause you to listen to TV or radio less often than you would like?	____	____	____
E-24.	Does a hearing problem cause you to feel uncomfortable when talking to friends?	____	____	____
E-25.	Does a hearing problem cause you to feel left out when you are with a group of people?	____	____	____

FOR CLINICIAN'S USE ONLY: Total Score: _____
Subtotal E: _____
Subtotal S: _____

From Weinstein & Ventry (1983). HHIE: Audiometric correlates. <u>Journal of Speech and Hearing Disorders</u>, <u>48</u>, 379-384.

Self Assessment of Communication (SAC)

Name _____

Date _____   Raw Score _____ x 2 = _____ - 20 = _____ x 1.25 _____ %

Please select the appropriate number ranging from 1 to 5 for the following questions.
Circle only one number for each question. If you have a hearing aid, please fill out the form according to how you communicate when the hearing aid is in use.

Various Communication Situations

1. Do you experience communication difficulties in situations when speaking with one other person? (e.g., at home, at work, in a social situation, with a waitress, a store clerk, with a spouse, boss, etc.)

   1) almost never   2) occasionally   3) about half of   4) frequently   5) practically
   (or never)   (about 1/4 of   the time   (about 3/4   always
                        the time)   of the time)   (or always)

2. Do you experience communication difficulties in situations when conversing with a small group of several persons? (e.g., with friends or family, co-workers, in meetings or casual conversations, over dinner or while playing cards, etc.)

   1) almost never   2) occasionally   3) about half of   4) frequently   5) practically
   (or never)   (about 1/4 of   the time   (about 3/4   always
                        the time)   of the time)   (or always)

3. Do you experience communication difficulties while listening to someone speak to a large group? (e.g., at church or in a civic meeting, in a fraternal or women's club, at an educational lecture, etc.)

   1) almost never   2) occasionally   3) about half of   4) frequently   5) practically
   (or never)   (about 1/4 of   the time   (about 3/4   always
                        the time)   of the time)   (or always)

4. Do you experience communication difficulties while participating in various types of entertainment? (e.g., movies, TV, radio, plays, night clubs, musical entertainment, etc.)

   1) almost never   2) occasionally   3) about half of   4) frequently   5) practically
   (or never)   (about 1/4 of   the time   (about 3/4   always
                        the time)   of the time)   (or always)

5. Do you experience communication difficulties when you are in an unfavorable listening environment? (e.g., at a noisy party, where there is background music, when riding in an auto or bus, when someone whispers or talks from across the room, etc.)

   1) almost never   2) occasionally   3) about half of   4) frequently   5) practically
   (or never)   (about 1/4 of   the time   (about 3/4   always
                        the time)   of the time)   (or always

6. Do you experience communication difficulties when using or listening to various communication devices? (e.g., telephone, telephone ring, doorbell, public address system, warning signals, alarms, etc.)

   1) almost never   2) occasionally   3) about half of   4) frequently   5) practically
   (or never)   (about 1/4 of   the time   (about 3/4   always
                        the time)   of the time)   (or always)

Feelings About Communications

7. Do you feel that any difficulty with your hearing limits or hampers your personal or social life?

   1) almost never   2) occasionally   3) about half of   4) frequently   5) practically
   (or never)   (about 1/4 of   the time   (about 3/4   always
                        the time)   of the time)   (or always)

8. Does any problem or difficulty with your hearing upset you?

   1) almost never   2) occasionally   3) about half of   4) frequently   5) practically
   (or never)   (about 1/4 of   the time   (about 3/4   always
                        the time)   of the time)   (or always)

Other People

9. Do others suggest that you have a hearing problem?

   1) almost never   2) occasionally   3) about half of   4) frequently   5) practically
   (or never)   (about 1/4 of   the time   (about 3/4   always
                        the time)   of the time)   (or always)

0. Do others leave you out of conversations or become annoyed because of your hearing?

   1) almost never   2) occasionally   3) about half of   4) frequently   5) practically
   (or never)   (about 1/4 of   the time   (about 3/4   always
                        the time)   of the time)   (or always)

Significant Other Assessment of Communication (SOAC)

Name _____

Form filled out with reference to _____ (client/patient)

Relationship to client/patient _____ (for example, wife, son, friend)

Date _____   Raw Score _____ x 2 = _____ −20 = _____ x 1.25 _____ %

Please select the appropriate number ranging from 1 to 5 for the following questions. Circle only one number for each question. If the client/patient has a hearing aid, please fill out the form according to he/she communicates when the hearing aid is in use.

Various Communication Situations

1. Does he/she experience communication difficulties in situations when speaking with one other person? (e.g., at home, at work, in a social situation, with a waitress, a store clerk, with a spouse, (boss, etc.).
   1) almost never (or never)   2) occasionally (about 1/4 of the time)   3) about half of the time   4) frequently (about 3/4 of the time)   5) practically always (or always)

2. Does he/she experience communication difficulties in situations when conversing with a small group of several persons? (e.g., with friends or family, co-workers, in meetings or casual conversations, over dinner or while playing cards, etc.)
   1) almost never (or never)   2) occasionally (about 1/4 of the time)   3) about half of the time   4) frequently (about 3/4 of the time)   5) practically always (or always)

3. Does he/she experience communication difficulties while listening to someone speak to a large group? (e.g., at church or in a civic meeting, in a fraternal or women's club, at an educational lecture, etc.)
   1) almost never (or never)   2) occasionally (about 1/4 of the time)   3) about half of the time   4) frequently (about 3/4 of the time)   5) practically always (or always)

4. Does he/she experience communication difficulties while participating in various types of entertainment? (e.g., movies, TV, radio, plays, night clubs, musical entertainment, etc.)
   1) almost never (or never)   2) occasionally (about 1/4 of the time)   3) about half of the time   4) frequently (about 3/4 of the time)   5) practically always (or always)

5. Does he/she experience communication difficulties when in an unfavorable listening environment? (e.g., at a noisy party, where there is background music when riding in an auto or bus, when someone whispers or talks from across the room, etc.)
   1) almost never (or never)   2) occasionally (about 1/4 of the time)   3) about half of the time   4) frequently (about 3/4 of the time)   5) practically always (or always)

6. Does he/she experience communication difficulties when using or listening to various communication devices? (e.g., telephone, telephone ring, doorbell, public address system, warning signals, alarms, etc.)
   1) almost never (or never)   2) occasionally (about 1/4 of the time)   3) about half of the time   4) frequently (about 3/4 of the time)   5) practically always (or always)

Feelings About Communications

7. Do you feel that any difficulty with his/her hearing limits or hampers his/her personal or social life?
   1) almost never (or never)   2) occasionally (about 1/4 of the time)   3) about half of the time   4) frequently (about 3/4 of the time)   5) practically always (or always)

8. Does any problem or difficulty with his/her hearing upset them?
   1) almost never (or never)   2) occasionally (about 1/4 of the time)   3) about half of the time   4) frequently (about 3/4 of the time)   5) practically always (or always

9. Do you or others suggest that he/she has a hearing problem?
   1) almost never (or never)   2) occasionally (about 1/4 of the time)   3) about half of the time   4) frequently (about 3/4 of the time)   5) practically always) (or always

10. Do you or others leave his/her out of conversations or become annoyed because of his/her hearing?
   1) almost never (or never)   2) occasionally (about 1/4 of the time)   3) about half of the time   4) frequently (about 3/4 of the time)   5) practically always (or always)

Amplification Profile

Hearing Aid Operation	All Time	Some of Time	Not at Al
1. Battery-Put In And Take Out Correctly	_____	_____	_____
2. On-Off Switch	_____	_____	_____
3. Other Controls "M" and "T" Switch	_____	_____	_____
4. Earmold Insertion	_____	_____	_____
5. Earmold Removal	_____	_____	_____
6. Place Aid Over Ear	_____	_____	_____
7. Volume Control-Adjust To Comfort	_____	_____	_____
8. Knows How to Clean Earmold And Aid	_____	_____	_____
Optional-Troubleshooting Minor Problems	_____	_____	_____

---

[7]Modified from Harlem Hospital, Columbia University.

Administrative Considerations in Implementation
of Service Delivery Models

Barbara B. Shadden
University of Arkansas, Fayetteville

As a profession, we still tend to cling to a rather narrow conceptual
model of service delivery that suggests that service provider and recipient
exist in a semivacuum, with the success or failure of intervention determined
primarily by client and clinician variables. Recently, Dowling (1981) has
argued convincingly that the service delivery model must be, at the very least,
tripartite--consisting of provider, recipient, and third party funding source.
It would be more realistic, however, to recognize that there are multiple
factors which interact to determine the success or failure of programming.

One of the key factors is the support of administrative personnel.
Administrators and their administrations are facts of life in the service
delivery world. The term administrative is used very loosely here to designate
those persons or agencies to whom speech-language pathologists and audiologists
are responsible or whose approval/support is required. Thus, administration
may refer to individuals in authority at hospitals, nursing homes, home health
organizations, universities, private or government-funded clinics, senior
citizen centers, community groups that represent sectors of the older
population, or even governmental agencies. The hard reality is that no single
professional can operate for long outside of the boundaries imposed by one or
more of these administrative frameworks.

The focus of this chapter is upon some of the administrative
considerations that influence service delivery to the older population. As
service delivery models expand in the gerontological arena, a whole new set of
problems arise with respect to implementation of these models. Ironically,
these problems are not separate from those encountered in the provision of more
traditional services. Instead, the newer problems are simply superimposed on
existing ones. For this reason, the chapter examines current communication
programming for older persons before attempting to summarize some of the more
pervasive administrative difficulties that might be anticipated with expanded

service delivery models. The chapter closes with an overview of possible strategies for resolving targeted problem areas.

In reviewing both problems and strategies, it is important to remember that administrative decisions concerning service provision are not made arbitrarily. On the contrary, an administrator is highly susceptible to external influences, some of which are identified in Figure 1. They may include (a) the availability of funding and the policies of funding agencies; (b) the attitudes, knowledge, and support of other health professionals; (c) the expectations and perceptions of needs on the part of older individuals; (d) the breadth of training and skills of the communication disorders professional; and (e) the diverse nature of specific services being proposed or provided. Figure 1 emphasizes the fact that multiple avenues exist for effecting administrative support of traditional or innovative service delivery models. If we focus exclusively on the administrator, we may reduce the likelihood of successful implementation of services.

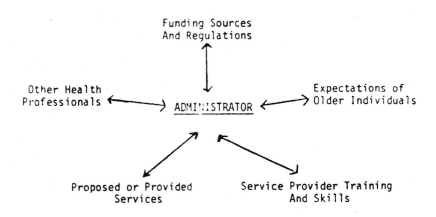

Figure 1. External influences impacting upon administrators and administrative decisions concerning service delivery.

Current Status of Service Delivery to Older Persons

Before the more critical administrative considerations in implementing communication for older individuals can be isolated, it is first necessary to describe briefly the current status of service delivery. Most available service delivery data pertains to traditional professional roles, intervention models, and settings. Lubinski (1981) describes these traditional roles and models as individual-oriented, with a heavy emphasis on specific communication disorders and relatively limited involvement in consultation and in-service. The literature focuses primarily upon service delivery within the context of long-term care facilities and home health agencies. The following summary documents the chronic underserving of older individuals within these settings, and details common barriers to service provision. Although administrative perceptions are stressed, observations pertinent to professional and older person variables are included in the discussion.

Incidence of Communication Disorders and Actual Service Needs

The incidence figures for speech-language and hearing disorders within the older population in the United States have been cited repeatedly in recent years. Most professional reports project that approximately one-third of all individuals over the age of 65 have a specific communication impairment (Sayles & Adams, 1979). This estimate has been confirmed by survey data from older persons themselves (Shadden, 1982) and by studies of nursing home populations (Long Term Care Facility Improvement Study, 1975).

Of greater interest, however, are figures describing the need for services or for programming consideration. Chafee (1967) reported that 92.5% of the 223 nursing home patients surveyed required special staff attention with respect to speech and hearing. More specifically, 60% of the extended care facility residents evaluated by Mueller and Peters (1981) were judged to have a communication impairment. It was determined that approximately one-half of these (29%) could benefit from intervention. Brody (1977) has estimated that one-third of the older adults in the community have a need for physical therapy, occupational therapy, and/or speech therapy.

Perceived Incidence on the Part of Administrators

Clearly, the incidence of communication impairment—and the need for professional services—is high within the older population. Do program administrators, however, perceive this incidence accurately? Dancer and Drummond (1982) asked nursing home and senior citizen center directors to estimate the percentage of their clients with communication problems. Mean estimates of speech-language problems were 7.2% and 0.5% and estimates of hearing problems were 17% and 4.6%, respectively, for nursing home and senior citizen center respondents. Nearly 90% of the nursing home administrators indicated they had recognized speech-language and hearing problems in their clients over the past 6 months. However, only 38% of the senior citizen center administrators acknowledged speech-language problems and only 64% had noted any hearing problems during the same time period.

These figures suggest strongly that administrators are vastly underestimating the incidence of speech-language-hearing problems. This conclusion is supported by Mueller and Peter's (1981) data from administrators of extended care facilities. Close to one-third of their respondents estimated the frequency of speech-language problems as falling within the 0-9% range, with a derived group mean of 20%. Responses with respect to hearing impairment were more evenly distributed up to 59%, but the derived group mean fell at the 34% level.

Levels of Service Provision in Varied Settings

Because institution or agency administrators appear to routinely underestimate the prevalence of communication disorders in their clientele, low levels of service provision might be anticipated. Certainly, 47% of the communication disorders professionals sampled in the state of Arkansas and across the nation feel that their services are being underutilized by the older population (Shadden & Raiford, 1984).

This impression of underutilization is supported by a fairly extensive body of literature. For example, survey data on long-term care facilities suggest that speech-language pathologists are employed full-time by 4%-7% of these facilities, part-time by 7%-27%, and as outside contracted services in 18%-73% of the settings (Chapey, Lubinski, Chapey, & Salzburg, 1979; Dancer & Drummond, 1982; Mueller & Peters, 1981). In the Mueller and Peters (1981) study, audiologists were employed full time by 1% of the facilities, part-time by 3%, and as outside consultants by 5.7%. Other percentages of facilities which provided any audiological services at all ranged from 15% to 57%.

To some extent, variability in levels of service provision across studies may reflect very real regional differences. However, unusually high figures may also be a product of classic misconceptions as to who is qualified to provide communication disorders services. In the Dancer and Drummond study, 76% of the senior citizen center directors reported provision of hearing services and 36% reported provision of speech-language services. However, the specified professionals cited included doctors, neurologists, hearing aid dealers, and (ironically) pediatricians.

This picture of chronic underserving of the long-term care facility population is underscored by professional demographic data. In a survey of speech-language pathologists and audiologists in Wisconsin, only 15% provided any services in such facilities, and only 2.5% were directly employed by the facility (Mueller & Peters, 1981). Similarly, in a more recent survey of communication disorders professionals in Arkansas and across the nation, between 0% and 16.4% reported employment within a nursing home context, with only 0%-4.1% of their time being committed to these settings (Shadden, 1982).

In the home health arena, there has been a slow but steady increase in the number of agencies employing a speech-language pathologist, from 20% in 1967 to 58% reported in 1981 (Hester, 1981b; Lubinski & Chapey, 1981). Eighty-nine percent of these professionals were employed part-time. Only 5% of the agencies sampled in the Lubinski and Chapey survey employed an audiologist in any capacity. These data suggest that older adults living independently may not be receiving adequate speech and hearing services. This conclusion is supported by a sampling of three communities of older individuals in northwest Arkansas (Shadden, 1982). As many as 41% of the communicatively impaired members of one community reported receiving no speech-language or hearing services at any time.

Barriers to Service Provision Reported by Administrators

Why are speech-language and hearing services not being provided to meet documented needs? This question must be answered first from an administrative viewpoint; the answers are relatively consistent across studies. In the Mueller and Peters (1981) survey of extended care facility administrators, almost 40% of the respondents indicated that speech-language pathology or audiology services were not provided because there was no need or because services were believed to be of no benefit. An additional 19% described budget constraints, 10% cited nonavailability of services, and fully 6% specifically indicated that physicians did not make referrals. These factors are similar to those described in the Dancer and Drummond paper surveying nursing home and senior citizen center directors. The top three barriers to service provision identified by their respondents were unavailability of finances, unavailability of services, and little or no knowledge of referral sources. Other factors included (a) patient refusal of services, (b) poor condition of patient, (c) negative recommendations by other professionals, (d) previous unsuccessful services, and (e) transportation.

Service provision in home health agencies appears to be limited by similar problems. The low supply of speech-language pathologists in the Hester (1981a) survey of home health administrators was attributed to lack of demand, low referral rates by doctors and nurses, and problems with a high rate of exclusion of speech therapy from reimbursement on the part of state Medicaid and private insurance plans. The top five problems reported by Lubinski and Chapey (1981), in order of greatest to least frequency, were:

1. travel time and parking;
2. personnel problems (including unavailability and use of moonlighting staff);
3. shortage of physician referrals, attributed to the physician's lack of understanding;
4. funding inadequacies;
5. lack of family involvement or follow-through.

The most common difficulties noted in all of these studies, therefore, can be summarized as follows. Funding is unavailable or difficult to obtain. Speech-language pathology and audiology services may be limited in availability or administrators may be unaware of where to look for such services. Other medical personnel, particularly physicians, do not make referrals for services. The need for services may be underestimated and misunderstood, or the services may not be viewed as being particularly valuable. All of these factors represent administrative realities. As such, they suggest areas that must be targeted for change if some of the administrative barriers to service provision are to be eliminated.

Problems in Service Utilization Identified by Others

Limited data are also available concerning professional and older person perceptions of service utilization. In a recent survey (Shadden & Raiford, 1984), speech-language pathologists and audiologists sampled nationally were asked to indicate how strongly they agreed or disagreed that certain factors influenced underutilization of communication disorders services by older clients. All subgroups agreed that the top two problems were inadequate referral from other professionals and the older persons' lack of awareness of service availability. Agreement was less consistent for the factors of (a) lack of awareness of communication disorders; (b) poor transportation; and (c) older persons being advised that services are of little or no use. Many of these concerns parallel those reported by administrators, although "problems in affording services" is conspicuously absent.

As part of the same study, older individuals living independently in northwest Arkansas were asked to indicate how strongly they agreed or disagreed that similar factors influenced their utilization of health services in general. Consistent agreement was found for only two items--one of which suggested an inability to afford health services, and the other reflected a lack of knowledge of services available. There appears to be some discrepancy here between the perceptions of older persons and communication disorders professionals, although both responding groups felt that lack of awareness of services was a problem.

Working Professional Factors Influencing Service Provision

A detailed analysis of the gerontological training and attitudes of audiologists and speech-language pathologists is beyond the scope of this chapter. However, several recent research findings merit a brief comment. First, at a recent ASHA convention (Committee on the Communication Problems of the Aged, 1983), it was reported that professionals in our field tend to rate the quality of their gerontological training less than favorably (mean rating of 2.9 on a 5-point scale with "1" equivalent to "very poor"). They also consistently rated the quality of their specific training in communication disorders lower for clients over age 65 than for preschool or elementary-school-age clients. Further, graduate programs in communication disorders appear to have made little progress in expanding course or practicum offerings in order to provide a broader-based gerontological focus. In essence, speech-language pathologists and audiologists continue to enter the work force with a somewhat restricted awareness of the communication needs of older persons, thus limiting the effectiveness of their advocacy of service delivery programs to administrators.

Second, the ageism attitudes of other health professionals have been documented in a variety of sources (cf., Davis & Holland, 1981; Solomon, 1982).

In a recent study, 495 communication disorders professionals across the nation completed a rating scale designed to reflect their beliefs and attitudes toward the communication behaviors of older persons. Analyses of scale data suggested that respondents were exhibiting a positive response bias, as reflected in an unwillingness to agree with statements defining "negative" communication attributes (Shadden, in press). Even statements pertaining to documented realities of physiological aging were denied. Although this may show a commendable degree of sensitivity to the issue of stereotype and bias, it creates other difficulties. Specifically, guilt or concern over ageism may result in an unrealistic assessment of needs or inappropriate interaction strategies (Davis & Holland, 1981). One further consequence might be a failure to present administrators with an accurate or complete "case" for a particular service delivery program.

Core Problems

It is possible to isolate a series of core problems in the implementation of service delivery to the older population, based on the preceding discussion. Each of these problems ultimately impacts upon administrative approval of and support for both traditional and innovative communication programming. Taken together, they may also act as guidelines for a broad plan of action designed to remove administrative barriers.

1. Administrators are not yet convinced of the need for and/or benefits of traditional communication disorders services...and have little or no knowledge of proposed expanded service delivery roles.

Within the past 10 years, efforts have been made to train administrators, among others, as to the nature and incidence of communication disorders and the need for appropriate services. ASHA's nationally disseminated workshop and brochure entitled Communication Problems and Behaviors of the Older American represents perhaps the most prominent of such efforts (Sayles & Adams, 1979). The final outcome of this training is not yet known and is dependent, in part, upon the support of local practitioners. The preceding overview of the status of service delivery, however, may suggest that efforts have been only partially successful. Moreover, the information presented in most training projects is outdated. Consequently, administrators have no real understanding of the fact that new approaches to ameliorating the communication behaviors of older persons exist. Without such an understanding, comprehensive and effective communication services of the aging cannot be planned and implemented.

2. Other health care providers, like administrators, are not convinced of the benefit of traditional communication disorders services and are uninformed concerning more innovative approaches to enhancing communication effectiveness in older persons.

Most professionals working with older clients can document instances where physician referral for speech-language pathology and audiology services was withheld due to lack of knowledge of availability of services or, more importantly, a belief that speech-language therapy in particular accomplishes nothing. Anecdotal reports suggest that many medical schools historically have taught that speech therapy is ineffective. Further, it appears that speech-language pathologists and audiologists who are respected members of health care teams are often valued because of their perceived individual strengths and skills, not their profession.

Whereas this presents numerous barriers to the daily delivery of quality programming, it also has a very direct impact upon administrative policy and priorities. Physicians in particular exert a powerful influence upon administrative policy-making. Other health care professionals shape the administrative view of a comprehensive health care package through their perceptions of client needs and their requests for services.

3. Funding sources for traditional speech-language pathology services continue to be inadequate and no mechanism exists at present for funding some of the newer, more innovative communication service delivery models discussed in this manual.

As clearly documented in a variety of sources (Dowling, 1981; Stryker, 1976; Wood & Martin, 1981), funding has been and continues to be a major problem in provision of services to the elderly. Not only is third-party reimbursement a constant source of frustration, but the regulations governing such reimbursement, at least with respect to Medicare and Medicaid, are in a state of constant change.

The topic of economic considerations has been addressed in detail in the preceding chapter. The critical issue here is that administrative personnel frequently cite inadequate funding as a barrier to provision of speech-language and hearing services. Understandably, administrators tend to utilize economic feasibility as a primary yardstick for evaluating proposed and existing programs. In attempting to solicit approval for expanded or innovative communication services, communication disorders professionals must be prepared to justify the associated expenses or to identify alternate mechanisms for funding. This may involve the collection of data useful in documenting need or perhaps the writing of grant proposals designed to solicit pilot or maintenance funding.

4. Older persons are relatively uninformed as to normal and disordered communication processes, the effects of aging upon such processes, and the kinds of services that may be of benefit to them. Further, many individuals may not perceive the need for services.

It has been documented that major segments of the population are not knowledgeable about our profession or about communication disorders (Killarney & Lass, 1981; Pearlstein, Russell, & Fink, 1977). There is no reason to believe that older individuals are better informed. In addition, preliminary research data suggest that the elderly tend to view their own communication skills and behaviors quite favorably, while simultaneously subscribing to the belief that the majority of "other" older persons possess less than adequate communication skills (Shadden, in press). Such attitudes might lead older individuals to expect that they personally would not benefit from some of the more innovative approaches to communication intervention ("It's not my problem!"). Further, older individuals have been described as reluctant to admit difficulties with hearing, presumably due to its stereotypical association with aging and senility (Pollack, 1978).

Although these are problems primarily affecting service utilization, they have an indirect impact upon administrative decisions. The older segment of the population is becoming an increasingly strong consumer force. If any community of older individuals can be convinced of the need for communication

289

services and can be directed to the appropriate policy-making administrative personnel, programming will be implemented. (In this context, the term "community" may refer to the narrow confines of a single nursing home or to a broader residential area or geographical region.) Professionals must be willing to become involved in this process of increasing levels of community awareness.

5. Speech-language pathologists and audiologists have not been trained adequately with respect to the impact of age-related physical, sociological, and psychological factors upon communication behaviors and disorders. Further, professionals have not traditionally received adequate training in funding sources, business management, public relations, and administration--training that might make them more effective in "selling" services and programs.

The lack of a broad-based gerontological education focus has already been addressed as the primary focus of this manual and needs no further comment.It is important to remember, however, that professional preparation influences more than the effectiveness and quality of any particular intervention program. In addition, it can directly impact upon the success or failure of program proposals to administrative individuals and groups.

In reviewing the core problems listed above, it is clear that considerable time and effort have been invested in efforts to resolve difficulties with respect to traditional communication disorders service delivery models--with limited success. As service delivery models are expanded, we may be forced to retrace some of our earlier footsteps in an attempt to re-educate health professionals, administrators, funding agencies, and monitoring governmental groups.

Fortunately, the very gaps in our awareness-enhancing programs in the past suggest that ideas about speech-language pathology and audiology can still be shaped. Many of the programming issues addressed in this manual emphasize a broadening of the role of the communication disorders professional and an expansion of the areas of older person's lives over which we can exert a positive influence. If successful in convincing others of the value of these new roles, improved opportunities for traditional service delivery should result. These changes also occur at a time when, as a profession, we are becoming more sensitive to the need for intelligent, skillful advocacy of ourselves, our services, and our clients. Continued professional growth and expansion, however, depend heavily upon the extent to which individuals are willing to invest their energies in this process.

Strategies for Overcoming Administrative Barriers

In this final section, educational, administrative, and professional strategies for overcoming or eliminating barriers to service delivery are presented. Recommendations are discussed with varying degrees of detail, since many address indirect avenues for administrative change that are covered more comprehensively in other chapters of this manual. Each strategy is intended to be simply one element in a broad-based plan of action whose basic focus is the improvement and expansion of communication services to older persons. The number one priority of every speech-language pathologist and audiologist must be to develop such a comprehensive plan of action for himself or herself—as an individual, team member with a professional setting, and a member of professional organizations at the local, state, regional, and national levels.

Educational Strategies

Our primary tool for improving service delivery continues to be the education of all concerned individuals, including other health professionals, administrators, and the older person as potential client. This education or information exchange, however, may take a variety of forms.

Traditional Inservice Training or Service Provider Workshops

The traditional vehicles for educating other professionals and administrators appear to be in-service training programs (staff education) within a particular facility or wider outreach workshops designed to provide information to a selected group of health care providers. In the past, these efforts have focused upon the training of participants to recognize common speech, language, and hearing disorders associated with aging in order to (a) encourage appropriate referral for treatment; and (b) facilitate staff interaction and communication with communicatively impaired clients. Another major goal has been the dissemination of information about speech-language pathologists and audiologists--their credentials, skills, and services. The ultimate intent, of course, is to improve the quality and availability of services to the older client.

Such training must continue in the future. Several areas for improvement can be identified. First, health care providers must be helped to develop an understanding of the centrality of communication to the life adjustment of all older clients, as a prerequisite to understanding more innovative service delivery models. We must therefore establish our credentials in the broader arena of communication and aging, as well as our specific expertise with respect to communication disorders.

Second, training must be highly experiential. Many presenters experience a need to overwhelm an audience with evidence of their technical expertise. Ironically, one tape recording, exercise, or role play will probably have a far greater and more lasting impact than a full hour of lecture (Shadden, Raiford, & Shadden, 1983). The goal should never be to make experts out of participants, but rather to heighten their awareness of and sensitivity to the consequences of any breakdown in communication.

Third, presenters should be prepared to make highly specific recommendations for needed programs and should emphasize the way in which proposed programming will benefit client and staff member alike. This implies a need for concrete examples, rather than abstract theory. It also suggests that services should never be recommended if they are not readily available, unless a clear plan of action for facilitating the implementation of services can be identified.

Dissemination of Information Within Gerontological Associations

A second avenue for impacting upon other professionals and program administrators is a somewhat neglected one--participation in gerontological associations at the state, regional, and/or national level. Although we are quick to claim that we are neglected as professionals within the aging network, we have made relatively few attempts to validate ourselves through presentations to or involvement with such associations. An examination of recent programs for the National Council on Aging and the Gerontological Society of America conventions is revealing. Very few presentations deal directly with specific communication disorders or even interpersonal communication, although research and programs with potential interpersonal

consequences abound. By our absence from such gatherings, we confirm the image
of speech-language pathology and audiology as ancillary services with limited
gerontological outreach. Through our presence, however, we can enhance
understanding and acceptance of our discipline, while simultaneously receiving
information that can improve our own professional services.

As members of the gerontological professional community, we can play a
prominent role in the development of a viable conceptual framework embracing
the full continuum of human communication and communication disorders, as
affected by the aging process. Few such models exist at the present time and
those that do exist need further evaluation (cf., Shadden, 1982). The
development and dissemination of appropriate communication models can be
extremely useful in several respects. With such models, it is possible to
identify those communication questions that need to be researched across
professional disciplines and to design intervention programs addressing the
communication needs of the elderly. An effective model can also define the
professional roles of the speech-language pathologist and audiologist and
should clarify our position within the aging network of service providers.
Most importantly, a model can be used to validate service delivery programs,
particularly the more innovative directions being suggested in this manual.

Training of Older Persons and Their Advocates
It has already been suggested that older persons wield considerable power
as the ultimate consumer of any services being offered. This suggests that
professionals must make an effort to convince the older community and their
advocates of the need for and value of varying forms of communication service
delivery. Workshops, newspaper articles, and public television presentation
are among the more common vehicles for reaching this population, with
television being particularly effective with the elderly (Davis, 1977).
Traditionally, we have used these vehicles to educate the older community about
communication disorders. In the future, a greater emphasis must be placed upon
the nature and benefits of communication services.

Administrative Strategies

Program Proposals to Administrators

Although administrators require the traditional kinds of education outlined in the section on in-service training, they are also in a relatively unique position of power with respect to decisions concerning provision of services. Programs are presented to them for approval or disapproval. Thus, an effective plan must be developed for any program proposal. Some of the ingredients of a successful plan of action (Hester, 1981a; Lubinski & Chapey, 1981; Walle & Newman, 1967) are outlined below. The concerns of any particular administrator should be anticipated and addressed throughout this process.

1. The administrator must be helped to understand clearly both the nature of the problem being addressed (e.g., the necessity of effective communication) and the ways in which improved communication will benefit staff, client, and facility alike. It is not sufficient to suggest that communication is central to all human endeavors. Specific examples must be provided to demonstrate more concrete gains. For instance, it may be possible to suggest that improved communication will be associated with less resident disorientation in a nursing home, adult day care, or senior center, thus reducing demands on staff time and attention.

2. The need for the proposed services within a particular facility must be well-documented. In addition to citations of current statistics, a survey or screening of the potential client body should be completed. It should be possible to tell the administrator that, "Roughly 40% of your residents/participants can benefit from communication services."

3. A highly specific, detailed explanation of the proposed program must be presented. "You need speech-language therapy for some of your clients" is an insufficient strategy.

4. It must be demonstrated that the proposed program (a) will be effective, (b) is financially feasible, (c) has the support of the staff and client groups involved, and (d) will not detract from other programming or unduly stress existing resources.

294

5. When possible, a demonstration project should be proposed, as a way of allowing the administrator to evaluate the merits of a program before approval for its full-scale implementation.

6. The professional should be capable of clearly summarizing points of agreement and disagreement in discussions with the administrator and must be willing to show "good faith" by negotiating a compromise, if necessary, or by offering to participate actively in seeking financial support.

Alternate Resources

Many administrative concerns can be overcome if the speech-language pathologist and audiologist can identify alternate resources that will absorb some of the financial or personnel burdens of implementing programming. In the financial arena, a variety of groups may be willing to contribute money and/or equipment, such as community service organizations (e.g., Kiwanis, Lion's Club, Sertoma), churches, local business and industry, organizations of older individuals such as American Association of Retired Persons (AARP), and area agencies on aging or similar agencies that are publicly funded to provide or support services for older persons. The advantages to different groups range from fulfilling a commitment to community service to improved public relations and tax write-offs. Support could be utilized to sponsor individual therapy, pay for renovations to a floor in a nursing home (Lubinski, 1981), provide a stipend for a student-in-training, or even absorb costs of a health professional workshop.

A second major source of alternate personnel resources is volunteerism. Volunteers may be local community residents, students, or even other older persons residing in the same facility (Lubinski, 1981). Retired speech-language-hearing professionals or other retired health professionals could be particularly useful. Ten hours of training provided by a communication disorders professional might ultimately expedite hundreds of hours of quality communication services to a particular population of older individuals. A third personnel resource would be other health care providers such as social service personnel who already interact with older clients in a given facility. Programs planned collaboratively with and implemented by such professionals can be highly successful. Finally, the potential contribution of family members to communication facilitation is frequently underutilized. In part, this reflects a concern that families should not be taken to be "therapists," even though their cooperation and assistance are critically important for maintenance and carry-over. As our service delivery models broaden to include a wider range of communication behaviors, however, the rewards to the family member for participation in programming will increase dramatically.

Professional Strategies

Enhanced Education

Within the communication disorders profession, the primary need is for more broadly-based gerontological training and recognition that the elderly are entitled to a wide range of services. Interest levels in obtaining training are high (Shadden, 1982), and earlier experiments with gerontological coursework suggest that perspectives on older clients are shaped by these educational experiences (Leutenegger & Stovall, 1971). Such education is provided by this manual and its associated conference; additional recommendations have been identified by Davis and Holland (1981). Speech-language pathologists and audiologists must also become better prepared to deal with the financial, political, and administrative realities that, in the final analysis, govern the successful implementation of programming.

Enhanced professional preparation has many advantages. First, a better understanding of aging and of the role of communication in the aging process will improve professionals' advocacy of services and education of others. Second, this understanding will increase the likelihood that service delivery models will be expanded and quality of services improved. This, in turn, may influence other professionals and administrators, because the benefits of such services will be more apparent (O'Connell & O'Connell, 1978). Third, the broadening of professional training in gerontology and in business realities can be expected to sharpen the skills necessary for defining and presenting program plans to administrators. Finally, a comprehensive grasp of current realities is necessary if alternative resources are to be identified and exploited.

Activism

Distasteful as it is to many, one of the realities of the world of service delivery is that administrative, and by extension, political lobbying is necessary. Planning agencies, funding agencies, and governing groups of other professional organizations simply will not recognize communication needs and take appropriate action without being advised properly. This is particularly true in the area of funding. The implication is that speech-language pathologists and audiologists must become directly involved in this process as individuals or, at the very least, must actively support our professional organizations in these endeavors. Appropriate individual actions include monitoring of state and federal legislation, contacting congressman, contacting and lobbying with private insurance companies, seeking representation at meetings such as the recent White House Conference on Aging, and so forth.

Summary

The major premise of this chapter has been that administrative decisions concerning implementation of services are influenced by a variety of factors. Any efforts to effect positive change in administrative policies must evolve out of a comprehensive plan of action that reflects an understanding of these multiple factors. With such an understanding, a number of educational, administrative, and professional strategies become available to us. The responsibility and the power rest in our hands.

Self-Study Questions

1. List as many external influences upon administrative decision-making as possible. Feel free to draw upon your own professional experience as well as information presented in this chapter.

2. Identify the five major problems identified in this chapter as having a negative impact upon the implementation of traditional and more innovative service delivery models.
   -- Describe the manner in which each of these directly or indirectly may influence administrative support for programming.

3.   Clarify what is meant by a "plan of action" for facilitating communication service delivery to older persons.

  -- Describe the strategies for influencing administrative consideration of communication programs that were discussed in this chapter.

  -- Develop your own personalized plan of action. Include all arenas in which you might ultimately be able to effect positive change.

  -- More specifically, select one particular program that you would like to see implemented and identify the series of steps needed to develop a successful proposal to a particular administrator in a particular setting.

REFERENCES

American Speech-Language-Hearing Association, Committee on the Communication Problems of the Aged. (1983). Professional competencies and training for working with the elderly. Miniseminar presented at the annual convention of the American Speech-Language-Hearing Association.

Brody, E. (1977). Long term care of older people. New York: Human Sciences Press.

Chafee, C. E. (1967). Rehabilitation needs of nursing home patients: A report of a survey. Rehabilitation Literature, 28, 377.

Chapey, R., Lubinski, R., Chapey, G., & Salzburg, A. (1979). Survey of speech, language, and hearing services in nursing home settings. Long Term Care and Health Services Admininistration Quarterly, 3, 307-316.

Dancer, J., & Drummond, S. S. (1982). Communication problems of the elderly: A survey. Unpublished manuscript.

Davis, G. A., & Holland, A. L. (1981). Age in understanding and treating aphasia. In D. S. Beasley & G. A. Davis (Eds.), Aging: Communication processes and disorders. New York: Grune & Stratton

Davis, R. H. (1977). The role of television. In R. A. Kalish (Ed.), The later years: Social applications of gerontology. Monterey, CA: Brooks/Cole.

Dowling, R. J. (1981). Federal health insurance for the elderly. In D. S. Beasley & G. A. Davis (Eds.), Aging: Communication processes and disorders. New York: Grune & Stratton.

Hester, E. J. (1981a). Health planning agencies and speech-language pathology. Asha, 23, 85-92.

Hester, E. J. (1981b). The status of speech-language pathology in the home health setting. Asha, 23, 155-162.

Killarney, G. T., & Lass, N. J. (1981). A study of rural public awareness of speech-language pathology and audiology. Asha, 23, 415-420.

Leutenegger, R., & Stovall, J. (1971). A pilot graduate seminar in speech and hearing problems of the chronically ill and the aged. Asha, 13, 61-66.

Long Term Care Facility Improvement Study. (1975). Washington, DC: Public Health Services Office of Nursing Home Affairs.

Lubinski, R. (1981). Programs in home heallth care agencies and nursing homes. In D. S. Beasley & G. A. Davis (Eds.), Aging: Communication processes and disorders. New York: Grune & Stratton.

Lubinski, R., & Chapey. R. (1980). Communication services in home health careagencies: Availability and scope. Asha, 22, 929-934.

Mueller, P. B., & Peters, T. J. (1981). Needs and services in geriatric speech-langruage pathology and audiology. Asha, 19, 323-328.

O'Connell, P., & O'Connell, E. (1978). Speech-language pathology services in a skilled nursing facility. Paper presented at the annual convention of the American Speech and Hearing Association.

Pearlstein, E., Russell, L., & Fink, R. (1977). Speech-language pathology and audiology: The public's view. Paper presented at the annual convention of the American Speech and Hearing Association.

Pollack, M. C. (1978). The remediation process: Psychological and counseling aspects. In J. G. Alpiner (Ed.). Handbook of adult rehabilitative audiology. Baltimore: Williams & Wilkins.

Sayles, A. H., & Adams, J. K. (1979). Communication problems and behaviors of the older American. Baltimore: American Speech-Language-Hearing Association.

Shadden, B. B. (1981). Communication and aging: A broader perspective. Miniseminar presented at the annual convention of the American Speech-Language-Hearing Association.

Shadden, B. B. (in press). Attitudes towards the communication skills and behaviors of the elderly. Aging and Society.

Shadden, B. B. (1982). Communication process and aging: Information needs and attitudes of older adults and professionals. Final report to the AARP Andrus Foundation.

Shadden, B. B., & Raiford, C. A. (1984). Factors influencing service utilization by older individuals: Perceptions of communication disorders, Journal of Communication Disorders, 17, 209-224.

Shadden, B. B., Raiford, C. A., & Shadden, H. S. (1983). Coping with communication disorders in aging. Tigaard, OR: C. C. Publications.

Solomon, K. (1982). Social antecedents of learned helplessness in the health care setting. The Gerontologist, 22, 282-287.

Stryker, S. (1976). Procedures relating to Medicare and other third-party payments. Asha, 18, 491-495.

Walle, E. L., & Newman, P. W. (1967). Rehabilitation services for speech, hearing, and language disorders in an extended care facility. Asha, 9, 216-218.

Wood, E. F., & Martin, D. H. (1981). A consumer perspective: The hearing aid delivery system. In D. S. Beasley & G. A. Davis (Eds), Aging: Communication process and disorders. New York: Grune & Stratton.

Suggested Readings

Required

Hester, E. J. (1981a). Health planning agencies and speech-language pathology. Asha, 23, 85-92.

Hester, E. J. (1981b). The status of speech-language pathology in the home health setting. Asha, 23, 155-162.

Lubinski, R. (1981). Programs in home health care agencies nad nursing homes. In D. S. Beasley & G. A. Davis (Eds.), Aging: Communication processes and disorders. New York: Grune & Stratton.

Mueller, P. B., & Peters, T. J. (1977). Needs and services in geriatric speech-language pathology and audiology. Asha, 19, 323-328.

Shadden, B. B., & Raiford, C. A. (in press). Factors influencing service utilization by older individuals: Perceptions of communication disorderws professionals. Journal of Communication Disorders.

Supplemental

Davis, G. A., & Holland, A. L. (1981). Age in understanding and treating aphasia. In D. S. Beasley & G. A. Davis (Eds.), Aging: Communication processes and disorders. New York: Grune & Stratton.

Lubinski, R., & Chapey, R. (1980). Communication services in home health care agencies: Availability and scope. Asha, 22, 929-934.

Shadden, B. B. (in press). Attitudes towards the communication skills and behaviors of the elderly. Aging and Society.

Walle, E. L., & Newman, P. W. (1967). Rehabilitation services for speech, hearing, and language disorders in an extended care facility. Asha, 9, 216-218.

Economic Considerations
in Implementing Service
Delivery Models

Richard M. Flower

University of California Medical Center, San Francisco

Although a discussion of economic considerations in serving older people with communication disorders might be developed from several points of view, we will restrict our purview to matters directly related to financial support for essential services. Few, if any, sources of that support are restricted to speech, language, and hearing services. However, our discussion will consider the application of those resources in the delivery of services to the segment of that population with communication disorders.

Economic Resources for Services to the Elderly

Two different types of support may be available for human services (a) support provided to underwrite services to individual consumers, and (b) broader support to underwrite human services programs. It is important to recognize however, that in any given instance both types of support may apply. For example, many community agencies receive programmatic support from United Fund campaigns and other benefactors. Yet they may also charge fees (often on a sliding scale) for the individual services they deliver to those individuals who are able to carry full or partial responsibility for the cost of services or who are covered by an insurance plan which provides third-party payment.

Support for Individual Services

Fees for services may be covered by individuals from their own or their family's resources or by third-party payment. Often all three resources are tapped to pay for services.

Consumer and Family Resources

Ever since our colonial and pioneer days, we Americans have professed that society as a whole should share in assisting citizens with special needs. These concepts were eventually expressed in statutory programs, many originating during the New Deal era of the 1930s, and, even more, in the Great Society movement of the 1960s. Care for the elderly has always figured prominently among the purposes of these programs. Despite public concern, however, the largest share of financial responsibility for that care continues to be borne by the elderly themselves and by their families. For example, even with America's renowned Medicare program, only about 45% of the costs of health care for the elderly are currently borne by Medicare, with the majority of the remaining costs paid by beneficiaries and their families either directly or through supplemental private insurance.

As the number of older Americans continues to rise, as the costs of health care and other human services escalate, and as taxpayers become increasingly reluctant to underwrite mounting federal and state budgets, the elderly must, themselves, bear more and more financial responsibility for whatever services they receive. Fortunately, in this affluent society some senior citizens are able to secure and pay for whatever services they require. It is eminently reasonable to expect those individuals to assume that responsibility so long as it does not exhaust the resources they have accumulated to maintain themselves with reasonable dignity. But a significant segment of older Americans live in poverty or at near-poverty levels, because their accumulated resources are insufficient in today's inflated economy, or because those resources have already been decimated by paying for treatment of major illnesses. Even they, however, must often assume at least a share of the costs if they are to receive whatever services they need.

Regardless of the source of payment for a given service, whether covered by public or private agencies or by the consumers themselves, every professional must be concerned for economy in the delivery of those services. In instances where the elderly pay for their own services, however, economy may be a much more immediate determiner of whether or not needed services are received.

Third-Party Payment

In terms of ultimate applicability to speech-language pathology and audiology services, third-party support for services to older people includes the governmental programs of Medicare and Medicaid (previously discussed in chapter four), and private health insurance.

Medicare

In discussing the politics of Medicare, ASHA's Health Insurance Manual (1984) states

> to understand Medicare, one must understand that it is the result of a long and bitter national debate regarding health insurance. That debate involved hundreds of interest groups and the most powerful political leaders and institutions.

Medicare is administered by the United States Department of Health and Human Services through the Health Care Financing Administration (HCFA), which promulgates the regulations that determine conditions of coverage and define reimbursement policies and procedures. Actual reimbursement of services, however, is primarily managed at regional levels through fiscal intermediaries—usually private corporations, commercial insurance companies, or Blue Cross or Blue Shield—which contract with HCFA to manage claims for Medicare coverage. Even though all intermediaries must process claims according to national regulations, substantial local differences may occur in the interpretation of those regulations.

Medicaid

Title XIX of the Society Security Act, which became law in 1965, established a medical assistance program for certain low-income groups. That program, now known as Medicaid, was designed to serve people eligible for cash benefits under such welfare programs as Aid to Families with Dependent Children (AFDC) and the Supplemental Security Income (SSI) program for the aged, blind, and disabled. Some states, albeit a dwindling number, also extend Medicaid coverage to people with sufficient income for basic living expenses but who are unable to afford medical care. Sometimes these are people who require such long-term expensive medical treatment as renal dialysis. These Medicaid beneficiaries, who are not welfare recipients, are sometimes referred to as medically indigent adults (MIAs).

Older people on very limited incomes who are Medicare beneficiaries may also receive assistance through Medicaid. The latter program may cover Part B premiums, annual deductibles, uncovered charges such as the 20% Part B co-payment, and some items excluded by Medicare such as prescription drugs, eye glasses, and hearing aids. Medicaid may also cover costs of services beyond the maximum limits of Medicare; this situation often obtains in instances of long-term placement in skilled nursing facilities—intermediate care or home health care.

Although fundamentally a federal program, a portion of Medicaid funds also derive from state treasuries. Nevertheless, all participating states must adhere to federal regulations with respect to coverage and eligibility and, to a much lesser degree, to procedures for reimbursement. Beyond these fundamental considerations, there are substantial interstate differences in the administration of Medicaid programs.

Federal law mandates that, to participate in Medicaid, all states mus provide certain essential services. These include (a) inpatient hospital services; (b) outpatient hospital services; (c) physician services; (d) services in skilled nursing facilities and certain home health services; early and periodic screening, diagnosis, and treatment of physical and mental defects for beneficiaries under age 21; rural health clinics and family planning services; and (e) laboratory and x-ray services. The Medicaid law also permits states to provide certain optional services, including these home health services that are not mandatory, prescribed prosthetic devices, physical and occupational therapy, and services for individuals with speech, hearing, and language disorders.

Private Insurance

In addition to its role as the model for both Medicare and Medicaid, private insurance may be a major factor in serving older people. There is a group of people, fortunately few, who do not meet eligibility criteria for either Medicare or Medicaid. These people may provide for their health care through private insurance plans in the same way younger people do. Of greater importance, however, is the private insurance most prudent senior citizens purchase to supplement their Medicare coverage. As we have already observed, Medicare beneficiaries still maintain substantial individual financial liability for the care they receive. Some of that liability can be covered by supplemental insurance plans.

Most private supplemental insurance policies cover deductibles and coinsurance. Many cover prescribed pharmaceuticals, and some extend the limits of coverage for acute and long-term care. Rarely, however, do they cover the portion of provider fees that exceed the UCR levels allowed by Medicare intermediaries. Few medical insurance supplemental plans cover dental services, but many older people purchase other insurance to cover those services. As health care costs continually increase and as a steadily growing segment of our population reaches the age for Medicare coverage, beneficiaries will inevitably be called upon to cover larger portions of their own health care costs. Private supplemental insurance will, as a consequence, become an increasingly important commodity. Unfortunately, the same forces that are reducing the extent of Medicare coverage are also effecting sharp increases in supplemental insurance premiums. Therefore, while finding supplemental insurance of greater importance, Medicare beneficiaries will simultaneously find it more unaffordable.

Economic Resources for Speech, Language, and Hearing Services

The authors of other chapters in this manual have discussed the types of services required by older people with speech, language, and hearing disorders. By way of review, the following assertions summarize the services the elderly may require:

1. They may require multiphasic, and often multidisciplinary, diagnostic services to establish the essential nature and extent of their communication disorders and to serve as a basis for planning intervention.

2. They may require individual prosthetic appliances to assist them in achieving optimal communication (e.g., hearing aids, electrolarynxes, and augmentative communication devices).

3. They may require therapeutic and other rehabilitation services to achieve optimal communication.

4. They may require services directed toward maintaining the communication proficiencies achieved in therapeutic and rehabilitation programs.

5. They may require adaptations in recreation and social activities if they are to enjoy opportunities to associate with other people.

6. They may require environmental adaptations and special devices if they are to live safely and maintain the highest level of

independence possible. This obtains whether they continue to live in their own homes or reside in special housing for the elderly, in board and care facilities, or in skilled nursing facilities.

7. Their families and significant others (often including other caregivers) may require counseling if optimal communication is to be maintained.

Finding support for these services involves consideration of all of the resources identified in the previous section of this chapter.

Multidisciplinary Diagnostic Services

Because most multidisciplinary diagnostic services for older people with communication disorders are administered within the context of the health care system, support is more readily available than for other services. Most health insurance plans, both private and governmental, cover substantial segments of these diagnostic services.

Virtually all physician services rendered in connection with establishing medical diagnosis related to communication disorders are covered by health insurance. (Remember, in view of deductibles, coinsurance, copayment, and less than full allowance for many physician and laboratory fees, "covered" often does not mean that the consumer assumes no personal financial liability.) Diagnostic services from professionals who are not physicians, (e.g., from clinical psychologists, may or may not be covered. Diagnostic services provided by speech-language pathologists and audiologists are often covered only if certain conditions are met:

1. The services must be considered "medically necessary." In practice this usually means that a physician states that the service is necessary and the insurer agrees with that conclusion.

2. The diagnostic services must generally relate to an illness or injury. This criterion is highly ambiguous, particularly when applied to conditions such as hearing loss and dysphonias that are commonly associated with the processes of aging. Whether such processes fall within the rubric of "illnesses" is obviously subject to different interpretations.

3. The service must be provided in a setting that is eligible for health insurance coverage. Among such settings are hospitals, skilled nursing facilities, home health programs, hospital outpatient clinics, rehabilitation centers, and physicians' offices. Sometimes, certain diagnostic services provided by audiologists in private practice are covered, but speech-language pathology services provided under similar circumstances usually are not.

4. The service must be provided by a qualified speech-language pathologist or audiologist. Statements of qualifications usually specify state licensure or the appropriate ASHA certificate in states that do not offer licensure. In many instances, services delivered by individuals completing CFY requirements are also covered.

5. The service must not exceed the maximum coverage allowed by the plan. This may be crucial when the client has suffered a serious illness or injury, requiring extensive treatment, immediately prior to referral for diagnostic services.

6. Under some plans, services must be provided by agencies with established contractual relationships with the insurance carrier. Such agencies are usually designated as preferred provider organizations (PPOs).

Medicare, because it is rooted in private health insurance plans, generally adheres to the conditions just cited. Further restrictions are also important, however. Under Part A, diagnostic speech-language pathology services may be covered while the beneficiary is in an acute hospital or while undergoing continued treatment either in a skilled nursing facility or through a home health agency immediately following discharge from the hospital. Those diagnostic services usually must bear some direct relationship to the illness or injury precipitating the hospitalization.

Medicare's earlier-mentioned, new prospective payment approach to coverage of in-hospital services may have major implications for diagnostic speech-language pathology and audiology services under Part A. Those services must be covered within the total payment allowed according to the patient's diagnosis related group. Hence, the hospital's administration and the physician in charge will determine whether the services are essential to the patient's care. It is already apparent that diagnostic speech-language pathology and audiology services will often be delayed until they can be provided in the skilled nursing facility, home health program, or outpatient center that will care for the patient immediately following discharge from the acute hospital.

Under Part B, Medicare beneficiaries may receive diagnostic speech-language pathology services provided in a hospital outpatient clinic, in a rehabilitation agency, in a medical clinic, or in a physician's office. In some instances, services provided under the auspices of home health agencies are also covered under Part B. Audiology services may be covered when requested by a physician to assist in the establishment of a medical diagnosis (so long as those services in no way relate to the selection of a hearing aid). Audiology services are covered when provided within the kinds of health care agencies specified above and when the audiologist is employed by a physician or by a physician-directed clinic. Unlike speech-language pathologists, audiologists may obtain Medicare provider numbers and be reimbursed directly for their services.

Medicaid also covers most diagnostic services provided directly by physicians. When offered to other patients within inpatient medical facilities, diagnostic speech-language pathology and audiology services are usually available to any Medicaid beneficiaries admitted to those facilities. Medicaid programs differ substantially among states with respect to their coverage of diagnostic services offered by speech-language pathologists and audiologists employed in other settings or engaged in private practice.

In instances where no private or governmental third-party coverage is available for diagnostic services for older people with limited financial resources, other options may be available. The Veterans Administration provides many such services for qualified beneficiaries. Services may also be available at community hospitals and at university-affiliated teaching hospitals that permit adjustment of fees according to patient means.

Thus far, we have emphasized support for multidisciplinary diagnostic services provided within single institutions. Often those services are offered by professionals practicing in different settings. Although single-institution services offer some advantages, high-quality services can also be achieved by coordinating the efforts of independent practitioners or separate agencies. Needed medical diagnostic services are covered when supplied by physicians in private practice, but as noted above, there are stringent limitations on third-party payment to speech-language pathologists and audiologists in private practice. Many freestanding community speech and hearing centers and incorporated groups of speech-language pathologists in private practice have qualified as rehabilitation agencies according to Medicare (and, often, Medicaid) regulations, even though they are primarily devoted to the delivery of speech-language pathology services. Most community speech and hearing centers, whether or not they have qualified as rehabilitation agencies, receive programmatic support beyond income from fees; consequently, they may provide free or low-cost diagnostic services for needy older persons with inadequate third-party coverage.

Prostheses

No other aspect of the delivery of services to older people with communication disorders presents as many financial problems as the procurement of prosthetic appliances. Most health insurance plans, both private and governmental, specifically exclude from coverage hearing aids and all services related to their selection, fitting, and maintenance. Most also exclude all augmentative communication devices. Among communication prosthesis, only electrolarynxes for laryngectomees are usually covered.

Hearing aids and attendant services can be offered by individual states as an optional benefit under Medicaid. In those states, Medicare beneficiaries who are also covered by Medicaid can sometimes obtain hearing aids. A 1980 survey, reported in ASHA's Health Insurance Manual (1984), showed that 28 states provided reimbursement for hearing aids for older beneficiaries through their Medicaid program. Private supplemental health insurance plans rarely cover hearing aids, but usually, only in instances where the supplemental insurance derives from employee health plans offering hearing aid benefits for both employees and retirees. Requests for coverage of other communication prostheses by Medicaid or by private supplemental plans are usually dealt with on a case-by-case basis.

The Veterans Administration has offered hearing aids and other prostheses to qualified veterans for many years (Newby, 1979). The VA hearing aid program has, in fact, often been identified as a model delivery system that should be emulated by other agencies serving people with hearing problems.

It is usually relatively easy to find private benefactors to assist in the purchase of prostheses for needy children. Unfortunately, it is much more difficult to find such assistance for older people. Many large medical centers and community agencies have prosthetic funds, so-designated by contributors. Seldom are these funds very affluent, however, and they must be used sparingly. Occasionally, assistance for individual clients is available from service clubs and fraternal organizations, but again, that assistance is much more likely to be available for children.

A steadily growing number of speech and hearing centers are directly dispensing prostheses, but usually only hearing aids. When all costs are considered for the sale of the instrument and the attendant professional services, the total price is probably essentially similar to the price charged for hearing aids by commercial dispensers. On the other hand, unbundling the cost of the instrument from fees for professional services may benefit needy senior citizens. Few agencies are able to dispense aids at less than manufacturer's prices. Yet, they may be able to adjust or even waive fees for attendant services by drawing on their program subsidies. Those services which constitute aural rehabilitation may even be covered by third-party payers.

When resources for purchasing hearing aids are unavailable, some communities provide hearing aid loan banks, usually through their speech and hearing centers. These banks stock reconditioned used aids or new aids that represent obsolete models, which are donated by individuals, families, commercial dispensers, and manufacturers. The best available hearing aid is loaned to a needy individual on either a short-term or permanent basis. Thus far, few, if any, similar loan banks are available for older people who need other communication prostheses.

Therapeutic and Rehabilitation Services

Many of the same restrictions cited for diagnostic services also apply to health insurance coverage of therapeutic and rehabilitation services provided by speech-language pathologists and audiologists (i.e., medical necessity as certified and recertified by physicians, relatedness to the consequences of illness or injury, and delivery of services within a covered setting by a qualified provider). However, some additional restrictions may be imposed.

Part A Medicare provides for reimbursement to hospitals, extended care facilities, and some health agencies for speech and language treatment services

310

(provided either by a member of the staff or by an independent contractor).
Aural rehabilitation services provided by audiologists may also be covered,
essentially as a speech therapy benefit. Part B Medicare covers speech and
language treatment services on an outpatient basis in a hospital outpatient
clinic, a medial clinic, rehabilitation agency, physician's office, or
sometimes through a home health agency. Once again, unless an independent
practitioner is able to qualify as a rehabilitation agency, he or she may not
be reimbursed directly for speech therapy or aural rehabilitation.

The Medicare law once specified that the plan for speech and language
treatment services must be written by a physician. In 1980, the law was
amended to specify that a treatment plan may be established by a physician or
"by the speech-language pathologist providing such services." Nevertheless,
the need for speech-language therapy must be certified initially by a
physician, and that need recertified by a physician at regular intervals
(usually every 30 days). The coverage of aural rehabilitation services by
audiologists is subject to essentially the same restrictions.

As observed with other services, states differ in their Medicaid coverage
of speech, language, and hearing services. With reference to mandatory
services, states usually adopt Medicare rules for coverage of speech, language,
and hearing services. If available to other patients in the same setting,
hospitals and skilled nursing facilities must usually provide speech, language,
and hearing therapy to Medicaid beneficiaries when "medically necessary."
Usually Medicaid does not pay separately for such services in those settings,
but includes them in the computation of overall reimbursement rates.

Outpatient speech, language, and hearing services are mandated under
Medicaid only insofar as they qualify as physician services. Physician
services are defined in federal law as those provided directly by physicians or
by other personnel working under a physician's personal supervision. States
differ in definitions of personal supervision, but many specify that the
nonphysician provider must be employed by one or more physicians and practice
in the same office or clinic.

Optional coverage of speech, language, and hearing services among state
Medicaid programs ranges from none to reasonably generous coverage (although
fewer and fewer state Medicaid programs are at the generous end of the
continuum). Commonly, the agencies that administer Medicaid reimbursement not
only require physician certification and recertification, but also prior

authorization for extended therapy programs. (Usually such authorizations cover a limited number of visits, with renewal of authorization required for additional visits.) Furthermore, in most instances providers are reimbursed for outpatient speech, language and hearing services to Medicaid beneficiaries at rates that are significantly lower than prevailing fees for the same services.

Some speech, language, and hearing services for older people may be covered by private insurance, either in lieu of or as a supplement to other medical coverage. However, such coverage will rarely, if ever, apply in instances where payment was disallowed by Medicare because the services failed to meet stipulated requirements.

Many of the earlier cited government-sponsored programs (the Veterans Administration, health departments, etc.) also support speech, language and hearing services for older people. Freestanding community speech and hearing centers provide these services, either within their centers or through satellite programs, and as do university speech and hearing clinics. Both community and university centers are usually able to offer services at reduced fees for needy older persons.

In some communities, adult education programs and community colleges offer what are essentially therapeutic programs. Most frequently offered are group instruction in alaryngeal speech, aural rehabilitation classes, and sign language instruction for people with recently acquired profound hearing impairments and for their families. In rare instances, these educational agencies may also offer individual clinical services.

As enumerated, it would seem that there are ample sources of support for speech and hearing therapy for older people. Clearly, the situation has improved substantially during the past 2 decades. Some very thorny problems remain, nonetheless. The stipulation in most third-party payment programs of physician certification and recertification can be a major obstacle. Two-thirds of the respondents to a recent omnibus survey of ASHA members identified this factor as a principal deterrent to the delivery of needed services (Fein, 1984). All too many physicians view survival from disease as the only goal of health care and do not consider the restoration or maintenance of social function to be appropriately covered by health insurance. Therefore, speech-language pathologists and audiologists must turn to other sources for support needed therapy and rehabilitation. When other sources of support cannot be found, older people are often excluded from the receipt of essential services.

Economic factors may also seriously restrict the availability of assistance to particular groups of older people. Services are unavailable to many residents of rural areas. They may also be difficult to obtain in central cities, particularly in areas primarily populated by members of minority groups. In virtually all areas, there are few services available for older people who do not speak English. We must, therefore, continue efforts to expand resources of support for all therapeutic and rehabilitation services for older people with communication disorders. But particular attention must be devoted to the availability of services to groups often identified as "hard to serve."

Maintenance of Proficiencies

There are two general circumstances under which services may be needed to assist older people to maintain optimal communication:

1. When they have achieved maximum benefits from rehabilitation services, it is important to ensure the maintenance of those benefits. Commonly, older people living in institutional settings, and even those who reside in their own home, withdraw from social contacts, particularly when they have limited proficiency in communication. Under these circumstances, whatever has been achieved through rehabilitation may be lost.

2. Older people with such degenerative conditions as Parkinson's disease may suffer unnecessary deterioration of their communication. With assistance, serviceable communication can often be maintained for a much longer time.

In most instances, maintenance programs are not covered by health insurance, because covered services are presumably "restorative." The following excerpt from a supplement to the Medicare Home Health Agency Manual,

313

dated October 1981 and identified as Transmittal Number 131, sets down typical restrictions:

> After the initial evaluation of the extent of the disorder or illness, if the restoration potential is judged insignificant or, after a reasonable period of trial, the patient's response to treatment is judged insignificant or at a plateau, an appropriate functional maintenance program may be established. The specialized knowledge and judgment of a qualified speech pathologist may be required if the treatment aim of the physician is to be achieved; (e.g., a multiple sclerosis patient may require the services of a speech pathologist to establish function). In such a as situation, the initial evaluation of the patient's needs, the designing by the qualified speech pathologist of a maintenance program which is appropriate to the capacity and tolerance of the patient and the treatment objectives of the physician, the instruction of the patient and supportive personnel (e.g., aides or nursing personnel, or family members where speech pathology is being furnished on an outpatient basis) in carrying out the program, and such infrequent reevaluations as may be required, would constitute covered speech therapy. After the maintenance program has been established and instructions have been given for carrying out the program, the services of the speech pathologist would no longer be covered, as they would no longer be considered reasonable and necessary for the treatment of the patient's condition and would be excluded from coverage.

Obviously, then, we must look outside the health care financing system to support most maintenance services. Among providers of clinical services, community speech and hearing centers have been the most likely sources of these services. As these centers have become increasingly dependent upon third-party reimbursement, however, many have discontinued their maintenance programs.

Despite the usual disallowance from third-party coverage, some inpatient long-term care facilities do offer maintenance programs. Day health care programs, designed to serve older adults who require long-term special care, but who can be maintained in their own homes at night and on weekends, represent an optimal setting for maintenance services.

Self-help groups for people with communication disorders have never been as prevalent as in other areas of disability. Nevertheless, such groups may offer excellent resources for maintenance services. Many communities offer self-help groups for the hearing-impaired, although they may primarily accommodate prelingually deaf adults. The American Hearing Society (a predecessor to the organization that eventually became the National Association of Hearing and Speech Action) had a network of chapters throughout the country that were usually supported from United Fund campaigns. (Many were progenitors of today's community speech and hearing centers.) These local chapters often sponsored self-help groups for the adventitiously hearing-impaired elderly. Some of these groups have survived within the context of community speech and hearing centers or other agencies. Lost Chord clubs, often affiliated with the International Association of Laryngectomees and sometimes abetted by chapters of the American Cancer Society, provide maintenance services for people using alaryngeal speech. Some communities have organized self-help groups for victims of stroke, Parkinson's disease, and other neurologic impairments. Specialized self-help groups and other maintenance services are becoming increasingly available to senior citizens.

Adult education and community college programs could represent an ideal setting for maintenance services. Usually these programs specify minimum enrollment requirements if a given "class" is to be offered; however, enrollment minimums may be greatly reduced when disabled people are served. Such requirements may interfere with offering therapeutic services in this setting, but they need not constitute a deterrent for maintenance services that may best be offered in group situations.

Obviously, maintenance services represent another neglected field of service to older people. Unfortunately, our profession must assume some responsibility for that neglect. It is also an area where students, paraprofessionals, and volunteers such as retired professionals can make substantial contributions. Professionals can offer whatever initial training and orientation is needed to prepare these paraprofessionals and volunteers, outline the activities to be pursued, and provide ongoing supervision so that these support personnel can carry out the actual maintenance programs. Such programs can be conducted either in residential facilities or in community agencies.

Adapted Social and Recreational Activities

Two general approaches may be taken to providing social and recreational activities for older people with communication disorders (a) special programs may be developed that are uniquely designed to serve these people; and (b) programs offered to the entire community may be equipped and adapted to enable participation by disabled people. Whenever possible, the second option is distinctly preferable. "Mainstreaming" may be as important in planning services for older adults with acquired disabilities as it is for handicapped children.

The special recreation programs designed for older people with communication disorders may be indistinguishable from the maintenance programs we have described. Most self-help groups offer both maintenance therapy and social opportunities. Occasional volunteer-based programs for stroke victims and victims of other neurologic diseases may offer a variety of recreational opportunities.

A few communities have organized special senior center programs for the elderly with hearing impairments. These special programs may be ideal for people whose severe hearing losses or associated deficits render them incapable of participating in regular senior center programs. Some accommodate people who rely on sign language for communication. Communities with special recreation centers for the handicapped that function either as private agencies or as divisions of their city recreation departments may offer special programs for the elderly within those centers.

Adapting Service Environments

The last decade has seen growing efforts to make the facilities and activities that are available to able-bodied citizens equally accessible to disabled citizens. This effort was codified in 1977 in Section 504 of the Rehabilitation Act of 1973 entitled "Nondiscrimination on the Basis of Handicap." The law specified that "no otherwise qualified handicapped individual in the United States shall, solely by reason of his handicap, be excluded from participation in, be denied the benefits of, or be subjected to discrimination under any program receiving federal financial assistance."

316

Throughout the efforts to facilitate Section 504, less attention has been paid to factors that limit accessibility for people with communication disorders than to the problems of people with restricted mobility. This situation may be attributable to a dearth of advocacy for people with communication disorders rather than to any general reluctance by facilities planners to consider the special needs of the communicatively handicapped.

The accessibility of facilities for older people with communication disorders usually involves two major modifications (a) the availability of high-quality amplification equipment which may either work in conjunction with or be entirely separate from the person's hearing aid, and (b) appropriate acoustical treatment to reduce reverberation and ambient noise levels. Sometimes these adaptations are covered by governmental funding for the construction and remodeling of public facilities. More often, however, support must come from the private sector. Many churches, theaters, and recital and concert halls have installed special equipment to serve the hearing-impaired. Some senior centers, fraternal lodge halls, and recreation facilities in retirement communities and other senior housing facilities also provide such equipment. These installations may be financed privately by the owners of the facilities; more often, service clubs, foundations, and private benefactors contribute the funding.

Making social and recreational resources in the community available to the elderly with communication disorders often involves more than adaptation of physical facilities. Staff members of these agencies must receive sufficient orientation to enable them to accommodate these people within the programs they conduct. Clearly, speech-language pathologists and audiologists must play a major role in these orientation programs. If they are to participate, however, it is usually necessary to find financial support to cover the costs of providing those professional services.

Despite the importance of ensuring the continuing participation of the disabled in the social life of their communities, many professionals have been relatively unconcerned about this important area of service. Regrettably, speech-language pathologists and audiologists often share this unconcern with respect to older people with speech, language, and hearing disorders.

Adapting Living Environments

Environmental adaptations may be necessary if older people with communication disorders are to live safely and happily, and as independently as possible, in their own homes, in special senior housing, or in board and care or skilled nursing facilities. As in the instance of public facilities, these adaptations usually involve special equipment or architectural modifications to reduce interferences to optimal communication.

Current regulations of the Department of Housing and Urban Development (HUD) covering the provision of funds for the construction and remodeling of large housing projects require that at least 5% of units be accessible to handicapped people. Once again, accessibility is usually interpreted to mean the absence of architectural barriers to access by people with impaired mobility or vision. Except for providing alarm systems that offer visual as well as auditory signals, few devices are installed to assist people with communication disorders. Although no HUD funds are specifically earmarked for adaptations for the communicatively handicapped, these adaptations would clearly be an appropriate application of those funds.

Most state licensure regulations for board and care and skilled nursing facilities require visual alarm systems when hearing-impaired persons live within those facilities. Although appropriate acoustic treatment of dining rooms, day rooms, and recreation areas may be recommended, it is seldom if ever required. Financial support for any of these adaptations must be provided by the individual or organization operating and facility.

A whole array of adaptive devices are now available to assist the hearing-impaired in their activities of daily living: special alarm clocks, visual-supplemented doorbell systems, amplifiers for radios and television sets, etc. These must be purchased by the people who use them or by their families. Occasionally the owners of board and care and skilled nursing facilities purchase such devices, often to assist their staff as much as to accommodate residents.

Partially as a result of the Telecommunications for the Disabled Act of 1982, there is now widespread interest in the availability of adapted telephone equipment for people with speech and hearing problems. That Act particularly emphasized the availability of hearing aid-compatible public telephones (especially telephones that are likely to be used in emergencies) and the availability of TTY equipment. In general, the various providers of telephones for residential use have tried to make adapted equipment available for those who need it. There are substantial differences among local communities with respect to the charges levied against consumers for such equipment, but in virtually all instances those charges represent less than the actual cost of supplying the equipment. Even those charges, however, may be a burden for people on limited incomes.

Through currently and soon-to-be available electronic technology, it is inevitable that other devices can be developed to contribute to the independent living of older people with speech, language, and hearing disorders. Two economic realities exist, however. First, the cost for developing such equipment must primarily be borne by commercial manufacturers. Because few of these devices will enjoy widespread sales, few manufactures can afford to invest in their research and development. Second, it is unlikely that any private or public third-party payer will assist in the purchase of such devices; consequently, they will be available only to the people who can afford them.

Family Counseling

As has already been observed, some of the most needed services for the elderly are those services for which the least economic support is available. This situation is readily apparent with respect to family counseling. Unquestionably, one of the most important determiners of success or failure in the rehabilitation of older people with speech, language, and hearing disorders is the understanding and assistance they receive from their spouses, their children, their caregivers, and the other close associates in their daily lives. Yet there are few resources available to cover the costs of these counseling services.

Third-party payment, based in the traditions of the most conventional approaches to medical care, only supports treatment to patients. Although limited segments of treatment visits may be purloined for family conferences, sessions spent primarily with families are virtually always excluded from coverage. Accreditation and licensure standards for health care institutions commonly require the availability of social workers, presumably to offer family counseling, among other services, but the cost for social work programs is usually included among the overhead expenses of these institutions, although fees may be charged to patients who can cover them. This establishes another perspective for third-party payers (i.e., necessary counseling is covered through the indirect expenses included in all fees and should not be reimbursed separately). Realistically, then, most speech-language pathology and audiology programs must do just that--include typical counseling services in computing their overhead expenses and add those costs to other indirect expenses in developing fee schedules. Unfortunately, however, even this measure may not solve the problem, because reimbursement levels often do not equal whatever fee schedules are developed. Even when services to clients are covered by third-party payers, agencies must usually subsidize counseling services from other sources.

Sometimes, in conjunction with the self-help programs described earlier, communities offer group programs for families of people with communication disorders. Because these programs not only offer counseling by professionals but also peer counseling by people confronting similar problems, they can be extremely valuable. Such programs are usually supported by community agencies, voluntary health associations, or, occasionally, by adult education programs.

Most communities offer counseling programs that are designed to serve broad segments of the population. These include family services agencies and mental health programs as well as religious-group-affiliated programs like Jewish and Catholic family services. Although the families or significant others of older people with communication disorders may be eligible for services from these agencies, their staff members are often unaware of the special problems that may attend these disorders and are consequently unable to provide effective counseling.

A growing number of writers in the speech-language pathology and audiology literature are identifying the limitations of medical-treatment-based models for the delivery of speech, language, and hearing services. If, in the final analysis, social competence is the ultimate goal of our efforts, it is difficult to fit that goal within conventional treatment-oriented frameworks. There may, consequently, be an ever-widening gulf between our professional practices and the contexts in which we engage in those practices. The eventual economic implications may be formidable. No better example can be found than that of providing needed counseling services to the families and significant others in the lives of older people with speech, language, and hearing disorders.

Summary

Health and human services of the elderly are supported by funding from both the public and private sector. These funds may be dispersed as third-party payment for individual services or as broader programmatic support. Despite the subsidies available to assist older people in obtaining the care they need, they must often maintain substantial personal liability for the costs of that care as well. As costs escalate and the elderly population grows, that personal liability will almost certainly increase.

Many diagnostic and therapeutic services for older people with speech, language, and hearing problems are covered by governmental and private third-party payment. However, coverage may be limited by typical requirements geared to the treatment of diseases rather than to the restoration and maintenance of social competence. It is particularly difficult to find support for the purchase of communication prostheses.

Older people with communication disorders also require many services that are not typically provided within the health care system, including adapted social and recreation activities, modifications in living environments to ensure safety and independence, and family counseling. Most economic support for these services must come from recipients or from the private sector. Every professional who is concerned about older people with speech, language, and hearing disorders must devote continuing effort to finding new sources of financial support and to developing innovative and economical approaches to the delivery of essential services.

Self-Study Questions

1. What are the essential differences between Part A and Part B Medicare? How do these differences apply to speech-language pathology and audiology services?

2. What factors may account for the substantial personal liability that Medicare beneficiaries may incur, even when the services they have received are presumably covered by Medicare?

3. Under what circumstances may older people be covered by Medicaid? When they are covered by Medicaid, what does this mean in terms of speech-language pathology and audiology services?

4. Why do many Medicare beneficiaries also carry private health insurance? How does that insurance apply to speech-pathology and audiology services?

5. What are the major sources of programmatic support for speech-language pathology and audiology services for older adults?

6. What are the major economic barriers to providing hearing aids and other communication aids for older people.

7. Why is it difficult to support maintenance programs for older people with irreversible communication disorders?

8. What are the potential sources of economic support for making residential and recreational facilities accessible to older people with communication disorders?

REFERENCES

American Speech-Language-Hearing Association. (1984). Health insurance manual. Rockville, MD: American Speech-Language-Hearing Association.

Fein, D. J. (1984). Findings from the 1983 ASHA omnibus survey. Asha, 26, 45-48.

Newby, H. A. (1979). Veterans administration. In L. J. Bradford & W. G. Hardy (Eds.), Hearing and hearing impairment. New York: Grune & Stratton.

Suggested Readings

American Speech-Language-Hearing Association Task Force on Private Health Insurance. (1980). A report on third-party reimbursement of speech-language pathology and audiology services. Rockville, MD: American Speech-Language-Hearing Association.

Brantman, M. (1973). The status and outlook for commercial health insurance coverage of speech and hearing services. Asha, 15, 183-187.

Flower, R. M. (1984). Delivery of speech-language pathology and audiology services. Baltimore, MD: Williams & Wilkins.

Prussin, J. A. & Wood, M. C. (1975). Private third-party reimbursement. Topics in health care financing, 2, 1-89.

Professional/Interdisciplinary
Considerations for Implementing Service Delivery Models

Jon K. Ashby

Abilene Christian University, Abilene, Texas

Inservice Education to Practitioners

An interesting perspective on the history of continuing education is presented by Schor (1981) in the context of nursing education. She suggests that in-service education evolved from a more general, voluntary, and informal history rather than from an ethical, strongly categorical, or accountability based system which appears to be developing now. Over the last 40 years the concept of staff education, staff development, in-service education, and continuing education has crystallized. It is based on the notion that professionals, on the job in which they are engaged as fulltime workers, need continuing education and training experience. This concept has become an integral part of most professional health care institutions and has been written into most licensure and certification standards. Questions continue to be raised about the feasibility of mandatory continuing education programs as to whether one can be legislated, enforced, or have adequate quality controls.

At a recent National Conference on Communication Disorders and Aging, one of the participants, a well-known neurologist, reflected on several of the presentations he had just heard. He appeared at once surprised and impressed that communication problems may be the basis for many of the most debilitating problems among aging patients. He further stated that many of the problems experienced by medical practitioners in diagnosis, treatment, and understanding of the quality of life in elderly persons were largely due to problems and breakdowns in communication. He seemed amazed that he had not been aware of this before.

Those in the audience were impressed with his intellectual honesty and became even more cognizant of the need for sharing with medical and other health care professionals the nature and character of communication disorders in aging.

At many meetings of caregivers and nonprofessional interest groups, concerns about the training of health service providers were discussed. Not infrequently the training of the physician is criticized for being lacking in coursework, specifically concerning gerontology. It is generally suggested that few medical schools offer required courses in the unique management of elderly patients. Most medical and dental schools have some curricular adjustment to a life cycle continuum but areas other than geriatrics are usually emphasized. This concern is well-known in the medical community since it has been voiced all the way to Washington by a variety of advocacy groups for the elderly.

Some unacceptable, inaccurate stereotypes held by physicians about their geriatric clients are assumed to lead to more perfunctory, second-rate medical treatment (Coccaro, Berube, Thornton, & Myerson, 1983). The criticism of medical training and the stereotypic (possibly less than proper) management of elderly patients is not without empirical support (Holtzman, Beck, & Ettinger, 1981).

Unfortunately, our own profession may have a similar character. At present the study of normal language development is required along with language disorders in children. The specification of coursework on the aging process is not delineated in the required education standard. It might well be that the communication disorders professional may be inadequately prepared to deal with persons with unique characteristics attributable to aging (Landy, 1983).

Conferences and seminars on aging and communication disorders are growing in popularity. It is evident that real interest is also being reflected also in the selection of in-service and continuing education programs.

There appears to be a good deal of literature on in-service training; however, it is not specific to the area of communication disorders. The bulk of published information focuses on teacher in-service or those programs involving nurses training. The basic elements are ostensibly the same regardless of the groups involved and therefore the considerations suggested would apply to our profession (Leutenegger, 1975).

There appears to be some confusion as to what constitutes an in-service program. One name or generic term has not been agreed upon. In-service training has been labeled professional growth, continuing education, management development training workshops, etc. This could be one reason why in-service programs are often lacking and are also too few in number (i.e., we are not exactly sure what constitutes in-service training or exactly what character it should take).

A number of resources are available for developing action plans and follow-up for professional in-service programs (Finley, 1981; Harris, 1980). These nuts and bolts type materials may provide the designer or developer of in-service programs access to quite a diversity of information. The U.S. Office of Education also provides a variety of materials and resources through federally-funded information and dissemination networks. These include the Education Research Information Center (ERIC), the National Diffusion Network, and the State Capacity Building Program (Finley, 1981). These general works on in-service education are quite helpful in the formation of functional programs that meet high instructional expectations.

A number of resources in in-service training are available specifically related to the area of aging that can be adapted to emphasize communication disorders. Slover and Greco (1975) authored a pamphlet intended to provide direction in planning workshops and in-service programs on aging. Another manual was developed to sensitize personnel in public welfare agencies by providing knowledge of the aging process, understanding of the needs of the elderly and encourage interest in aging services (Spear, 1979). Ernst and Shore (1975) wrote an excellent manual geared to training persons concerned with the provision of nursing home care. This latter publication provides a wide variety of experience-oriented instruction that can be adapted quite easily to stress communication disorders. Asha (1977) published an in-service training module, "Breaking the Silence Barrier, an In-service Program for Nursing Home Staff Working with Communicatively Handicapped Geriatric Patients." This manual includes suggested visual aids, glossary, and helpful suggestions for experimental activities. Those activities may be enhanced by further exploring environmental barriers through simulating age-related losses (Hickey, 1975; Hubbard & Santos, 1981; Pastalan, Mantz, & Merrill, 1973). Asha (1980) also published "Resource Materials for Communication Problems of Older Persons". These materials are well-organized and presented in a format to facilitate planning and allocation of materials, aids, and information sources. Shadden, Raiford, and Shadden (1983) produced an excellent in-service manual with a wide variety of guides and resource materials for presenters. This workshop text on "Coping with Communication Disorders in Aging" integrates training material with training experience. The authors suggest that the program has been targeted for three specific presentation formats.

1. precrisis intervention workshops for older persons;
2. an in-service training program for health professionals;
3. supplemental classroom materials for professional coursework in gerontology.

Developing In-service Programs

The focus of much of the literature has been on the development of in-service programs (Grimes, 1975; Kirkpatrick, 1979; Ray, 1977). The basic elements of program development relate most specifically to identifying and assessing the needs of the individuals to be trained. This may be accomplished by a variety of sampling techniques including the often overlooked questionnaire. From the sampled information, the in-service developer is able to identify areas of strengths and weaknesses for the prospective trainees, perceived priorities of the prospective trainees, and detailed suggestions for goals and content. This initial planning stage may be the most important and significant in goal-setting and achievement because in-service programs in the past have too often been based on what the trainer felt was important and not based on the real needs of trainees (Ray, 1977).

Meeting needs of the identified group of potential trainees should be considered in the goals. These should not necessarily be generated from outside the group. Otherwise the presenter will set up a program, formulate his or her own goals, and recruit trainees to participate. Many will come expecting outcomes not addressed, and others needing the experience may be missed. Some in-service programs are required and become routine or perfunctory, so that it is often difficult to gain and maintain attention. If the goals are to bring about change, real needs of trainees must be an integral part of all aspects of the program.

A second element of developing an in-service program might be to assess the needs of the group to be studied (in this case the elderly). This could be done by evaluating services already in existence for this population and also providing questionnaires for service recipients. Specific goals and objectives may be developed from direct observation of the groups identified (Seldin, 1979).

The elderly are often critical of service providers because of a perceived lack of knowledge about their particular plight. They stress our need for better training of practitioners to deal with the uniqueness of their health, communication, and social patterns. Advocacy groups also help to inform professional groups about who is falling between the crack, or where they are not perceiving the significance of our efforts in a larger picture.

Based on the needs assessments, a sufficient time frame should be developed. Too many programs in the past have attempted to cover every aspect of the topic in a very short time instead of having specific goals and objectives which could be more easily discussed in the time limits allotted.

Because participation in the program is necessary for real behavioral change, this aspect should be factored in as an indispensible element in successfully reaching our goals. A balance including information and participation is obviously important but experience should not be overlooked or reduced in favor of more academic pedagogy. Maximizing behavioral change in an in-service program is not a product of the amount of information provided in the time constraints; learners must also be participants (Moore & Campbell, 1978).

Selecting appropriate methodology for in-service programs is another major area of concern. The Ohio Department of Education (1978) identified eight different formats--lecture, interview, observation, brainstorm, demonstration, buzz sessions, group discussions, and gaming. When subjected to effectiveness analysis the lecture, demonstration and observation formats (where trainees are passive learners) were low in achieving behavior change, whereas the other formats are high in both behavior and attitude change. Although more popular the traditional pedagogical formats but may be less efficient in producing desired goals. A common statement following a lecture format by 10 experts is that "she really knows what she is talking about, but I still don't understand." This will not bring on the behavior change appropriate to alter attitudes toward, or the treatment of, the elderly. It is comforting to know others are more knowledgeable about some matters but this will only indirectly effect the performance of trainees.

Cross and Westbrook (1979), state that an appropriate relationship between colleges and in-service programs is lacking in all fields. He identifies four problems which exist between these organizations.

1. Problems with college credit;
2. the move to grant certificates for noncollege local programs;
3. the power of certain groups within the organization to control the in-service education format content, process, and access; and
4. lack of college support and cooperation in the field.

The politics involved in developing in in-service program also appear to be an important element in the developmental stages. The literature suggest this aspect of program formulation is quite important. Policies and public relations must be established at a variety of professional, interprofessional, and intraprofessional levels in any community.

Community Presentations for Public Education

Heisel, Darkenwald, and Anderson (1981) studied patterns of participation in organized educational programs among the elderly. They found that elderly people do not exhibit a high level of participation in educational activities when compared with younger adult age groups. This should not have been unsuspected because those who are elderly now did not, as a group, have the educational opportunities of younger persons. Many elderly people have and will fight for educational opportunities for all age groups, but having established the need do not choose to participate themselves. It seems they are locked into a pattern of developing those opportunities for others, and not for themselves. Therefore, they might not be expected to participate in learning procedures outside their range of experience. This lack of participation is particularly acute among the very old, women, and blacks. Elder-hostel programs have been extremely successful but cater almost exclusively to those who have a history of participation in learning activities, patticularly the well-educated and relatively affluent (Ward, 1984). New ideas and programs are being developed in this extraordinary field of older adult education.

Price and Grigsby (1981) report that all students in life-long learning courses were concerned about their future development, regardless of their

328

chronological age. Those who have enrolled in preretirement educational programs were better able to handle the life changes of aging, particularly the acute ones following retirement. The positive results seem to have followed the exploring of options because subjects were made aware of many existing and potential alternatives. It is fortunate that so many positive training effects can be realized from such programs, but unfortunate that communication disorders professionals and content are usually ignored or are presented in a cursory manner.

Silverstein (1984) found that knowledge of available services varied widely in her sample of urban elderly. Only a minority were able to demonstrate a high level of social awareness. She found that informal sources and media were more likely to inform the elderly of available services than formal ones. The elderly used a number of primary and secondary sources to obtain knowledge of services. The formal sources were more likely to bring about a use of services, but poorest in providing information about service availability. Strategies suggested to improve the informal network included holding workshops for the middle-aged children of elderly persons, instituting gerontology units into elementary and high-school curricula, in-service training for health care providers, and public information seminars. These are areas in which communication disorders specialists can be active in providing information and advocacy.

One of the criticisms of our profession is that we have been vocal only on issues and programs that could be considered self-serving. Berry (1984) recently stated that "we cannot live as just a speech teacher; we have to live first of all as world citizens." She encouraged community volunteer efforts that will increase the respect and support of the profession. Her statements were related to public school speech-language pathologists but were appropriate in this context as well. We must become active in programs and issues that affect the lifestyle, life quality, and health of all elderly before we can credibly comment on only one of its aspects.

In an effort to inform the public of available services, one should emphasize (a) advertising media for public awareness; (b) informal networks which surround the person in everyday life; and (c) formal networks of professional persons and organizations that serve the elderly (White House Conference on Aging, 1981). Making quality services available must be coupled with an active public information and education thrust. Not emphasizing this dimension will leave large portions of the communicatively handicapped unserved.

We all know that an impairment in the ability to communicate can become one of the greatest burdens for aging persons. We are also fully aware that reduction of visual and auditory acuity can impair the aging individual's reception of written or spoken language and severely strain social interaction when viewed in a communicative context. This often results in patterns of confusion, anxiety, depression, withdrawal, and isolation (Leutenegger, 1975). Even in cases of limited impairment, as in a mild hearing loss, the fatigue which results from constantly straining to hear and understand can lead to apathy and withdrawal from group interaction. Yet this obviously important information has not been adequately communicated to the general public.

In addition, family, friends, and others who regularly interact with the aging individual who has communication disorder may further add to the burden of the impairment by their lack of sensitivity and understanding. Family members or professionals interacting with the elderly person who has a hearing loss often repeat the worn-out statement, "he hears what he wants to hear!" Actions such as this indicate a lack of understanding of the changing interaction between communicative impairment and environment. In another instance, a person's seeming belligerence or inattention may be ascribed to a nasty disposition or senility rather than being recognized as part of the communication disorder complex (Leutenegger, 1975). With the markedly negative effects that communication disorders can have on social interaction, the public would certainly benefit from education about the nature of these impairments as they affect the aging.

Those in the aging population need to be encouraged to maintain good health and to seek professional assistance and guidance with the onset of any communication disorder. Some may be reluctant to do so, because of the cost, lack of confidence in professional treatment, or the seriousness of the condition. Others may be unaware of an impairment due to lack of information or possibly because of its gradual onset. Still others may be confused about what types of impairments can be helped by medical or rehabilitative effort, or may not be informed about the availability of resources in their community. Many elderly people have been raised with a tough-it-out, self-sufficient attitude. They may not view the idea of receiving treatment as a strength but a sign of weakness. Some are not confident of the rehabilitation community and confuse our efforts with others. "We in the health professions need to be concerned about maintaining the maximal use of sensory and physical capabilities that decrease with age, or the goal of extended life loses meaningfulness" (Clark & Mills, 1979). This will require not only providing the service, but informing the public about the availability and need for services (Singer & Brownell, 1984).

Various approaches have been used to educate the public regarding various health and rehabilitation issues. Radio and television have been used with some success to present spot announcements such as commercials and short health education programs. Foulk and Young (1982) offer some practical and specific guidelines for implementing health education broadcasts primarily for public information. Bartman, Mummery, Poppe, Robbins, & Robertson-Palmer (1982) describe what could be accomplished in a store-front health information center in a suburban mall. Visitors were encouraged to browse through the literature and exhibits, to ask questions, and take advantage of information and referral resources offered there. Health fairs have enjoyed success in drawing large crowds for a variety of health screening tests and health education (Faris, 1979; Mason & Calvacca, 1982). Gerardi (1982) described a novel concept called an Outreach and Health College, consisting of mini-courses which lasted from 5 to 8 weeks and which dealt with pertinent health issues. Access to the courses was provided to the public through local senior centers. Under the supervision of a qualified health educator, students from affiliated universities assisted with instruction.

A variety of group instructional programs are available to reduce negative stereotypes about the elderly and to facilitate improved communication between the generations (Freimuth & Jamieson, 1979). Conter and Schneiderman (1982) also discuss the need to develop and market new educational programs for and about the older adult. Robichaud and Brown (1979) describe a unique experience by which people learn what it's like to fill the shoes of the impaired elderly. The "As Parents Grow Older" program is an educational and group therapy program for the adult children of aging parents, which provides information and sensitivity toward problems of their elderly parent as well as the participants own aging.

Without public education the many changes brought on by aging will be seen only as physical and mental deterioration and unfortunately may be misunderstood. This insensitivity and lack of understanding can only increase the stressfuless and deterioration of relationships between the communicatively impaired elderly and the family, or rehabilitation professionals involved. Health education can help both the elderly and others in the community move toward a better quality of life along with the length of years.

It has long been a tenant of the hearing aid industry that hearing aids must be sold. The product must be marketed to the public in such a way as to gain the attention of the targeted group, and be received in such a manner that learning can take place. Private practitioners in communication disorders are now marketing services. Public education may inform, but it must also attempt to do a quality job of recruiting clients for needed services (Singer & Brownell, 1984).

Use of Volunteers as Adjuncts to Service Delivery

Voluntarism has a rich history in American history. Much of the uniqueness of our way of life has been fostered by the freedom of all individuals to choose activities at one's own discretion. Our high level of prosperity and advanced civilization has produced more available time for those who desire such activities. Voluntarism continues to be changing and adaptable to meet the needs of society. This proud heritage will lead to regeneration and reinstitution of powerful leadership, advocacy, and opportunities for service for those who care enough to give of themselves. It is not possible to view the American way of life apart from the voluntary efforts and seemingly unlimited generosity of its people (Manser & Cass, 1976).

The role of the volunteer is a dynamic one, changing with the imperatives of society (Marts, 1966). During the past decade numerous criticisms have been directed toward the whole concept of voluntarism (Manser & Cass, 1976). Much of the negative comment appears to be directed at the decline in the traditional volunteer groups and their functions, and the institutionalization of many formal volunteer agencies. The critics do not seem to be taking into account the changing character of the society or where the spontaneity of the volunteer movement is directed. The volunteers are working but in more nontraditional and more widely divergent roles (Bernard, 1984; Ward, 1984).

Acting as a volunteer in nearly any context may be perceived with both positive and negative reactions. It appears that there may be as many disadvantages for the volunteer as there are advantages for the senior citizens who receive the services, particularly when untrained or unsupervised persons are used.

Many successful service programs have originated from volunteer groups that have been rigorously trained, monitored, and supervised. Organizational techniques must be incorporated in order for volunteer work to be successful; they cannot be expected to function on their own. When volunteers are organized and well-trained, studies have shown that institutions tend to respect their services (Manser & Cass, 1976). Otherwise volunteers may be rejected or unappreciated by administrators and staff. Reasons for lack of acceptance are varied from a fear that volunteers will misinform the elderly about the professional services they receive, that they might second guess service providers, or a fear that inadequacies of the institution might be revealed to the public (Butler & Lewis, 1977). There is some support for this view as demonstrated in Detroit where community volunteers involved in a visitation program to nursing homes revealed that these groups were more effective in serving a watch-dog function than formal systems of government (Vincent, 1976). Many institutions are uneasy about such scrutiny.

It also appears that those who volunteer to assist the elderly are for the most part senior citizens themselves. This could be due in part to the assumption that no one understands a senior's difficulties better than other seniors (Kruger-Smith, 1973). It might also be suggested that retired persons have more time and opportunity for volunteer work. It appears that by providing service to the community and to other older persons, senior citizens may gain considerable self-satisfaction while at the same time serving community needs.

Aurthur (1970) suggests that "people who stay young despite their years do so because of an active interest that provides satisfaction through participation" (p. 26). Numerous local, state, and federally-funded volunteer programs perform unique, fulfilling, and needed community services. Federally-funded senior volunteer programs are varied and can be used to develop the skills of the volunteer or provide services. Not all of these programs are limited exclusively to elderly volunteers; some provide financial assistance or reimbursement for expenses but all encourage and strongly recruit the elderly.

1. Volunteer Clearinghouse - Many communities have such programs organized under a variety of sponsors such as a Junior League, United Way Agency or RSVP.

   Volunteer c/o
   National Center for Citizen Involvement
   1111 North 19th Street, Suite 500
   Arlington, VA 22209

2. American Association of Retired Persons (AARP) - The largest service and advocacy group with volunteer opportunities of many types. This is a primary community resource for volunteerism.

   Volunteer Bank c/o
   AARP
   1909 K Street N.W.
   Washington, DC

3. Area Agencies on Aging - Opportunities on a regional level coordinating government agencies. A wide variety of services are available and accessible through the AAA. The impact of these organizations has been greater than probably any other government-related service program in the solicitation, organization, and functional use of volunteers.

4. Senior Centers - Local senior centers usually provide multipurpose services within and beyond the confines of the facility. These centers have had a profound impact on many aspects of the community life and services for the elderly.

5. Religious Groups and Institutions - Elderly programs initiated and administered by religious groups are among the most popular and successful in the private sector.

6. Governor's Office - In nearly every state the office of the Governor has a commission, agency, department, or office dealing with aging. Many also have offices for volunteer organizations. Opportunities and referral information can usually be obtained by contacting these governmental services in your state.

7. ACTION - Domestic Volunteer Services Act - 1973
   806 Connecticut Ave., N.W.
   Washington, DC 20525

   a. Retired Senior Volunteer Program (RSVP) - Extensive opportunities for a wide variety of volunteer services in public and nonprofit institutions and community service programs. Travel and meal expenses are reimbursed.

   b. Foster Grandparents - Volunteers serve handicapped or special needs children under programs initiated in each community to meet community needs.

   c. Senior Companion Program - Similar to Foster Grandparents Program. Volunteers serve adult or elderly special needs or handicapped persons who may or may not be institutionalized. Compensation is provided in the same manner as in Foster Grandparent Programs. In some communities these two programs have been combined.

d. Service Corps of Retired Executives (SCORE) - A program using retired persons with business experience to advise those in new business ventures. The small Business Administration administers this popular program.

e. Volunteers in Service to America (VISTA) - Places volunteers for 1-2 years in domestic impoverished areas of the country in community projects. Small salary to assist in living expenses is provided.

f. Peace Corps - Volunteers spend 2 years in overseas service in a developing nation.

8. Senior Community Service Employment Program (SCSEP) "Project Agenda" - A community service employment program for senior citizens. This program has been sponsored by the National Association for Spanish-Speaking Elderly.

Senior Community Service Employment Program
1801 K Street, N.W., Suite 1021
Washington, DC 20006

9. Job Training Partnership ACT (JTPA) - 1983, PL 300
Addresses the need among the elderly and others for job training and also retraining. This employment-oriented program, although not based on voluntarism, has potential to provide manpower in other programs serving the elderly.

This selected list is provided to demonstrate the myriad of opportunities open to the elderly for training and functioning in important community service roles. Many provide financial incentives and all have the potential of high personal satisfaction. These programs are only a small number compared to state and local opportunities from both public and private sectors. This list also suggests a wide variety of skills, interests, and abilities the elderly have as resources, which have remained relatively untapped by programs and institutions for the communicatively handicapped (Asha, 1980). A number of creative suggestions for developing programs, particularly intergenerational ones, leave open many options for the communicatively impaired of all ages to serve others (Rothstein, 1983; Salmon, 1979). Seguin (1972) has developed a thought-provoking position paper which includes a discussion of training modules, issues, and volunteerism.

Volunteers have been used extensively in fundraising and community relations throughout the history of both private and public institutions.

Speech-language pathology and audiology clinics and programs have not extensively used volunteers in service delivery or supportive service. Some question about the motives of volunteers is often raised by administrators. There seems to be a lack of openness or hesitancy about being scrutinized by nonprofessionals. It should be acknowledged that most volunteers seek an altruistic reward, in the form of some personal satisfaction, or have a desire to pay back a perceived debt of gratitude. It is also true that some seek and receive secondary benefits such as job skill experience, information on employment opportunities, learning of new skills, and may gain attention of prospective employers. Others appear to be power hungry or out to prove something that appears nebulous, to the dismay of all concerned. In any case, this used to be a viable method for many people to secure training. Others, such as displaced homemakers and the elderly, still use volunteer experiences as a foot in the door for future employability. In any case, these conditions generally make for quality, experienced, dependable, and reliable manpower. There appears to be an enormous potential for the use of volunteers as adjuncts to treatment in communication disorders, particularly among the elderly.

Self-Study Questions

1. In selecting a format for an in-service program, which ones would be the most effective in changing the behavior or attitudes of staff toward the elderly? Which would be least effective?

2. What considerations should be included in public education programs if the goal is to inform the elderly of available services.

3. How has volunteerism changed in recent years to become a more attractive alternative as a source of meaningful activity for the volunteer, and manpower for service agencies?

4. What are some of the federal, state, and local opportunities for volunteer service that an elderly person may consider?

5. Discuss the possible disadvantages or dangers of using untrained or unsupervised volunteers in a service delivery system.

6. Can the criticisms of medical profession education about inadequate training in gerontology for physicians also be consistent with Communication Disorders training programs?

7. How should meeting the needs of a particular group of potential trainees for an in-service program be considered in goal setting?

8. What are some of the resource materials available for in-service training in the area of aging and communication disorders?

REFERENCES

American Speech-Language-Hearing Association. (1980). "Breaking the silence barrier between you and your patient, an inservice program for staff development." American Speech and Hearing Association.

Aurthur, J. K. (1970, April). "Retire to action: A guide to voluntary service. Aging, 13, 26.

Bartman, S., Mummery, V., Poppe, M., Robbins, B., & Robertson-Palmer, K. (1982, February). Shopping for health? Maybe this storefront health information centre can help." The Canadian Nurse, 78, 48.

Bernard, M. (1984, April). Volunteer care for the elderly mentally infirm and their relatives: A British example. The Gerontologist 24(3).

Berry, M. (1984, March). Asha, 26(3).

Clark, C. C., & Mills, G. C. (1979). "Communicating with hearing impaired elderly adults. Journal of Gerontological Nursing, 5(3), 40-44.

Coccaro, E. G., Berube, L., Thornton, J., Myerson, A. T. (1983). Gerontological geriatric training in medical school: Preferences of students, educators, and practitioners of medicine in regard to curricular content. Educational Gerontology, 9, 293-306.

Conter, R. V., & Schneiderman, S. T. (1982, March). Using interdisciplinary networks to rush new audiences through strategic out-reach. Paper presented at Western Gerontological Society.

Cross, J., & Westbook, D. (1979). Inservice education: The state of the scene. North Texas State.

Ernst, M., & Shore, H. (1975). "Sensitizing people to the process of aging: The in-service educator's guide. North Texas State University, Denton, TX: Center for Studies in Aging.

Faris, J. B. (1979, March/April). Nationwide health fair projects to mark Older Americans month. Aging, 2-3.

Finley, S. (1981, November). Providing technical assistance in the location of information resources to designers and developers of professional inservice programs. U. S. Office of Education Publication #ED 212276 p. 29.

Foulk, D., & Young, M. (1982, May). Radio: A tool for health educators. _The Journal of School Health_, _52_, 312.

Freimuth, V. S., Jamieson, L. (1979). Communicating with the elderly: Shattering the stereotypes. _Theory and research into practice series_. American Speech Convention Association.

Gerardi, G. E. (1982). An outreach program for the urban elderly. _Journal of Gerontological Nurse_, _8_, 440-442.

Grimes, J. (1975). _In-service: A how-to-book._ Des Moines: Iowa State Department of Public Instruction.

Harris, B. M. (1980). _Improving staff performance through inservice education._ Boston: Allyn & Bacon.

Heisel, M. A., Darkenwald, G. G., & Anderson, R. E. (1981). Participation in organized educational activities among adults age 60 and over. _Educational gerontology: An international quarterly_, _6_, 227-240.

Hickey, T. (1975). Simulating age-related sensory impairments for practitioner education. _The Gerontologist_, _15_(5), 457-463

Holtzman, J. M., Beck, J. D., & Ettringer, R. L. (1981). Cognitive knowledge and attitudes toward the aged of dental and medical schools. _Educational Gerontology_, _6_, 195-207.

Hubbard, R. W., & Santos, J. F. (1981). Empathy training as a instructional tool for geriatric health professionals. _Educational Gerontology_, _6_, 191-194.

Kirkpatrick, R. (1979). The development of a model to guide the practitioner in continuing education programs: Learning theory and applications module. Unpublished manuscript, Nova University, FL.

Kruger-Smith, B. (1973). _Aging in america._ Toronto, Canada: Beacon Press.

Landy, M. (1983, January/February). Redefining the role of the speech-language pathologist in relation to the elderly population. _Human Communication-Canada_, _7_(1), 5-9.

Leutenegger, R. R. (1975). _Patient care and rehabilitation of communicative-impaired adults._ Chicago, IL: Charles C. Thomas.

Manser, G., & Cass, R. H. (1976). _Voluntarism at the crossroads._ New York: Family Service Association of America.

Marts, A. C. (1966). _The generosity of Americans._ Englewood Cliffs, NJ: Prentice-Hall.

Mason, D. J., & Calvacca, L. R. (1982, June). Health fair: Providing a learning experience through a community service project. _Journal of Nursing Education_, _21_, 35-47.

Moore, W., & Campbell, R. (1978, November). A pilot training program, and evaluation of training for an area agency on aging. Paper presented at the Conference of Gerontological Society.

Ohio State Department of Education. (1978). Focus on inservice education. Columbus.

Pastalan, L. S., Mantz, R. K., & Merril, S. (1973). The simulation of age related losses: A new approach to the study of environmental barriers, In W. E. Preiser (Ed.), Environmental design research, monograph, Vol. 1.

Price, W. T. & Grigsby, T. (1981). Continuing education: A factor in preparing for retirement. Educational Gerontology, 6,(2).

Ray, B. H. (1977). A need-based inservice training workshop for the clerical staff of the state of Florida health and rehabilitation services. Unpublished doctoral dissertation, Nova University, FL.

Robichaud, M. P., & Brown, M. L. (1979, November). A simulation experience to sensitize persons to the sensory losses of the elderly. Paper presented to the Gerontological Society.

Rothstein, D. G. (1983). Developing a voluntary neighborhood intergenerational program, Journal of Gerontological Social Work, 6, 99-106.

Salmon, R. (1979). The older volunteer: Personal and organizational considerations, Journal of Gerontological Social Work. 2, 67-75.

Schor, I. (1981). The continuing nursing education and adult education movements in the United States, Nursing Forum, 20, 86-101.

Seldin, C. A. (1979, December). Taking inservice education off the back burner. Phi Delta Kappan, 61, 266.

Sequin, M. M. (1972). Older volunteer training program: A position paper. Los Angeles: Ethel Percy Andrews Gerontology Center, University of Southern California.

Shadden, B. B., Raiford, C. A., & Shadden, H. S. (1983). Coping with communication disorders in aging. Tigaard, OR: C. C. Publications.

Silverstein, N. M. (1984). Informing the elderly about public services: The relation between sources of knowledge and service utilization. The Gerontologist, 24.

Singer, J., & W. Brownell. (1984, April). Assessment of hearing health knowledge. The Gerontologist, 24,(2), 160-166.

Slover, D., & Greco, C. M. (1975). Analysis and selection of training resources in aging. University Gerontology Center, Syracuse University, NY.

Spear, M. (1970). Guide for inservice training for developing services for older people. U.S. DHEW.

Vincent, E. (1976). The care of the geriatric patient. St. Louis: C. V. Mosby.

Ward, R. (1984). The aging experience: An introduction to Social gerontology, (2nd d.), New York: Harper & Row.

Whitehouse Conference on Aging. (1981). Community forums handbook. Washington, DC: The White House Conference on Aging.

Suggested Readings

Atchley, R. C. & Seltzer, M. M. (1977). "Developing education programs in the field of aging." Oxford, OH: Scripps Foundation Gerontology Center.

Beigel, D. & Naparstek Arthur, (Eds.). (1982). Community support systems and mental health. New York: Springer.

Burnside, I. (1984). Working with the elderly: Group processes and techniques (2nd ed.). Wadsworth Health Sciences Divison.

Butler, R. N., & Lewis, M. I. (1982). Aging and mental health: Positive psychosocial and biomedical approaches (3rd ed.).

Dackenwald, G., & Larson, G. (Eds.). (1980). Reaching the hard-to-reach adults. San Francisco: Jossey-Bass.

Dancer, J., & Thomas, W. E. (1983, July). Interdisciplinary health care for the elderly: Beyond the boundaries, Asha, 28(7).

Dowd, J. J. (1984). Beneficience and the aged. Journal of Gerontology, 39(1), 102-108.

Duncan, M. E., & Bass, R. K. (1981). "Attitudes toward educational media: Implications for educational gerontology," Educational Gerontology, 6, 77-91.

Flanagan, J. (1981). The successful volunteer organization. Chicago, IL: Books.

Friedman, J. K. (1977). A manual for the beginning practitioner in the field

Howard R. (1975, January). Inservice education for volunteers working in the field of gerontology. Monograph. San Jose State University.

Jacobs, B. (1976). Working with the impaired elderly. The National Council on the Aging.

Manachem, D. (1982). Preference for age homogenous versus age heterogenous social interaction. Journal of Gerontological Social Work, 4, 41-53.

Netting, F., & Hinds, H. (1974, February). Volunteer advocates in long-term care: Local implementation of a federal mandate. The Gerontologist. 24,(1).

Norback, C, & Norback, P. (1977). The older American's handbook. Van Nostrand Reinholt.

Seltzer, M. M. (1978). Gerontology in higher education: Prospective and issues. Wadsworth Publishing.

Somers, A. R., & Fabian, D. R. (1981). The geriatric imperitive: An introduction to gerontology and clinical geriatrics. New York: Appleton-Century-Crofts.

Spilich, G. J. (1983). Implications for cognitive change for gerontological pedagogical practice. International Journal and Human Development, 18, 31-37.

Silverstone, B., & Hyman, H. K. (1982). You and your aging parent. Pantheon.

Ward, R. A. (1984). The aging experience: An introduction to social gerontology. Harper & Row.

Wilson, P. A. (1983). Towards more effective intervention in natural helping networks. Social Work in Health Care, 9, 81-88.

Wolinsky, F., & Coe, R. (1984, May). Physician and hospital utilization among noninstitutionalized elderly: An analysis of the health interview survey, Journal of Gerontology, 39(3), p. 334-341.

Resource Materials

American Speech-Language-Hearing Association. (1977). Breaking the silence barrier: Inservice training module. American Speech-Language-Hearing Association.

American Speech-Language-Hearing Association (1980). Resource materials for communicative problems of older persons (rev ed.). American Speech-Language-Hearing Association.

Ernst, M., & H S., (Eds.). (1978). Sensitizing people to the processes of aging: The inservice educators guide. North Texas State University, Denton TX: Center for Studies on Aging.

Sayles, A. H., Adams, H., & Adams, S. K. (Eds.) (1978). Communication problems and behaviors of the older American. American Speech-Language-Hearing Association.

Accessing the
Federally-Legislated
Aging System

Linda Jacobs-Condit

and

Alina C. Otal

American Speech-Language-Hearing Association, Rockville, Maryland

Aging, as a process of the life cycle, is normal and universal, crossing cultural, sexual, racial, ethnic, and class lines. Furthermore, as a subgroup of the general population, the aging (or elderly) have very special needs. Many professionals, such as nurses, social workers, occupational/physical therapists, pharmacists, physicians, and dentists provide interventional services to the elderly.

What, specifically, are some of the avenues by which we can better integrate ourselves into the service delivery system for the elderly? The opportunities include, but are not limited to:

o broadening our own base of knowledge about the process and effects of aging;

o becoming aware of and actively participate in organizations which represent or serve the aging in other capacities;

o broadening the knowledge of other professionals, allied health service providers, and consumer public about communication and aging; and

o becoming informed advocates for the rights and needs of all aging persons.

Some of these approaches, specifically, in-service activities, have been discussed previously. Therfore, this section will address the aging service delivery system which is mandated by federal legislature, as well as accessing into this system of service provision to the elderly.

One avenue speech-language pathologists and audiologists can follow in order to become effective advocates for the needs and concerns of the elderly is to increase awareness and knowledge about the federal legislation which impacts upon the aging and, in effect, mandates the existence of the "aging network."

The major federal legislation is the Older Americans Act (OAA), enacted in 1965 (PL 89-73) and subsequently strengthened by numerous amendments. Of particular interest to communication disorders specialists is the Older Americans Act Amendments of 1975 (PL 94-135). The PL 94-135 added four new special-emphasis programs (transportation services, home care and health services, residential renovation and repair, and legal services) and contained authority for the establishment of model projects to confront hearing problems of the elderly.

The 1975 Amendments further authorized the Commissioner of the Administration on Aging to make grants and contracts with any public or nonprofit private agency for the development or operation of statewide, regional, metropolitan area, county, city, or community model projects designed to promote the well-being of older persons. Included among the projects authorized were model projects designed to inform hearing-impaired elderly citizens of the need for and availability of appropriate professional evaluation, diagnosis and aural rehabilitation, and model projects designed to expand or improve the delivery of aural rehabilitation services to the hearing-impaired elderly.

The 1978 Amendments to the Older Americans Act, in addition to extending the Act through 1981, allocated funds for the Federal Council on the Aging, the National Information and Research Clearinghouse for the Aging, research, training, model or demonstration projects, and programs for older American Indians.

As defined by law, and as amended in 1981 (PL 97-115), the Objectives of the Older Americans Act of 1965 (Title I) are as follows:

> The Congress hereby finds and declares that, in keeping with the traditional American concept of the inherent dignity of the individual in our democratic society, the older people of our Nation are entitled to...secure equal opportunity to the full and free enjoyment of the following objectives:

1. An adequate income in retirement in accordance with the American standard of living.

2. The best possible physical and mental health which science can make available and without regard to economic status.

3. Suitable housing, independently selected, designed, and located with reference to special needs and available at costs which older citizens can afford.

4. Full restorative services for those who require institutional care.

5. Opportunity for employment with no discriminatory personnel practices because of age.

6. Retirement in health, honor, dignity--after years of contribution to the economy.

7. Pursuit of meaningful activity within the widest range of civic, cultural, education and training, and recreational opportunities.

8. Efficient community services, including access to low-cost transportation, which provide a choice of supported living arrangements and social assistance in a coordinated manner and which are readily available when needed.

9. Immediate benefit from proven research knowledge which can sustain and improve health and happiness.

10. Freedom, independence, and the free exercise of individual initiative in planning and managing their own lives.

    (U.S. Senate, PL 97-115, March 1982, p. 403)

The following information regarding the Administration on Aging is reproduced from Reorganizational Plan for the AoA, DHEW (October 1978).

Title II of the Act establishes the Administration on Aging (AoA) as the principal agency designed to carry out the provisions of the Older Americans Act of 1965 as amended. The AoA serves as an advocate at the federal level for the needs, concerns, and interests of older people. Headed by a Commissioner who develops and directs the program of the Administration on Aging and reports directly to Secretary of Health & Human Services, the organizational structure of the AoA is depicted in Figure 1. Specifically, the Administration on Aging consists of:

The Office of the Commissioner establishes priorities, sets policies, and directs plans and programs conducted by the AoA. The Commissioner advises the

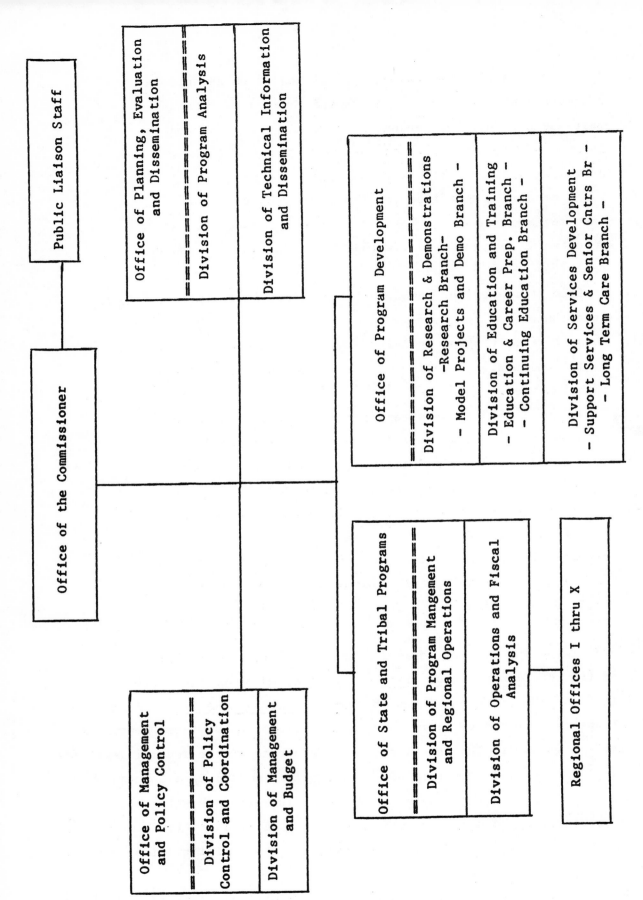

Figure 1. Administration on aging organizational chart.

Assistant Secretary and heads of DHHS agencies administering programs which impact on the lives of older people. In addition, the Commissioner serves as an advocate for older people with other departments and agencies of the Federal government and with voluntary organizations, and undertakes plans to coordinate activities on behalf of the aging. Finally, the Office of the Commissioner assures affirmative action throughout the federally-mandated aging system.

The Office of Management and Policy Control is responsible for policy analysis and development, long- and short-range planning, development of legislation, preparation of required reports, budget development and preparation of justification for the annual budget request, and provision of management services.

The Office of Public Information, in coordination with the Office of Public Affairs, develops and distributes professional and lay publications, as well as audiovisual materials about older people and programs and services for older people. It prepares and issues brochures, fact sheets, news releases, exhibits, and films on the needs and concerns of the aging, and measures to improve the circumstances, available services, and environment for the older population. In addition, it fosters the annual Senior Citizen Month (May).

The Office of Program Operations is responsible for supervising and directing the activities of the 10 Regional Offices of the AoA in response to their responsibilities under the Older Americans Act.

The Office of Program Development develops policies and program plans, regulations, and program instructions to improve facilities, programs, and services available to the nation's older population for service programs administered by the AoA under the AoA. The Office fosters, oversees, assists, and assesses the development of state-administered community-based systems as authorized under Title III, Title V, and Title VII of the OAA and related Acts.

The Office of Education and Training administers programs to increase the supply of trained personnel in the field of aging; to increase the knowledge in other professional fields of the processes of aging and the circumstances and requirements of older people; and to increase the availability, accessibility, and adequacy of training and educational programs on aging within educational institutions throughout the country. The Office conducts continuing studies and periodic reviews of manpower needs and resources in the field of aging; develops and monitors a national plan for increasing these resources; and prepares reports thereon for the Administration on Aging, the

Federal Council on Aging, the Office of the Secretary, the President, and the Congress.

The National Clearinghouse on Aging facilitates access of teachers, students, researchers, practitioners, and interested members of the general public to rapidly growing literature and basic data in the field of aging.

The Office of Research, Demonstration, and Evaluation develops strategies and conducts activities to develop adequate knowledge for developing and testing facilities, programs, and services calculated to improve the environment for older people. The Office promotes coordination of research and evaluation activities in the field of aging. The Office oversees the grant and contract activities designed to carry out research, development, and evaluation programs, and develops AoA policies and criteria for monitoring grants and contracts supported through the office.

The Regional Offices on Aging are headed by regional program directors who are responsible to the Commissioner through the Associate Commissioner for Field Operations. Regional Offices (see Appendix A) provide information for and contribute to the development of national policy dealing with the elderly. Based on national policy and priorities, they establish regional program goals and objectives, and provide direction and assistance in the administration of mandated programs.

State and area agencies on aging, under the jurisdiction of the Regional Offices, were first established with the 1973 amendments to the OAA. As part of the federally mandated "aging network," the state agencies on aging have the responsibility to coordinate the provision of "health services, transportation, education, employment, and income maintenance programs which could provide assistance to the elderly" (U.S. Senate, Report #96-55, March 30, 1979, p. 107). The area agencies on aging, in turn, are responsible for making funds available to senior centers, nutrition sites, churches and schools, for example, which are the sites of service provision to the elderly.

Title II of the Older Americans Act of 1965 also provided for a White House Conference on Aging, based on congressional findings that the size of the elderly population was growing at a tremendous rate and that, because millions of the elderly lived below the poverty level, improved economic well-being for the elderly was essential. In addition, Congress identified several factors which warranted improvement in order to effect improved quality of life for the elderly. These factors are (a) comprehensive and available quality health

347

care; (b) availability of suitable and reasonably priced housing; (c) comprehensive and effective social service delivery system, and comprehensive long-term care policy; (d) greater employment opportunities for middle-aged and older individuals who want or need to work; (e) national retirement policy; (f) national policy aimed at expediting biomedical research on aging; and, (g) need for national policies aimed at eliminating false stereotypes about aging and the process of aging (U.S. Senate, 1979).

It was the intent of Congress that the Federal government work jointly with the states and their citizens to develop recommendations and plans for action to meet the challenges and needs of older individuals consistent with the objectives of the Title II. In developing programs for the aging pursuant to the Conference, the right and obligation of older individuals to free choice and self-help in planning their own futures was emphasized.

Title III of the AoA provided allocation of funds for Grants for State and Community Programs on Aging based on the population of elderly within each state. It was the purpose of Title III to encourage and assist state and local agencies in developing comprehensive and coordinated service systems for older individuals (i.e., supportive services, nutrition services, and multipurpose senior centers). The ultimate goals of service to the elderly unter Title III were to:

1. Secure and maintain maximum independence and dignity in a
    home environment for older individuals capable of self-care
    with appropriate supportive services;
2. Remove individual and social barriers to economic and
    personal independence for the older individual; and
3. Provide a continuum of care for the vulnerable elderly
    (U.S. Congress, 1965, p. 1517).

Title IV addresses Training, Research, and Discretionary Projects and Programs. Part A directs attention to a national manpower policy for the field of aging by supporting training programs at all academic levels. Part B supports research projects related to meeting the needs of public officials and service procedures. Part C is concerned with demonstration projects and programs such as comprehensive long-term care, legal services for older persons, utility costs, and other national priorities. Part D provides grants to assist in developing comprehensive long-term care systems and upgrading multipurpose senior centers. Part E supports multidisciplinary centers of gerontology. Within Title IV is an emphasis on the development of services for impaired persons, including homebound older persons.

Title V authorizes Community Service Employment for Older Americans. There is a 90/10 federal/non-federal match of funds for these programs.

Title VI provides Grants for Indian Tribes. Eligible tribal organizations can receive grants to pay for the delivery of social and nutritional services for Indians aged 60 and over. Surplus Indian educational facilities are made available for use by the tribes as multipurpose senior centers, extended care facilities, community center activities, and nutritional services.

Thus, the Older Americans Act of 1965 and its amendments have far-reaching implications for service delivery to the aging throughout the nation for state, regional, and local communities.

Social Security Act

The following information regarding the Social Security Act is reproduced largely from Organizations & Agencies in the Area of Aging, Asha (1980).

One of the most widespread benefit programs for older adults is the Old Age, Survivors, and Disability Insurance Program which pays social security benefits to millions of Americans because of retirement, disability, or death. Benefits are based on a percentage of average monthly earnings over the time period when the worker contributed to the system and on the age when the worker starts to receive benefits. Recent legislative action has made payments contingent upon inflation as well.

- o If you reach 65 in 1983, your retirement benefit can be as much as $709.
- o If you reach 62 in 1983, your monthly retirement benefit at age 62 can be as much as $526.
- o If you become disabled in 1983, the monthly benefit to you as a disabled worker can be as much as $795, depending on your age and past earnings.
- o If you have eligible dependents, the total monthly family benefit payable can be as much as $1,192.

o Survivors of a worker who dies in 1983 can expect to
   receive as much as $1,393 a month for a family of three or
   more. (U.S. DHHS, April 1983, p. 20-21).

Social Security benefits will increase as the relationship between social
security payment levels and the cost of living index stabilizes.

Three additional provisions of the Social Security Act have been added in
more recent years. The Supplemental Security Income (SSI) Program, Title XVI,
offers a standard minimum cash amount to blind or disabled persons and to
persons over age 65. Three sources of assistance may contribute to the
payment--basic Federal benefits, mandatory supplements from the state, and
voluntary additional state supplements. To be eligible for SSI, persons must
meet the income and assets test.

Medicare and Medicaid were enacted over 10 years ago as Title XVIII and
Title XIX of the Social Security Act. Medicare is a medical insurance program
open to all those who receive Social Security retirement benefits and others
who meet certain requirements. Benefits under Medicare are uniform throughout
the United States. Part A Medicare is a Hospital Insurance program that pays
cost above a deductible amount for in-hospital care and post-hospital care in a
skilled nursing facility or for home health care. Part B is a voluntary
supplemental program that pays for out-patient physician fees and other
services. Money to pay for Medicare hospital benefits comes from trust funds
financed by payroll contributions.

Medicaid furnishes medical assistance to most low-income people who meet
SSI standards. Available in every state except Arizona, Medicaid can pay for a
wide range of in- and out-patient hospital services, physicians' fees,
diagnostic tests, home health, and family planning services, and the deductible
costs under Medicare, if the person is eligible for both. Benefits, which vary
from state to state, are financed by federal, state, and sometimes local taxes.

There are innumerable national, state, and local organizations whose goals
include service to and/or support of the elderly. Congressional committees
with jurisdiction over areas related to the aging can be found in Appendix B.
A list of federal programs benefitting the elderly can be found in Appendix C,
and Appendix D lists federal resources and services for health care for the
elderly. A list of federal and nongovernmental agencies or organizations

interested in or responsible for service to the elderly can be found in Appendix E. An abridged list of other resources can be found in Appendix F.

Accessing the System

There exists in many communities an interagency committee which meets on a regular basis. Comprised of personnel from various disciplines that provide service to the elderly (i.e., Agencies on Aging, public health, social services, mental health, recreation), the committee serves to provide up-to-date information on aging. This would be an excellent forum by which speech-language pathologists and audiologists could interact with others who provide service delivery to the elderly the end result of which could be improved knowledge regarding communication changes as well as an increase in the provision of speech, language, or hearing services to the elderly.

In order to access the aging system at the ground level, one thing a speech-language pathologist or audiologist needs to determine is how the local Agency on Aging functions. The local Agency on Aging which may have city, county, or regional jurisdiction receives its funds from the State Office on Aging. The State Office, in turn, is funded through the Regional Office of the Administration on Aging (see Appendix A).

The majority of senior citizen centers fall under the jurisdiction of the local Agency on Aging. However, in some instances, individual centers may be church-affiliated or receive monies from sources other than the Federal government (i.e., the United Way or the United Black Fund); even so, some linkage with the local Agency on Aging always exists.

Once the jurisdiction and operation of the local Agency on Aging in a given locality has been ascertained, an appointment could be made with its director. The purpose, at this point, would be for the speech-language pathologist or audiologist to discuss what the communication disorders specialist could offer in the form of time or services. The name of the facility, its staff and services provided could be listed in the Agency on Aging's Information and Referral Guide. Presentations could be made to the staff at senior citizen centers as part of their in-service training, for example, on how to recognize changes in speech, language, or hearing functions. Free hearing, speech or language screenings could be provided to the participants of the local senior citizen centers.

There are many ways in which the elderly population could become more aware of the services of speech-language-hearing professionals. Most Agencies on Aging publish a monthly newsletter for distribution to all senior citizens in their jurisdiction. A short informative article on communication impairments common to the elderly could be submitted for publication. Also, many Agencies sponsor a Senior Citizens' I.D. Discount Program, by which participating elderly may receive discounts from participating sponsors for services or products. A guide of participating sponsors is updated periodically and mailed to all elderly who have discount cards. Thus, if it is possible to offer services at a reduced rate to these senior citizens, the name of the facility and percentage of reduction in fees could be listed in the guide. This exposure could be highly beneficial in increasing the delivery of speech, language, and hearing services to the elderly.

The senior citizens center is one place to reach a large audience of elderly on a regular basis. The senior center is operated by a center director or coordinator whose responsibilities are numerous: (a) oversees the day-to-day operations of the center; (b) provides counseling, information and referral; (c) and coordinates scheduling, programming, as well as a myriad of other activities. In this respect, the center director or coordinator is a key person in accessing the elderly population and would, in all likelihood, be delighted if a lecture or service delivery program could be included in activities on a volunteer basis.

Most directors of senior citizens' centers circulate among themselves a list of suggested programs that are of an educational and/or recreational nature provided by individuals or organizations either for free or at a minimal cost. Most centers have no budget for programs, so it is very important to stipulate fee requirements from the outset.

Senior citizens' centers are multiservice centers. In addition to their on-going programs of glaucoma testing, blood pressure screening, cancer detection, and nutrition information, some also provide transportation to/from the center, to doctors, or to essential shopping, whereas others may also serve as nutrition sites. It would be mutually beneficial to include the services of speech, language, and hearing professionals among these activities. This public information service would improve the public's awareness of changes in hearing, speech, and language functions as an aspect of aging. More importantly, these recipients of knowledge could be given specific strategies which could be used to facilitate improved communication with and among the aging. Only by staying in touch with themselves, their peers, the community, and the world at large can the elderly be in a position to maintain a life of quality and independence.

Self—Study Questions

1. Why is the 1975 amendment to the Older Americans Act particularly important to our profession?

2. Which federal agency serves as a advocate for the needs, concerns and interests of older people?

3. According to the 1973 amendments to the Older Americans Act, under whose jurisdiction are the state and area agencies on aging?

4. What is the basis for allocating grant funds to state and community programs for the aged.

5. Based on findings of the White House Conference on Aging, what was the emphasis of program development for the elderly?

6. On what are Social Security benefits based?

7. What are some ways in which speech—language pathologists and/or audiologists can access into the aging network?

8. Give some examples of the services you, as a communication disorders specialist, can suggest to the director of the local agency on aging. Use examples from the manual as well as activities from our own experiences.

REFERENCES

American Speech-Language-Hearing Association. (1980). <u>Organizations & agencies in the area of aging</u>. American Speech-Language-Hearing Association, Rockville, MD.

U.S. Congress (1965, July). <u>Enactment of the Older Americans Act of 1965.</u> (PL 89-73).

U.S. Congress (1975, November). <u>Amendments to the Older Americans Act</u> (1975), (PL 94-135).

U.S. DHEW (1978). <u>Reorganizational plan for the administration on aging.</u> U.S. DHEW.

U.S. DHHS (1983, April). <u>Social security strengthened: 1983 social security amendments,</u> (SSA Pub #05-10345). U.S. Government Printing Office #381-795/4045.

U.S. Senate (1979, March). <u>Developments in aging: 1973-1978</u>. (PL 95-478). U.S. Government Printing Office.

U.S. Senate (1982, March). <u>Development in aging: 1981</u>. Volume 1, PL 97-115). U.S. Government Printing Office #89-509.

Appendix A

Administration on Aging

Regional Offices

Regional Program Director
Administration on Aging
Department of Health & Human Services
Region I
John F. Kennedy Federal Building
Boston, MA   02203

Regional Program Director
Administration on Aging
Department of Health & Human Services
Region II
26 Federal Plaza
New York, NY   10007

Regional Program Director
Administration on Aging
Department of Health & Human Services
Region III

P.O. Box 13716
Philadelphia, PA   19101

Regional Program Director
Administration on Aging
Department of Health & Human Services
Region IV
101 Marietta Towers
Suite #901
Atlanta, GA   30323

Regional Program Director
Administration on Aging
Department of Health & Human Services
Region V
15th Floor
300 South Wacker Drive
Chicago, IL   60606

Regional Program Director
Administration on Aging
Department of Health & Human Services
Region VI
1200 Main Tower Building
Room 2060
Dallas, TX   75201

Regional Program Director
Administration on Aging
Department of Health & Human Services
Region VII
Federal Office Building
601 East 12th Street
Kansas City, MO   64106

Regional Program Director
Administration on Aging
Department of Health & Human Services
Region VIII
19th& Stout Streets, Rm. 7430
Federal Office Bldg.
Denver, CO   80202

Regional Program Director
Administration on Aging
Department of Health & Human Services
Region IX
406 Federal Office Building

50 Fulton Street
San Francisco, CA 94102

Regional Program Director
Administration on Aging
Department of Health & Human Services
Region X
Third & Broad Bldg. MS-412
2901 Third Avenue
Seattle, WA 98121

Appendix B
Congressional Committees
House and Senate

House Committees and Subcommittees with Jurisdiction Over Areas Related to the Elderly

Information concerning "House Committees and Subcommittees with Jurisdiction over Areas Related to the Elderly" was taken from Federal Responsibilities to the Elderly (Executive Programs and Legislative Jurisdiction), January 1979, published by Superintendent of Documents, U.S. Government Printing Office, Washington, DC 20402.

Select Committee on Aging

Conducts studies and investigations on problems of the elderly; primarily a fact finding body; advises committees listed below which have the responsibility to act on bills benefiting the elderly.

Full Committee Staff: Responsible for oversight investigations, special studies and hearings by full committee, and staff administration.

Subcommittee on Retirement Income and Employment: Income maintenance and employment.

Subcommittee on Health and Long-term Care: Health care programs.

Subcommittee on Housing and Consumer Interests: Housing and consumer interests.

Subcommittee on Human Services: Social services for the elderly.

Committee on Agriculture

Subcommittee on Domestic Marketing, Consumer Relations, and Nutrition: Food Stamp Program, and certain other nutrition-related programs.

Committee on Banking, Finance, and Urban Affairs

Subcommittee on Housing and Community Development: Housing programs which serve the elderly.

Committee on Education and Labor

Education programs; programs under the Older Americans Act; employment programs for the elderly administered by the U.S. Department of Labor; Older American Volunteer programs administered by ACTION; age discrimination in employment; senior opportunities and services administered by the Community Services Administration; private pensions plans.

Subcommittee on Select Education

Subcommittee on Economic Opportunity

Subcommittee on Employment Opportunities

Subcommittee on Manpower, Compensation, and Health Safety

Subcommittee on Elementary, Secondary, and Vocational Education

Committee on the Judiciary

Subcommittee on Crime: Law Enforcement Assistance Administration (Crime Prevention).

Committee on Interstate and Foreign Commerce

Subcommittee on Health and Environment: Grants to states for medical assistance programs (Medicaid), National Institute on Aging, nursing home and intermediate care facilities authorized under the National Housing Act of 1959, Section 232.

Subcommittee on Transportation and Commerce: Railroad Retirement Act.

Committee on Post Office and Civil Service

Subcommittee on Compensation and Employee Benefits: Civil Service Retirement Act.

Committee on Public Works and Transportation

Subcommittee on Surface Transportation: Services for the elderly authorized under the Urban Mass Transportation Act.

Committee on Veterans Affairs

Subcommittee on Compensation, Pension and Insurance: Veterans pension programs.

Subcommittee on Medical Facilities and Benefits: Health care programs.

Committee on Ways and Means

Full committee has jurisdiction over taxation and private pension plans.

Subcommittee on Social Security: Old-age, Survivors, and Disability Insurance Program (Social Security).

Subcommittee on Health: Health insurance for the aged and disabled (Medicare).

Subcommittee on Public Assistance: Supplemental Security Income (SSI), social services for low income individuals authorized under Title XX of the Social Security Act.

Senate Committees and Subcommittees with Jurisdiction Over Areas Related to the Elderly

Special Committee on Aging

Conducts studies and investigations on problems of the elderly; primarily a fact finding body; advises committees listed below which have responsibility to act on bills benefiting the elderly. Has oversight and investigative responsibilities on all matters relating to elderly.

Committee on Agriculture, Nutrition and Forestry

Subcommittee on Nutrition: Food Stamp Program and other certain nutrition-related programs.

Committee on Banking, Housing and Urban Affairs

Subcommittee on Housing and Urban Affairs: Housing programs which serve the elderly; nursing home and intermediate care facilities authorized under the National Housing Act of 1969, Section 232; services for elderly under Urban Mass Transportation Act.

Committee on Finance

Old Age, Survivors, and Disability Insurance Program (Social (Security); grants to states for medical assistance (Medicaid); health insurance for the aged and disabled (Medicare); private pension plans; social services for low-income individuals authorized under Title XX of the Social Security Act, Supplemental Security Income program (SSI); taxation. Subcommittees primarily have oversight functions.

Subcommittee on Health: Health care programs.

Subcommittee on Private Pension Plans: Private pension programs.

Subcommittee on Social Security Financing: Old-Age Survivors and Disability Insurance (Social Security).

Subcommittee on Supplemental Security Income: Supplemental Security Income (SSI).

Committee on Human Resources

Subcommittee on Aging: Programs under the Older Americans Act.

Subcommittee on Health and Scientific Research: Health care programs.

Subcommittee on Employment, Poverty and Migratory Labor: Senior opportunities and services administered by the Community Services Administration; older Americans volunteer programs administered by ACTION.

Subcommittee on Labor: Private pension plans; Railroad Retirement Act; manpower programs; age discrimination in employment.

Subcommittee on Education, Arts and the Humanities: Education programs.

Committee on Governmental Affairs

Subcommittee on Civil Service and General Services: Civil Service Retirement Act.

Committee on the Judiciary

Subcommittee on Criminal Laws and Procedures: Law Enforcement assistance Administration (Crime Prevention).

Committee on Veteran Affairs

Subcommittee on Compensation and Pensions: Veterans pension programs.

Subcommittee on Health and Readjustment: Health care programs.

Types of Federal Assistance

The types of Federal assistance programs include: formula grants; project grants; direct payments for specified use; direct payments with unrestricted use; direct loans; guaranteed/insured loans; insurance; sale, exchange, or donation of property and goods; use of property, facilities, and equipment; provision of specialized services, advisory services and counseling; dissemination of technical information; training; investigation of complaints; federal employment; and research contracts.

Appendix C
Federal Programs Benefiting the Elderly

Employment and Volunteer

Employment Standards Administration (LABOR) Age Discrimination in Employment

Employment and Training Administration (LABOR) Community Based Employment and Training Programs

Community Service Employment for Older Americans

Employment Programs for Special Groups ACTION (Independent Agency)

   Foster Grandparent Program

   Retired Senior Volunteer Program (RSVP)

   Senior Companion Program

   Volunteers in Service to America (VISTA)

Health Care

Health Care Financing Administration (HHS)

   Grants to States for Medical Assistance Programs (Medicaid)

   Program of Health Insurance for the Aged and Disabled (Medicare)

National Institute of Mental Health (HHS-Public Health Service) Community

   Mental Health Centers

Veterans Administration (Independent Agency)

   Veterans Domiciliary Care Program

   Veterans Nursing Home Care Program

Housing

Farmers Home Administration (AGRICULTURE)

    Rural Home Repair Program (Sec. 504)

Rural Rental Assistance (Sec. 521)

Office of Insured and Direct Loan Programs (HUD)

    Housing for the Elderly (Sec. 202)

    Low and Moderate Income Housing (Sec. 8)

    Low Rent Public Housing

Office of Assisted Housing (HUD)

  Housing for the Elderly (Sec. 202)

  Low and Moderate Income Housing (Sec. 8)

  Mortgage Insurance on Rental Housing for the Elderly (Sec. 231)

  Low Rent Public Housing

Community Planning and Development (HUD)

  Community Development

Income Maintenance

Food and Nutrition Service (AGRICULTURE)

  Food Stamp Program

Social Security Administration (HHS)

  Old Age Survivors Insurance Program (Social Security)

  Supplemental Security Income Program

Railroad Retirement Board (Independent Agency)

  Railroad Retirement Program

Office of Personnel Management (Independent Agency)

  Civil Service Retirement

Veterans Administration (Independent Agency)

  Veterans Pension Program

Social Service Programs

Administration of Aging (HHS)

  Multipurpose Senior Center Facilities

  Nutrition Programs

  State and Community Social Service Programs

    (Title III)

Administration for Public Services (HHS)

  Social Services for Low Income Persons and Public Assistance Recipients

    (Title XX)

Office of Revenue Sharing (TREASURY)

Revenue Sharing

Legal Services Corporation (Independent Agency)

Legal Services Corporation

Training and Research Programs

Administration on Aging (HHS)

Model Projects

Personnel Training (Title IV-Older Americans Act)

Research and Demonstration Program (Title IV-Older Americans Act)

National Institute of Aging (HHS-Public Health Service)

Research on Aging Process and Health Problems

Federal Council on Aging

Transportation

Urban Mass Transportation Administration (DOT)

Capital Assistance Grants for Use by Public Agencies

Capital Assistance Grants for Use by Private Non-Profit Groups

Reduced Fares

Capital and Operating Assistance Grants

Appendix D

Federal Resources and Services for Health Care

Medicare

Program of Health Insurance for the Aged and Disabled (MEDICARE), Social
Security Act., Title XVIII, (42 U.S.C. 1395, et seq.)

This Act provides coverage of specified health care services for persons aged
65 or older and eligible disabled persons.

Part A (Hospital Insurance), covers hospital and post-hospital skilled
nursing home care and home health services. Part B (Supplementary Medical
Insurance) is subject to premiums and covers physicians and other specified
outpatient services.

Field Liaison and Division of Technical Policy programs may be contacted at
Bureau of Health Insurance, Health Care Financing Administration, Department of

Health and Human Services, 6401 Security Boulevard, Baltimore MD 21235. The Chief Administrative Law Judge and the Appeals Council are located at the Bureau of Hearings and Appeals, Social Security Administration, Department of Health and Human Services, 3833 North Fairfax Drive, Arlington, VA 22203. The Congressional and Public Inquiry Section is located in the Bureau of Hearings and Appeals, Social Security Administration, Department of Health and Human Services, 801 North Randolph Street, Arlington, VA 22203.

Medicaid

Grants to States for Medical Assistance Programs (MEDICAID), Social Security
  Act, Title XIX, (42 U.S.C. 1386, et seq.).

Federal grants to states cover 50-83% of costs of medical care for eligible low-income families and individuals. Within federal guidelines, states establish eligibility and scope of benefits.

Information concerning Medicaid may be obtained from: Branch of Reimbursement, Branch of Policy and Legislation, Branch of Health Service, Division of Long Term Care, Division of Fraud and Abuse Control, Utilization Control Division, and Consumer Advocate. These Medicaid offices may be addressed at the Division of Policy and Standards, Medicare Bureau, Health Care Financing Administration, Department of Health and Human Services, 330 C Street, NW, Washington DC 20201

Health Care Facilities

Health Resources Development Construction and Modernization of Facilities
  (Hill-Burton Program), Public Health Services Act, Title XVI, (42 U.S.C.
  291).

Federal formula grants and loans are made to public and private agencies and to state governments for construction, expansion, or modernization of long-term care institutions and other outpatient and inpatient facilities. The federal share of project cost is determined by designated state agency.
Community Mental Health Centers, Community Health Centers Act, (42 U.S.C.
  26181, et seq.).

Federal grants are provided to States to establish community mental health centers that provide comprehensive mental health services to low-income persons of all ages.

Construction of Nursing Homes and Intermediate Care Facilities, National Housing Act, as amended 1959, Section 232 (12 U.S.C. 1715 Z -1).

The federal government insures loans to non-profit agencies or individual sponsors to finance the construction, rehabilitation, or equipment supply of certified nursing homes or intermediate care facilities.

Directory: Nursing Home Ombudsman Program.

Nursing Home Interests Staff, Administration on Aging, 330 Independence Avenue, SW, Washington, DC 20201.

The Administration on Aging initiated an ombudsman program in 1975 to respond to concerns of residents of nursing homes and other interested people about the quality of care in nursing homes. A directory of State Ombudsman Developmental Specialists is available and gives the appropriate contacts for information describing how to obtain further details of the program and how to register complaints. Distribution: General.

General Programs

Directory: State Agencies on Aging and Regional Offices.

DHEW Publication No. (OHD) 77-20283. The Administration on Aging, Office of Human Development, US Department of Health and Human Services, Washington, DC 20201.

In a brief pamphlet the address for each State Agency on Aging is listed as well as the 10 regional offices of the Administration on Aging. Distribution: General.

The Health Service Administration, Public Health Service, Department of Health and Human Services, offers comprehensive Public Health Services Formula grants to State Health and Mental Health Authorities as well as Heath Services Department Project grants that serve a broad spectrum of the population. Older adults also benefit from these programs. Information is available at Bureau of Community Health Service, Parklawn Building, 5600 Fishers Lane, Rockville, MD 20852.

Mental Health-Hospital Staff Development Grants and Community Mental Health Centers-Staffing and Construction (Community Mental Health Centers) are programs under the Alcohol, Drug Abuse, and Mental Health Administration, Public Health Service, Department of Health and Human Services. Information may be obtained at Division of Mental Health Service Programs, National Institute of Mental Health, 5600 Fishers Lane, Rockville, MD 20852.

Information concerning nursing homes may be requested from the Office of Long Term Care, Health Care Financing Administration, Department of Health and Human Services, 5600 Fishers Lane, Rockville, MD 20852; from the Nursing Home Interests Staff, Administration on Aging, Office of Human Development, Department of Health and Human Services, 400 Sixth Street SW, Washington, DC 20201; and from the Model Projects Division, Office of Research, Demonstration on Aging, Office of Human Development, Department of Health and Human Services, 330 C Street, Washington, DC 20201.

U.S. Civil Service Commission

Civil Service programs concerned with medical benefits include: Health and Life Insurance Section, Government Wide Plans, Employee Organization Plans, and Comprehensive Health Plans. Contacts may be made with these programs at the Bureau of Retirement, Insurance and Occupational Health, U.S. Civil Service Commission, 1900 E Street, NW, Washington, DC 20415.

Railroad Retirement Board

The Health Insurance Operations Section may be addressed at Division of Disability and Health Insurance Operations, Bureau of Retirement Claims, Railroad Retirement Board, 844 Rush Street, Chicago, IL 60611.

CHAMPUS (Civilian Health and Medical Programs for Uniformed Services)

The various CHAMPUS Programs are located at the following addresses: Directorate for Champus Policy, Office of Assistant Secretary for Health and Environment, Department of Defense, The Pentagon, Washington, DC 20301; Liaison Activities, Office of CHAMPUS, Fitzsimmons Army Medical Center, Denver, CO 80240; Policy Coordination Branch, Office of Medical Services, Bureau of Medical Services, Health Services Administration, Public Health Services, Federal Center Building, No. 3, 6525 Belcrest Road, West Hyattsville, MD 20782; Office of Activities, Retiree Section, Air Force Military Personnel Center, Randolph Air Force Base, Texas 78148; Retired Activities Division, Personal Affairs Directorate, TAG Center, Forrestal Building, 1000 Independence Avenue, SW, Washington, DC 20314; Retired Activities Section, Personal Affairs Branch, Personnel Service Division, Headquarters MSPA 3, U. S. M. C., Washington, DC 20380; Retired Personnel Support Section, Services and Benefits Branch, Personal Services Branch, Personal Services Division, Office of Personal

Affairs, Department of the Navy, Washington, DC 20370; <u>Commissioned Personnel Division</u>, NOAA Corps, National Oceanic and Atmospheric Administration, Department of Commerce, Rockville, MD 20852; <u>Employment Operations Branch</u>, Commissioned Personnel Operations Division, Public Health Service, Department of Health and Human Service, Department of Health and Human Services, 5600 Fisher's Lane, Rockville, MD 20852.

Rehabilitation Services Administration (DHHS)

In 1975 the Rehabilitation Services Administration (RSA) shifted from the Social and Rehabilitation Services Administration to the Department of Health and Human Services, taking over the research and development functions relating to the elderly. The RSA works closely with state vocational rehabilitation agencies to help hard-to-place and disabled persons find employment and to improve their skills through rehabilitation training services. Within the RSA, a Research and Development unit awards grants and supports counselor training programs. Inquiries about direct services in the area of daily living, special medical devices or rehabilitation and psychosocial services should be directed to the state vocational rehabilitation agency. The RSA, through its Research Information System, provides program information to professional persons and agencies who are interested in research, demonstration and training programs. The RSA also sponsors 19 Rehabilitation and Training Centers situated regionally across the country. Among these is the Helen Keller National Center for Deaf-Blind Youths and Adults.

Veterans Administration

The Federal government had only marginal responsibilities for health care when the Veteran's Administration (VA) system was established. The VA health care system now includes 172 hospitals in a health care system that provides services for 13 million inpatients and 17 million outpatients a year. These veterans are treated by the Federal facilities and by contracted services in non-VA facilities.

Eighty-nine medical schools have affiliation agreements with 109 VA hospitals; thousands of health professional students are trained in these facilities each year.

One of the goals of the Veterans Administration is to provide comprehensive care for aging veterans by continued development of a full spectrum of alternatives to hospitalization (nursing homes, domiciliaries and alternatives to institutionalization (day care centers, personal care home placement, hospital-based home care).

The VA is aware of the problems that will arise as the result of the aging of large numbers of veterans of World War II and the Korean War. Present planning is predicated on the premises that there will be no major new wars, no technological developments that will significantly prolong life and reduce the incidence of chronic diseases between the present time and 1985, and that the socioeconomic characteristics of veterans who will apply to the VA for long-term care services will not change significantly.

Some of the other considerations include the siting and sizing of VA installations based on present veteran migration patterns and that the veterans from World War II and the Korean War were mainly males --only 373,000 (2.1%) were women. Veterans will make up a sizeable segment of their age cohort, thus affecting community planning when efforts are made to determine the total resources available to the veteran population.

The Aging Veteran: Present and Future Medical Needs, October 1977, is available from the Veterans Administration, 810 Vermont Avenue, NW, Washington, DC 20420.

Appendix E
Agencies/Organizations
Serving the Aging

Accent on Information, Inc.
P. O. Box 700, Bloomington, Il 61701 (309)-378-2961

Provides computerized information retrieval system of the handicapped and those who work with the handicapped.

Alexander Graham Bell Association for the Deaf
Volta Bureau, 3417 Volta Place N.W., Washington, DC 20007
(202)-337-5220

Promoted education options for deaf and hard-of hearing through advocacy, information center, publications and continuing education; serves deaf persons, parents, professionals, and the general public.

American Academy of Family Physicians

   1740 West 92nd Street, Kansas City, MO   64114   (800) 821-2512

American Alliance For Health, Physical Education, Recreation and Dance

   Unit on Programs for the Handicapped

   1900 Association Drive, Reston, VA   22091   (703) 476-3400

Provides information, publications, consultive and related services on physical education, recreation and health programs involving handicapped persons.

American Association for the Advancement of Science

   Project on the Handicapped in Science

   1776 Massachusetts Avenue, N.W., Washington, DC   20036   (202) 467-4497

Encourages the elimination of career and educational barriers to disables scientists; publishes a variety of materials concerning disabled persons in science.

American Association for Continuity of Care

   1101 Connecticut Avenue, N.W., Washington, DC 20036

American Association of Homes for the Aging

   1050 17th Street N.W., Suite 770, Washington, DC   20036   (202) 296-5960

Nonprofit LTC institutions that provide housing, congregate housing, skilled nursing and related services to more than 300,000 elderly in USA.

American Association of Public Health Dentists

   11800 Sunrise Valley Drive Suite 808, Reston, VA   22091   (703) 476-5437

American Association of Retired Persons

   1909 K Street, N.W., Washington, DC   20049   (202) 872-4700

American Association of Workers for the Blind

1511 K Street n.W., Washington, DC 20005 (202) 347-1559

Includes individuals and agencies working for the general welfare of blind persons.

American Coalition of Citizens With Disabilities

1200 15th Street, N.W., Suite 201, Washington, D.C. 20005 (202) 785-4265

Helps to enhance the human and civil rights of disabled people through research and training on education, vocational rehabilitation and Section 504 of the Rehab Act of 1973; disseminates information.

American College of Health Care Administrators

4650 East West Highway, P.O Box 5890, Bethesda, MD. 20814 (301) 652-8384

Professional society for those who administer LTC facilities, designed to promote, preserve and sustain the well-being of the aged and chronically ill.

American Council of the Blind

1211 Connecticut Avenue, N.W., Suite 506, Washington, DC 20036 (202) 833-1251

Consists primarily of blind persons; promotes the independence and dignity of all blind people through effective and meaningful citizenship in all facets of our society.

American Dental Association

211 E. Chicago Avenue, Chicago, IL 60611 (312) 440-2500

American Dental Hygienists Association

444 N. Michigan Avenue, Chicago, IL 60611 (312) 440-8900

American Diabetes Association

600 Fifth Avenue, New York, NY 10020 (212) 541-4310

Promotes medical research and disseminates information on diabetes

Amerian Dietetic Association

    430 N. Michigan Avenue, Chicago, IL 60611 (312) 280-5000

American Federation for Aging Research (AFAR)

    335 Madison Avenue, New York, NY 10017 (212) 503-7600

AFAR's objectives are to encourage and support basic and clinical biomedical research in the field of aging and to develop public support for research in aging.

American Foundation for the Blind

    15 West 16th Street, New York, NY 10011 (212) 620-2000

Serves as a clearinghouse for information about blindness; offers professional consultation to governmental and voluntary agencies for the blind; publishes extensive material on blindness; sells consumer products for blind persons.

American Geriatrics Society, Inc.

    10 Columbus Circle, New York, NY 10019 (212) 582-13333

Comprised of health care professionals from all parts of the world who are devoted to the clinical care of the elderly.

American Health Care Association (AHCA)

    1200 15th Street N.W., Washington, DC 20005 (202) 833-2050

AHCA is a nonprofit federation of 48 state associations serving almost 8,000 licensed nursing homes and allied facilities providing long-term health care to convalescent and chronically ill elderly.

American Library Association

    Association of Specialized and Cooperative Library Agencies
    50 E. Huron Street, Chicago, Il 60611 (312) 944-6780

Promotes library services to persons with visual, physical , health, and/or behavioral problem; furthers development of standards for materials, services and personnel; encourages cooperation among agencies and organization in publicizing and implementing library services to handicapped persons.

American Lung Association

1740 Broadway, New York, NY 10019   (212) 245-8000

American Medical Association

535 N. Dearborn Street, Chicago, IL 60610   (312) 751-6390

Responsible for the interface of the AMA with other long-term care organizations.

American Medical Directors Association

2192 Ingleside Avenue, P.O. Box 2098, Macon GA 31203   (912) 745-9880

Nonprofit organization of physicians dedicated to improving medical care i long-term care facilities.

American Nurses' Association Inc.

2420 Pershing Road, Kansas City, MO 64108   (816) 474-5720

Division on Gerontological Nursing Practice recommends and implements ANA policy related to improving health care for older adults and develops standards of gerontological nursing practice.

American Occupational Therapy Association

1383 Piccard Drive Suite 300, Rockville, MD 20850   (301) 948-9626

American Osteopathic Association

212 E. Ohio Street, Chicago, IL 606111   (312) 280-5800

American Physical Therapy Association

1156 15th Street, N.W., Washington, DC 20005   (202) 466-2070

Promotes development of physical therapy education and services.

American Printing House for the Blind Inc.

 1139 Frankfort Avenue, Louisville, KY 40206 (502) 895-2405

Provides textbooks at less than college level, literature and educational aids for the blind; conducts research in specific problems relating to the selection and preparation of textbooks and educational aids.

American Psychiatric Association

 1400 K Street N.W., Washington, DC 20005 (202) 682-6000

American Red Cross

 17th & D Streets N.W., Washington, DC (202) 737-8300

American Society for Geriatric Denistry

 271-11 76th Avenue, New Hyde Park, NY 11040 (212) 343-2100 ext 260

American Society for Training and Development

 600 Maryland Avenue, S.W., Washington DC 20024 (202) 484-2390

Leader in human resource development field.

American Society of Allied Health Professionals

 One DuPont Circle N.W., Suite 300, Washington DC 20036-1174
 (202) 293-3422

American Society of Consultant Pharmacists

 2300 9th Street South, Arlington, VA 22204 (703) 920-8492

National professional society of pharmacists providing pharmacy and consultant services to nursing homes, home health care facilities.

Arthritis Foundation

 1314 Spring Street, Atlanta, GA 30309 (404) 872-7100

Asociacion Nacional Pro Personas Mayores

    1730 W. Olympic Blvd. Suite 401, Los Angeles, CA 90015 (213) 487-1922

    2025 Eye Street N.W., Suite 219, Washington, DC 20006 (202) 293-9329

Assembly of Ambulatory and Home Care Services (AAHCS)

    American Hospital Association

    840 N. Lake Shore Drive, Chicago, IL 60611

    Goals of AAHCS are to provide leadership to the hospital industry in the
    development and expansion of services which will be responsive to
    community needs; and to maintain and promote liaison with outside
    organizations interested in home care services.

Association for Education of the Visually Handicapped

    919 Walnut Street 7th Floor, Philadelphia, PA 19107 (215) 923-7555

    Professionals and parents interested in education and guidance of blind
    and partially sighted children and adults; cooperates with educational
    institutions to expand opportunities for the visually handicapped.

Association for Gerontology in Higher Education

    600 Maryland Avenue S.W., Washington, DC 20024 (202) 484-7505

    Member colleges and universities whose purpose is to foster development of
    and increase the commitment of higher education in the field of aging
    through education, research, and public service.

Association of University Programs in Health Administration

    1911 N. Fort Myer Drive Suite 503, Arlington, VA 22209 (703) 524-5500

Beverly Foundation

    1445 Huntington Drive, South Pasadena, CA 91030 (213) 441-1114

    Commitment to creative aging with a national outreach involving continuing
    professional education and materials, community services/education
    projects, and research and development.

Blinded Veterans Association

   1735 DeSales Street, N.W., Washington, DC 20036 (202) 347-4010

   Assists blinded veterans in obtaining federal, state, local benefits and
   general rehabilitation; works with employers and blinded veterans in
   obtaining jobs.

Braille (Louis) Foundation for Blind Musicians

   215 Park Avenue South, New York, NY 10023 (212) 982-7290

   Helps blind musicians become established professionally; auditions,
   evaluates and counsels musicians and composers; sponsors concerts.

Bureau of Health Care Delivery and Assistance

   Health Resources and Services Administration

   5600 Fishers Lane Rm 7A-55, Rockville, MD 20857 (301) 443-2270

Catholic Health Association of the U.S.

   4455 Woodson Rd, St. Louis, MO 63134 (314) 427-2500

   Educational institutes, symposia, publications, research, consultation.

Combined Federal Campaign

   95 M Street S.W. Washington, DC (202) 488-2043 or 2075

Concerned Seniors for Better Government

   1346 Connecticut Avenue, N.W., Washington, DC 20036 (202) 466-6140

Connecticut Hospice Institute

   61 Burban Drive, Branford, CT 06405 (203) 481-6231

   Created to promote the development of the hospice concept in communities
   to care for people whose death from serious illness is imminent.

Consultant Dietitians in Health Care Facilities

   8235 Stoneridge, Wichita, KS 67206 (316) 688-1605

An ADA practice group whose members work in nursing homes and long-term care facilities.

Dept. of Health & Human Services
200 Independence Avenue S.W., HHS Humphrey Bldg. Rm 716G, Washington, DC 20201 (202) 245-7694

Foundation of ACHCA, Inc.
c/o American College of Health Care Administrators,
4650 East West Highway, P.O. Box 5890, Bethesda, MD 20814 (301) 652-8384

To serve charitable, educational, research and scientific purposes related to the field of LTC and LTC administration.

Disabled American Veterans
807 Maine Avenue S.W., Washington D.C. 20024 (202) 554-3501

Gerontological Society of America
1411 K Street N.W. Suite 300, Washington, DC 20005 (202) 393-1411

Multidisciplinary organization devoted to bettering the condition of the aged through research and education.

Goodwill Industries of America
9200 Wisconsin Avenue, Washington DC 20014 (301) 530-6500

Provides vocational rehabilitation services and employment opportunities for the handicapped.

Gray Panthers
2480 16th Street, N.W. Suite 903, Washington, DC 20009
(202) 332-6117

Hadley School for the Blind
700 Elm Street, Winnetka, IL 60093 (312) 446-8111

Offers correspondence courses in braille and recorded forms to blind and deaf-blind students and adults. Service is free and worldwide.

Handy-cap Horizons

3250 East Loretta Drive, Indianapolis, IN 46227 (317) 784-5777

Conducts group tours for handicapped persons interested in worldwide and domestic travel.

Health Care Financial Managers Association

1050 17th Street N.W., Washington, DC (202) 296-2920

Health Care Financing Administration (HCFA)

200 Independence Avenue, S.W., HHS Humphrey Building Rm 314G, Washington, DC 20201 (202) 245-6727

Health Resources & Services Administration

5600 Fishers Lane Parklawn Bldg, Rm 14-05, Rockville, MD 20857 (301) 443-2216

Helen Keller International, Inc.

22 West 17th St, New York 10011 (212) 924-0297

Establishes projects to prevent blindness. Conducts low-cost, self-help training programs for blind children and adults in which they laarn vital daily living and vocational skills.

Helen Keller National Center for Deaf-Blind Adults Youths

111 Middle Neck Rd, Sands Point, NY 11050 (516) 944-8900

Assess physical and psychosocial functioning of deaf-blind youths and adults; provides comprehensive individualized rehabilitation training; trains workers of other agencies and community education programs; acts as a resource center; develops registry of deaf-blind youths and adults; develops and designs research programs and sensory aids for the deaf-blind.

Hillhaven Foundation

    1835 Union Avenue Suite 100, Memphis, TN 38104-3994 (901) 274-8428

Sponsors educational and research programs and conferences; provides educational materials and publications for providers of LTC. Aim is maintenance of quality standards and improvement of quality of services in LTC facilities.

Home Health Services & Staffing Association

    2101 L Street N.W. Suite 800, Washington, DC 20037 (202) 775-4707

Hospital Research & Education Trust

    840 N. Lake Shore Drive, Chicago, IL 60611 (3120 280-6620

Office on Aging and Long-Term Care was established to help hospitals respond to the health needs of the changing population.

Hospital, Institution & Education Food Service Society (HIEFSS)

    4410 W. Roosevelt Rd., Hillside, IL 60162 (312) 449-2770

Indoor Sports Club

    1145 Highland Street, Napoleon, OH 43545 (419) 592-5756

Arranges recreation and sports activities for disabled persons.

Intercare

    P.O. Box 8561, Moscow, ID 83843 (208) 882-7551

International organization dedicated to improving the state of the art of long-term health care.

Joint Commission on Accreditation of Hospitals

    875 N. Michigan Avenue, Suite 2201, Chicago IL 60611 (312)-642-6061

Legal Research & Services for the Elderly

    925 15th Street N.W. Washington, DC 20005 (202) 347-8800

Lions Clubs International

    300 22nd Street; OakBrook, IL 60570 (312) 986-1700

Promotes community service, supports sight conservation and work for the blind.

Mainstream, Inc.

    1200 15th Street N.W., Washington, DC 20005 (202) 833-1136
    Toll-free #1-800-424-8085

Counsels consumers, businesses, schools, and government on affirmative action for disabled persons, barrier removal and attitude change.

Muscular Dystrophy Association

    810 Seventh Avenue, New York, NY 10019 (212) 586-0808

Supports research into cause and cure of muscular dystrophy and related diseases; offers patient services through 200+ chapters nationwide.

Myasthenia Gravis Foundation

    18 East 26th Street, New York, NY 10010 (212) 889-8157

Promotes research and conducts professional and public education programs.

National Accreditation Council for Agencies Servicing the Blind & Visually Handicapped

    79 Madison Avenue, New York, NY 10016 (212) 683-8581

Develops standards and administers voluntary program of accreditation for organizations that provide direct services for blind and visually handicapped persons. Produces self-study and evaluation guides.

National Amputation Foundation

    12-45 150th Street, Whitestone, NY 11357 (212) 767-0596

Aids all amputees in employment, social, and mental rehabilitation.

National Association for Home Care

519 C Street, N.E. Stanton Park, Washington, DC 20002 (202) 547-7424

National Association for Practical Nurse Education & Service Inc.

254 W. 31st Street, New York, NY 10001 (212) 736-4540

NAPNES accredits schools offering practical nursing programs. Provides guidance and assistance to initiate and carry out a wide range of programs aimed at increasing LPN, VN professional competence.

National Association for Retarded Citizens

2709 Avenue E, East, P.O. Box 6109, Arlington TX 76011 (817) 261-4961

Promotes research, legislation and public understanding through local chapters of parents, professionals, and others interested in the mentally retarded.

National Association for Visually Handicapped

305 East 24th Street, New York, Ny 10010 (212) 889-3141

Distributes large print textbooks and other reading materials for the partially sighted; educates the public of the needs of the partially sighted; serves as a national clearinghouse of information about available services.

National Association for Spanish Speaking Elderly

1424 K Street N.W., Washington, DC (202) 393-2206

National Association of Meal Programs

604 W. North Avenue, Box 6959, Pittsburgh, PA 15212 (412) 231-1540

Members active in delivery of meals to older persons, both in the home and in group settings; provides technical assistance, information exchange, leadership in legislative action.

National Association of Nutrition and Aging Services Programs
  c/o Aging Project, Inc., Reno County Courthouse,
  Hutchinson, KS 67501 (316) 669-8201

National Association of Social Workers
  7981 Eastern Avenue, Silver Spring, MD 20910 (301) 565-0333

National Association of State Units on Aging
  600 Maryland Avenue, S.W. West Wing 208, Washington, DC 20024
  (202) 484-7182

National Association of the Deaf
  814 Thayer Avenue, Silver Spring, MD 20906 (301) 587-2788

National Association of the Physically Handicapped
  76 Elm Street, London OH 43104 (614) 852-1664

  Promotes the welfare of physically handicapped persons through local
  chapters.

National Braille Association
  654A Godwin Avenue, Midland Park, NJ 07432 (201) 447-1484

  Braille Book Bank provides college students braille copies of textbooks at
  less than cost; maintains a Reader-Transcriber Registry to provide blind
  readers with personal items helpful in work, recreation and daily living;
  maintains a braille collection of standard tables found in math and
  related disciplines.

National Caucus and Center on Black Aged
  1424 K Street, N.W. Suite 500, Washington, DC 20005 (202) 637-8400

National Center for a Barrier Free Environment
  1140 Connecticut Avenue, N.W. Suite 1006 Washington, DC 20036
  (202) 466-6896

Provides information, education, and technical assistance on the creation of physical facilities accessible to persons with disabilities. Services include information clearinghouse, national network of technical assistance providers, conferences and seminars, and public information programs.

National Center for Health Statistics
Statistics Branch, 3700 East West Hwy, Center Building Room 263, Hyattsville, MD 20782 (301) 436-8522

National Citizens Coalition for Nursing Home Reform
1309 L Street N.W. Washington, DC 20005 (202) 797-8227

The National Committee, Arts for the Handicapped
1701 K Street N.W., Suite 905, Washington, DC 20006 (202) 223-8007

Disseminates information about arts for disabled persons; promotes education in the arts; provides funds for model sites, special projects, and the Very Special Arts Festival Programs.

National Committee on the Treatment of Intractable Pain
P.O. Box 9553 Friendship Stn, Washington, DC 20016 (301) 983-1710

National Congress of Organizations of the Physically Handicapped Inc.
101 Lincoln Park Blvd., Rockford IL 61102

Promotes employment, legislation, rehabilitation, and equal rights for physically handicapped persons through member organizations.

National Council of Health Centers
2600 Virginia Avenue N.W. Suite 1100, Washington, DC 20037
(202) 298-7393

National Council of Senior Citizens
925 15th Street N.W., Washington, DC 20005

National Council on the Aging

> 600 Maryland Avenue S.W., West Wing 100, Washington, DC 20034
> (202) 479-1200

National Easter Seal Society

> 2023 W. Ogden Avenue, Chicago, IL 60612 (312) 243-8400

> Administers service programs for persons with disabling conditions,
> including public education, production and distribution of
> rehabilitation-related publications, research into cause, prevention and
> treatment of handicapping conditions, and advocacy efforts to insure the
> rights of people with handicaps.

National Eye Institute

> NIH, Bethesda, MD 20205 (301) 496-5248

> Supports and conducts fundamental and clinical studies on the eye and
> visual system and on the causes, prevention, and treatment of visual
> disorders.

National Federation of the Blind

> 1800 Johnson Street, Baltimore, MD 21230 (301) 659-9314

> Goal is complete integration of blind persons into society through state
> and local organizations of blind persons.

National Foundation for Hospice and Home Care

> 519 C Street N.E., Stanton Park, Washington, DC 20002 (202) 547-7424

National Foundation for Long Term Health Care

> c/o Robert Deane, 1200 15th Street, N.W., Washington, DC 20005
> (202) 833-2050

> Nonprofit organization; objective is to develop programs in research and
> education in LTHC

National Homecaring Council (NHC)

235 Park Avenue S, 116h Floor, New York, NY 10003 (212) 674-4990

Council encourages the organization of homemaker services, serves as a central source of information, administers an agency approval accreditation program, and publishes and distributes educational and promotional materials.

National Hospice Organization

1901 N. Fort Myer Drive, Suite 402, Arlington, VA 22209 (703) 243-5900

NHO promotes the concept of hospice care for dying people, and provides information and education to member hospices, the health care community and the general public.

National Indian Council on Aging, Inc.

P.O. Box 2088, Albuquerque, NM 87103 (505) 766-2276

National Institute of Neurological & Communicative Disorders & Stroke (NINCDS)

NIH, Bethesda, MD 20014 (301) 496-4000

Supports and conducts research on neurological, sensory, and communicative disorders.

National Institute on Aging (NIA)

NIH, 9000 Rockville Pike, Bldg. 31, Rm 2C-02, Bethesda, MD 20205 (301) 496-9625

National League for Nursing

10 Columbus Circle, New York, NY 10009 (212) 582-1022

Develops and improves the standards for quality nursing education, service and health care delivery in the U.S.

National Library Service for the Blind & Physically Handicapped

Library of Congress, 1291 Taylor Street, N.W., Washington, DC 20542

(202) 287-5100

Provides free library service to visually and physically handicapped persons through a network of cooperating regional and subregional libraries nationwide.

National Multiple Sclerosis Society

205 E. 42nd Street, New York, NY 10017 (212) 674-4100

Supports and coordinates research on multiple sclerosis and related disorders; provides services and aid to disabled multiple sclerosis patients and their families; offers public information services.

National Rehabilitation Association

1522 K Street, N.W., Washington, DC 20005 (202) 659-2430

Members concerned with all aspects of rehabilitation of the physically and mentally handicapped and the socially disadvantaged.

National Rehabilitation Information Center

4407 Eighth Street, N.E., The Catholic University of America, Washington, DC 20017 (202) 635-5826.

National Retinitis Pigmentosa Foundation

8331 Mindale Circle, Baltimore, MD 21207 (301) 655-1011

National Society to Prevent Blindness

79 Madison Avenue, New York, NY 10016 (212) 684-3505

Sponsors programs of public and professional education, research, and community services in the area of sight conservation.

National Spinal Cord Injury Foundation

369 Elliot Street, Newton Upper Falls, MA 02164 (617) 964-0521

Works to improve physical and vocational rehabilitation of persons with spinal cord injuries; promotes legislation of benefit to the handicapped; promotes research into a cure of paralysis through regeneration.

National Student Nurses' Association
  10 Columbus Circle, New York, NY 10018 (212) 581-2211

National Therapeutic Recreation Society
  1601 N. Kent Street, 11th Floor, Arlington, VA 22209 (703) 525-0606

  Promotes recreation and leisure activities for all persons, including the ill, disabled, and aged.

National Wheelchair Athletic Association
  40-24 62nd Street, Woodside, New York 11377 (212) 424-2929

  Organizes wheelchair sports; provides both rehabilitative and competitive opportunities for the handicapped

New Eyes for the Needy
  549 Millburn Avenue, Short Hills, NJ 07078 (201) 376-4903

  Collects used eyeglasses for redistribution; provides free prescription glasses to the needy on request.

Office for Handicapped Individuals
  Education Dept., Mary E. Switzer Bdg, Rm 3106, Washington, DC 20202
  (202) 245-0080

Office of Special Education & Rehabilitative Services
  Rehabilitative Services Administration, Education Dept., Washington, DC
  20201 (202) 245-0918

  Develops the federal-state programs of vocational rehabilitation for the disabled and programs for those with developmental disabilities.

Oncology Nursing Society

   3111 Banksville Road Suite 200, Pittsburgh, PA   15216   (412) 344-3899

Paralyzed Veterans of America

   4350 East West Hwy Suite 900, Washington, DC   20014   (301) 652-2135

   Sponsors improved benefits and legislation, employment opportunities, and
   wheelchair sports programs for paralyzed veterans.

Parkinson's Disease Foundation

   William Black Medical Research Building
   640 W. 168th Street, New York, NY   10032   (212) 923-4700

   Raises funds to support research into the cause, cure, and prevention of
   Parkinson's disease; distributes information on patient care and
   rehabilitation.

President's Committee on Employment of the Handicapped

   Washington, DC   20210   (202) 653-5044

   Promotes maximal employment opportunities for the handicapped; sponsors
   the annual Employ-the-Handicapped Week.

President's Committee on Mental Retardation

   Washington, DC   20201   (202) 245-7634

   Recommends federal action where needed, promotes coordination and
   cooperation among public and private agencies, and encourages better
   public understanding of mentally retarded persons.

Recording for the Blind

   215 East 58th Street, New York, NY   10022   (212) 751-0860

   Supplies taped educational material free of charge to blind, perceptually
   and physically handicapped.

Regional Resource and Information Center for Disabled Individuals

Moss Rehabilitation Hospital 12th Street & Tabor Road,

Philadelphia, PA 19141 (215) 329-5715

Provides information and documents relating to physical disabilities, services and programs for people with disabilities, professionals, and the general public.

Rehabilitation International U.S.A. (RIUSA)

20 W. 40th Street, New York, NY 100018 (212) 869-9907

Member organizations concerned with the rehabilitation of the physically handicapped; collects, compiles, and disseminates international information relative to rehabilitation; operates the International Rehabilitation Film Review Library which rents and sells rehabilitation films from the U.S. and foreign countries.

Self Help for Hard of Hearing People, Inc.

Howard E. Stone, Jr., President

P.O. Box 34889

Washington, DC 20034

Senate Special Committee on Aging

Senator John Heinz, Russell Senate Bldg Rm 443,

Washington, DC 20510 (202) 225-6343

John Rather, Dirksen Bldg Rm G-233 (Staff Director),

Washington, DC 20510 (202) 224-5364

Social Security Administration

6401 Security Blvd, Baltimore, MD 21235

Administers the federal retirement, survivors and disability insurance programs and the supplemental security income program. Also provides information on Medicare.

Society of Teachers of Family Medicine

    1740 W. 892nd Street, Kansas City, MO 64114 (816) 333-9700

Telephone Pioneers of America

    195 Broadway, Rm C-1837, New York, NY 10007 (212) 393-2512

    Active and retired senior telephone employees perform volunteer services such as repair of talking book machines, braille transcription, and hospital services.

The Third Age Center

    Fordham University at Lincoln Center, 113 W. 60th Street, New York, NY 10023 (212) 841-5547

United Way Headquarters

    95 M Street, S.W., Washington, DC (202) 488-2000

U.S. Dept. of Health & Human Services

    Administration on Aging, 330 Independence Avenue, S.W., Rm. 4759 Washington, DC 20201

Urban Elderly Coalition

    600 Maryland Avenue S.W., West Wing 205, Washington, DC 20024 (202) 554-2040

Veterans Administration (VA)

    810 Vermont Avenue N.W., Washington, DC 20420

    Administers laws authorizing benefits for former members of the Armed Forces and their dependents, including compensation payments for disabilities or death related to military service; pensions based on financial need for totally disabled veterans, or certain survivors for disabilities or death not related to military service; burial; comprehensive medical program including a system of nursing homes, clinics, and medical centers.

Western Gerontological Society

833 Market Street, Suite 516, San Francisco, CA 94130 (415) 543-2617

National, nonprofit membership organization of practitioners, educators, researchers, and others in the field of aging.

Appendix F
Resource Materials

American Speech-Language-Hearing Association. (1980). Organizations & Agencies in the area of aging.

American Speech-Language-Hearing Association. (1980). Resource materials for communicative problems of older persons.

Beasley, D. S., Davis, G. A. (Eds) (1981). Aging: Communication processes & disorders. New York: Grune & Stratton.

Bollinger, R. L., Waugh, P. F., Zatz, A. F. (1977). Communication management of the geriatric patient. Danville, IL: Interstate.

Butler, R. (1975). Why survive? Being old in America.

Byerts, T. O., Howell, S. C., Pastalan, L. A. (Eds). (1979). Environmental context of aging: Life styles, environmental quality and living arrangements. New York: Garland STPM Press.

Craik, F. I. M., Trehub, S. (1982). Aging & cognitive processes. New York: Plenum Press.

Davis, R. H. (Ed). (1981). Aging: Prospects & issues. Los Angeles: USC Press.

Henoch, M. A. (Ed). (1979). Aural rehabilitation for the elderly. New York: Grune & Stratton.

Hull, R. H. (Ed). (1981). The communicatively disordered elderly. New York: Thieme-Stratton.

Leutenegger, R. R. (1975). Patient care and rehabilitation of communication-impaired adults, Springfield, IL: Thomas.

Mace, N., Rabins, P. J. (1981). The 36 hour day. Baltimore: Johns Hopkins Press.

Maurer, J. F., Rupp, R. R. (1979). Hearing & aging: Tactics for intervention. New York: Grune & Stratton.

Obler, L. K., Albert, M. L. (Eds). (1980). Language and communication in the elderly. Lexington, MA: Lexington Books.

Ordy, J. M., Brizzee, K. R. (Eds). (1979). Sensory Systems and communication in the Elderly. New York: Raven Press.

Oyer, H. J., Oyer, E. J. (Eds). (1976). Aging and communication. Baltimore: University Park Press.

Rowles, G. D., Ohta, R. J. (Eds). (1983). Aging and milieu: Environmental perspectives on growing old. New York: Academic Press.

Schow, R. L. (1978). Communication disorders of the aged: A guide for health professionals. Baltimore: University Park Press.

Shadden, B. B., Raiford, C. A.; Shadden, H. S. (1983). Coping with communication disorders in aging. Tigaard, OR: C. C. Publications.

Tamir, L. M. (1979). Communication and the aging process: Interaction throughout the life cycle. New York: Pergamon Press.

Wilder, C. N., Weinstein, B. E. (Eds). (1984). Aging and communication: Problems in management. New York: Haworth Press.

Conclusion

Rosemary Lubinski
SUNY Buffalo, New York

It would be fitting to have an elderly person reflect upon the contents of this manual and write the conclusion, but I write this as an aging person and as one professionally and personally devoted to caring about the communication of older persons. We have come to study the aged as though they are a group of people to be analyzed, diagnosed, and eventually "therapized." But they are us. Each of us reading this manual, is one of "them." Each day we are creeping and leaping toward being an older person, and that realization should help us to understand that aging is not an abstraction that happens to other people. Getting old is a reality, if only we live long enough.

In reading this manual, you should have found several themes: (a) There is a growing number of older people, who are diverse in their characteristics, skills, and needs, and (b) who have a strong need to maintain their communication skills and opportunities. The ability to communicate is a life-long process and the need to communicate is intimately intwined with our self-identity, socialization, independence, and self-maintenance. In fact, I will go so far as to state that being able to communicate through any means possible is the most crucial skill needed by the elderly.

As communication specialists, we have just awakened to the challenge this premise presents. This manual helps us to identify the complexity of factors, both within and outside the older person which affect communication. Our older patients or clients present us with personal histories, varied and multifaceted communication disorders, complicating internal and external sequelae, and a persistent need and desire to communicate. It is this final point that must guide our work with this population.

It has been very easy for us to reject older aphasic clients from therapy on the basis that they are old, their problems are too severe, and progress will be minimal. Older hearing-impaired persons are not always referred for audiological consultations, because of such misconceptions that a hearing aid would be of little value at this age, it might get lost, or the older person might forget to turn off the battery. I repeatedly hear the phrase, "You're not working with someone that old, are you?" This clearly implies that our efforts should only be directed toward younger, potentially productive clients. It does not take into consideration that communication is an important need, in fact, a necessity for older persons.

This manual stresses in great part the receptive and expressive communication skills of the elderly. The communication profile of the elderly must also reflect the opportunities they have for communication. This manual would be incomplete if we stressed only the skills of communication without placing those skills in context. The study of pragmatics has helped us to understand that communication must occur for some reason, and that the situations in which communication occurs greatly affect the process itself. Our job as communication specialists is not done following diagnostics or therapy. It is only complete when we realize that older people must have someone with whom to communicate who values them and reinforces their communication efforts. Similarly, older persons must have interesting activities as well as a stimulating physical and social environment which provide them with communication topics. Working with elderly patients or clients and sending them back to an institutional setting or to a family context which discourages communication cancels the benefits of our therapy. Thus, the environment in which the elderly person communicates must be considered as part of our intervention concept.

As communication specialists we sit on a challenging frontier in working with the aged. If we are to meet their needs, several issues must be faced:

1. better training to understand the nature and process of aging, our attitudes toward aging, and the role of the communication specialist with this population in home, hospital, and institutional settings;

2. development of a variety of service delivery models in each of these settings;

3. reassessment of our concept of progress in therapy;

4. working with other disciplines to underscore the communication of older persons and how these might be met through a needs multidisciplinary approach;

5. community education concerning the communication skills of the elderly and the professionals available to meet these needs;
6. federal, state, and agency understanding of the role of the communication specialist with this population.

If you have burrowed through this manual, you have taken the first step toward meeting the communication needs of the elderly—the step of sensitivity and knowledge. The next step is commitment and experimentation. Our older population provides us with the raw material for creative approaches in traditional direct therapy and in environmental intervention. The creativity we expend in developing better approaches to improving the communication skills and opportunities of today's elderly will be reaped in our own future.